THE WAYS WE LOVE

THE GUILFORD FAMILY THERAPY SERIES

Michael P. Nichols, Series Editor

The Ways We Love
A Developmental Approach to Treating Couples

Sheila A. Sharpe

THE GUILFORD PRESS
New York London

© 2000 The Guilford Press
A Division of Guilford Publications, Inc.
72 Spring Street, New York, NY 10012
www.guilford.com

Printed in the United States of America

This book is printed on acid-free paper.

Last digit is print number: 9 8 7 6 5 4 3 2 1

Library of Congress Cataloging-in-Publication Data

Sharpe, Sheila A.
  The ways we love : a developmental approach to treating couples /
    Sheila A. Sharpe.
      p. cm. — (The Guilford family therapy series)
  Includes bibliographical references and index.
  ISBN 1-57230-530-4 (hardcover)
    1. Marital psychotherapy—Case studies. 2. Love—Case studies.
  I. Title. II. Series.

RC488.5 .S488 2000
616.89′156—dc21   00-035389

In memory of my parents,
Thomas Elfred Hogan and Virginia Pettit Hogan

And for Michael and Colin

About the Author

Sheila A. Sharpe, PhD, specializes in psychotherapy with couples and individuals and is in private practice in La Jolla, California. She has published and presented several papers on a developmental object relations approach to couple therapy as well as writing on other topics. Most recently she has written two papers on sibling relationships. She teaches in the Advanced Psychoanalytic Psychotherapy Program of the San Diego Psychoanalytic Society and Institute. She is also on the guest faculty of New Directions in Psychoanalytic Thinking, a program of the Washington Psychoanalytic Foundation. She is a member of the San Diego Psychoanalytic Society and Institute, the American Psychological Association, Division 39, Section VIII, and the San Diego Psychological Association.

Preface

When I first set out to write this book, I had no idea what was in store for me. At the end of a tumultuous six years, I have come to find that my experience bears a certain resemblance to the ups and downs of the love relationships described on subsequent pages. I began this project feeling excited, energized, and more than a little in love with my ideas. Some of this unrealistic, initial inflation stemmed from my particular background.

Books, and especially the writing of books, were idealized in my family. My father always aspired to be a playwright or novelist, and for him writers and writing held an exalted status. I can remember him striding through the house, reading aloud from a book or play he particularly admired, his voice booming, his eyes alive with excitement. Since childhood, I thought the most important thing to be was a writer, or to help people, like my mother did as a psychotherapist. This book clearly embodies an expression of those values, wishes, and dreams passed on to me by both of my parents. I only wish they were alive to receive this acknowledgment of their tremendous influence on me.

Inspiration for the subject matter of this book came most directly from working with my patients over many years and finding that unhappiness in their love relationships, if not the obvious cause of trouble, so often underlay many other kinds of complaints. I give profound thanks to all of my patients for letting me into their lives, for putting up with my experimental interventions and odd bursts of enthusiasm whenever I thought we had stumbled onto something important in our work, and for sharing their humor and responding to mine, so that we had some times of laughter and fun to offset the painful, hard work of therapy.

Needless to say, the high excitement and idealism with which I began writing this book soon gave way to the reality of actually trying to give form and shape to my thoughts and produce a coherent first draft. The conceptual scheme I had once thought to be so enlightening became more confused and less convincing as one chapter limped its way into the next. Like the first round of disillusionment in a love relationship, my initial love affair with my fantasied book turned quite sour as I settled into the hard work of writing day-to-day, an activity that mainly seemed to produce reams of terrible prose. My mood plummeted. I began brooding that I was wasting my life with a worthless book.

Many people were vitally important in helping me through this long, difficult period of clarifying my ideas and reshaping my conceptual framework to be truer to my own and others' clinical experience.

I owe tremendous gratitude to Kitty Moore, Senior Editor at The Guilford Press, and Michael Nichols, Editor of The Guilford Family Therapy Series, for their unflagging faith in the project, for their patience with my many setbacks and different directions, and their line-by-line help, teaching me to write more clearly and concisely, and less like an enthusiastic disciple of Henry James.

Fred Sander and Robert Winer, cochairs of the Interdisciplinary Seminar (on couple and family therapy) of the American Psychoanalytic Association, were particularly important in the initial development of my concepts. For three years, they invited me to present first drafts of certain chapters at the winter meetings. In addition to their belief in the value of my ideas, both also provided ongoing astute criticism and key suggestions. To all of the participants in those seminars I give my thanks for their helpful input, but especially to Deborah Luepnitz, who presented a critical discussion of my early theoretical framework that led to substantial revision of my thinking.

I am also grateful to Robert Winer, as director of the Psychoanalytic Object Relations Couple and Family Therapy Training Program of the Washington School of Psychiatry, for inviting me to present my work at two of this unique program's conferences. For their enthusiastic support and thoughtful commentaries, I thank all of this program's remarkable faculty and students, in particular Joyce Lowenstein, Dee Stern, Sharon Alperovitz, John Zinner, Roger Shapiro, Charles McCormack, Justin Frank, Kristina MacGaffin, and Ann Devaney.

I have long admired the work of James Framo and envied his ability to express himself in writing and in person with such charm, eloquence, and clarity. I am especially grateful for his support of my earliest efforts, when I had little confidence as a couple therapist and writer.

It is a pleasure to also thank Judith Siegel and Marion Solomon, both exceptional clinicians and authors, for supporting my early contributions.

By the ninth or tenth revision, I began to get a better grip on what I wanted to say and how to say it. The book started to look like something that had theoretical consistency and clinical value. I started to feel more hopeful about it, even a little proud of certain parts, while still recognizing its shortcomings. I was now approaching a more balanced, realistic perspective (as occurs in the maturing of a love relationship). At this point, I believed in the book enough to present a chapter at a conference sponsored by the San Diego Psychoanalytic Society and Institute. I am particularly thankful for the chance to exchange ideas with the other presenters: Ethel Person, Judith and Robert Wallerstein, Otto Kernberg, and Robert Tyson. I have long admired these authors and clinicians, and their enthusiastic reception of my talk gave me a real boost and the temporary feeling that I had finally arrived.

I now had the confidence to expose a revised draft and certain chapters to the discerning eyes of a few of my colleagues and friends. I am very thankful to you all for your helpful critiques and advice: Shelly Satterfield, Haig and Sue Koshkarian, Lynn Corrin, Stephanie Nigh, Susan Richards, Allan Mallinger, Elizabeth Zinner, Marcia Krill, Fred Sander, and especially Marty Graner, who generously read more than one draft. Her keen intelligence and unerring good sense have contributed greatly to the book's clarity and clinical utility.

I also wish to give thanks to the many important friends who have not yet read the book, but have kindly listened to me complain, worry, and obsess about this project for many years and provided meaningful support and many useful suggestions: Joy Tilton, Julie Tilton, Kristen Lee, Mara Carrico, Ada Burris, DeDe Herst, Claudia Andrews, Felice Levine, Gina Livesay, Sharon Weld, Fran and Bill Fenical, Sally and Patrick Ledden, Gil and Ann Williamson, and Pam and Norm Estabrook.

To Allan Rosenblatt, my longtime friend, colleague, coauthor, editor, supervisor, and teacher, I owe more gratitude than I can ever express. Countless drafts of every page of this book have passed under his keen scrutiny and received his invaluable criticism. Many of the ideas were generated and clarified by our clinical and theoretical discussions, making this work, in many respects, a collaborative effort. A few meager sentences cannot begin to thank him for his extraordinary contribution.

There is no doubt that writing a book causes great stress to family life and a love relationship. The impact is like the arrival of a baby, but one that keeps requiring the constant care of a newborn. My husband, Michael, and my son, Colin, have been profoundly supportive in both emotional and practical ways in spite of the fact that they have had to endure the continual hardship of my frequent unavailability over a long period of time. Both entered the process with me, contributing ideas, encouragement, comfort, and crucial help especially with the computer, my constant companion and tormentor. This book could not have been written without their support. Furthermore, they have earned my lifelong gratitude and affection by giving their love when I was not so good at giving mine.

Contents

PART II. PATTERNS OF SEPARATENESS

DEVALUING

CONTROLLING

COMPETING

Introduction

"How has love failed me? Let me count the ways," quipped a sad young man I was helping through the death throes of his relationship. His cynical takeoff on the first line of Elizabeth Barrett Browning's famous love sonnet is a telling expression of current disillusionment in romantic love. Even the ideal of a good marriage has come under attack. Judith Wallerstein reported that her first audience burst into derisive laughter when she asked for volunteers to participate in her research on *The Good Marriage* (1995).

I first learned about love and marriage at my mother's knee. She told me that falling in love was a wonderful experience, but it did not last and you could not build a life on it. Real love and marriage meant a lot of hard work and sacrifice. After one of her "marriage is hard work" lectures, I toyed with the idea of not getting married. It seemed like a lot more fun to just stay in love. When I fell in love for the first time, a new idea entered my mind—maybe Mother was wrong. Maybe there was a way to make the enchantment of love last.

I would never have guessed then that this seed of rebellion would turn into a career devoted to understanding love relationships and trying to make them happier for my patients, as well as myself. It's a difficult job, it turns out, one that involves a good deal of hard work, but also great rewards. If she were alive, my mother would say, "I told you so."

Our culture has steeped us in two dichotomous ideals of love and marriage. The first is the ideal of romantic love. In this fairy tale, you fall in love, marry joyously, and live happily ever after. The second is the ideal of devoted love. The couple, in this saga, also falls in love, but only as a brief interlude of madness before getting down to the real business of loving, which is to struggle side by side through years of

1

hard work, raising children, self-sacrifice, and compromise. A recent version of this ideal is the two career, equal partnership marriage. Falling in love is not so relevant in this version. The intensity of passion and devotion quickly goes to the partners' careers more than to each other or their children.

Who would want to say "yes" to any of these marriage proposals? The first is an adolescent fantasy that disappoints time and time again, the second sounds like signing up for boot camp for the rest of your life, and the third looks like a phobic attempt to avoid intimacy with your family and find true love with a career (something over which you may have more control). No wonder many people are choosing the single life, or any other kind of life but the "ideal" married life.

A tenacious myth keeps our understanding of marriage from advancing. It could be called the myth of Athena, because Athena sprang from the head of Zeus as a fully grown, perfectly formed goddess—fully armed as well. We view the marital relationship similarly, as springing into being, fully formed, when two people marry.

This lack of a developmental perspective can be attributed not only to the ideals of romantic and devoted love but also to early psychoanalytic theory that viewed individual development as essentially completed by late adolescence. While psychoanalytic theory is in the process of integrating the concept of adult development, society is still under the influence of the earlier version. Most conceptions of adult development[1] focus on the individual adult's journey through the life cycle and not on the marriage relationship as having a distinct evolution of its own.

This book presents a formulation of how love relationships develop and a treatment approach for therapists working with couples based upon this conception. Marriages and other committed love relationships[2] are viewed as consisting of multiple patterns of relating that develop in parallel over time in an interrelated fashion. In working with couples in therapy over the last thirty years, I have identified seven central relationship patterns that appear to be universally expressed in adult love relationships in our society. These patterns include nurturing, merging, idealizing, devaluing, controlling, competing for superiority, and competing in love triangles. While other relational patterns exist, these are the most fundamental. Each of these patterns has its own developmental course, subject to

---

[1]See Erikson (1963); Gould (1978); Levinson, Darrow, Klein, Levinson, and McKee (1978); Colarusso and Nemiroff (1981); and Nemiroff and Colarusso (1985, 1990).

[2]Commited love relationships are the subject of study whether the partners are married or unmarried. Marriage is used to refer to both situations, in order to avoid repetition of more cumbersome terms such as "commited partnership " or "commited love relationship."

certain derailments, and also recapitulates childhood themes[3] and is reflected in our cultural expressions of love and marriage.

These patterns reflect everyone's relational needs. We need to be nurtured and to nurture, to feel cared for, and to care for others. We need to be able to merge, at times, to feel fundamentally connected and part of a greater whole. We need to idealize our partners and to be idealized to stay attracted and to feel cherished. We need to devalue at times of serious disappointment in our partners and ourselves, so that necessary changes and greater acceptance can be integrated. Sometimes, we need to control, dominate, and oppose to feel powerful and independent. At other times, we need to compete with our partners to define and test our strengths and weaknesses. We also may need to contend with outsiders (e.g., children, parents, work) in order to preserve the priority of the bond with our partners.

However, there is also a downside to each of these patterns, a painful, potentially destructive aspect. A relatively sturdy relationship that continues to grow in spite of difficulties can usually tolerate the stress of these negative potentials. However, when one of these patterns dominates and rigidifies into a primarily defensive form, a couple relationship will become stagnant or actively destructive.

Seeking a good metaphor for this conception, Athena again comes to mind, because of her unsurpassed skill as a weaver. The way a marriage develops is like weaving a tapestry that is never completed, but always evolving. The marriage tapestry begins with early forms of the basic patterns. Over the years, these patterns become more elaborate and intertwined. As each pattern of relating evolves and interweaves with all the other patterns, the partners create a more richly hued and distinctive relationship tapestry. (Figure 1 at the end of the Introduction [p. 10] displays and summarizes the evolution of each pattern in relationship with all of the other patterns.)

This metaphor describes a relatively good intimate relationship that manages to sustain growth, in spite of the inevitable setbacks and conflicts. Love relationships that become more than temporarily stuck are like a weaving that may progress a little during one day but comes undone the next, so that no progress is ever made. Whatever steps forward the partners may take are quickly reversed, so that the relationship stays stalled in repetitive, painful interactions.

There are several authors who have made important contributions to a developmental conception of marriage, notably Ellen Berman and Har-

---

[3]In my effort to distinguish the major relational themes and their interrelated evolution, I was influenced by Anna Freud's (1963) concept of developmental lines.

old Lief (1975, 1981), Carol Nadelson, Derek Polonsky, and Mary Mathews (1984), David McWhirter and A. Mattison (1984), Daniel Wile (1985), Ellyn Bader and Peter Pearson (1988), Barry Dym and Michael Glenn (1993), Stephan Goldbart and David Wallin (1994), Judith Wallerstein and Sandra Blakeslee (1995), as well as my own previous work in this area (Sharpe, 1981, 1990, 1997, 1998).[4] These authors conceptualize marriage as one entity that develops in stages, each stage involving the partners' mastery of certain psychological and interpersonal tasks.[5] This book builds on these contributions but aims to capture the greater complexity of couple relationships. Rather than a single developmental progression evolving in serial stages, I conceptualize multiple developmental lines evolving in parallel, though interrelated, ways.

In earlier efforts, I applied the stages in a child's development of object relations described by Mahler, Pine, and Bergman (1975) to the evolution of couple relationships. Bader and Pearson (1988) also advanced a similar formulation. Working with this model for several years, I have found it to be limited in its overemphasis on a single developmental process, separation–individuation, with insufficient regard for couples' needs for varying kinds of connection. Viewing troubled couples solely in terms of pathological syndromes also began to seem restrictive. Partners are more responsive to the theoretical and clinical framework elaborated here. This approach focuses on the positive, normal aspects of relationship development and incorporates a balanced view of couples' ongoing needs both to create a deeper connection and to be separate individuals.[6]

Each pattern of relating expresses an aspect of this polarity—how to be connected with our partners and yet be a separate individual within the relationship. Optimal development of each pattern leads to partners' feeling more deeply attached and, at the same time, comfortably separate. Although the book explores what can go wrong in the development of each relationship pattern, the theory and clinical approach underscore couples' adaptive, as well as defensive, efforts. I have found a clinical focus on dysfunction to interfere with the creation of a safe, growth-promoting environment.

---

[4]This group of authors does not include the many who have contributed to a differently focused but also related developmental conception of the family. See Zilbach (1968, 1989), Duvall (1971), Solomon (1973), Hoffman (1980), Terkelsen (1980), Sander (1979), and so on.

[5]Many of these conceptions are derived from Erik Erikson's (1959, 1963) eight-stage formulation of the individual's development throughout the life cycle.

[6]In a series of papers, Sidney Blatt and Rachael Blass (1990; Blass & Blatt, 1992, 1996) have responded to this lack of theoretical integration by charting the developmental lines of attachment and separateness, as they interact throughout the life cycle of the individual.

Take mind reading, for example. Many therapists view a couple's wish to communicate in this fashion as a symptom of pathological fusion, symbiosis, or merged relatedness. Directly or indirectly, couples are prevailed upon to give up mind reading. They may be encouraged to clarify verbally their needs and expectations, or specifically directed to make "I" statements. Communication training may be instigated. Many couples then feel criticized and pressured to correct this supposed flaw or risk disappointing the therapist. Many try to give up mind reading for the therapist's sake, but this kind of compliance in sessions rarely advances a relationship, let alone the partners' self-esteem. Clinical approaches of this kind reflect a singular emphasis on separation–individuation of the partners, without adequate understanding of their equal or greater (in this instance) needs for attachment.

In the approach advanced here, mind reading and merging are considered to be universal and normal ways couples relate. These essential features of romantic love are fundamental to feeling deeply and empathically connected. However, if such patterns continue to *dominate* a relationship well beyond the romantic phase, a disruption in development has likely occurred, and these patterns have become defensive. In treatment, I would initially seek to understand with a couple the wishes and fears (often unconscious) that motivate their mind reading.

Partners often reveal that mind reading and other forms of merging are felt to be necessary to keep them safely attached, rather than feeling abandoned and alone. They preserve fantasies of oneness that seem vital to feeling loved. When these needs and fears are understood and worked with to whatever depth is necessary, a couple can usually move forward developmentally and change the dysfunctional aspects of these patterns, while improving the functional aspects.

The theoretical framework just described is summarized as follows:

- A couple relationship is a system that develops over time in a way that is distinct from, though related to, development of the individual partners.
- A couple relationship consists of multiple patterns of relating that develop in an interwoven, interdependent fashion throughout the life of a relationship.
- Seven universal patterns of intimate relating have been identified: *nurturing, merging, idealizing, devaluing, controlling, competing for superiority, and competing in love triangles.*
- Each pattern of relating has its origin in an individual's early relationship development and can be viewed as an ongoing developmental theme that is reworked in different ways throughout life.

- Each pattern expresses a distinctive facet of the partners' needs to be connected yet separate.
- The optimal result of the developmental progression of these patterns is the couple's increasing ability to create a mutual relationship that also supports individual development.
- In a couple relationship, each pattern thus undergoes a normative developmental progression that may become derailed at any point in the couple's life, causing temporary or long-term problems. Thus, the patterns can take either growth-promoting or growth-inhibiting forms.
- These patterns become destructive in a couple relationship when one or more dynamics become too dominant or rigidly fixed in form, so that development halts and a functional balance is lost between the partners' needs to be connected and to be separate.
- Effective couple therapy focuses on understanding the protective meanings of the couple's particular defensive patterns, as reflecting each partner's wishes for and fears of intimacy and self-development. The general therapeutic aim is to aid the couple in restoring an optimal developmental process and balance between relationship and personal growth.

This theoretical and clinical approach also incorporates the contributions of those authors who have applied object relations concepts to couple and family relationships, beginning with the pioneering work of Henry Dicks (1963) and subsequently followed by many others, including John Zinner (1976), James Framo (1970/1982b, 1982a, 1992), Jurg Willi (1982), Deborah Luepnitz (1988), Samuel Slipp (1988), David and Jill Scharff (1991), Judith Siegel (1992, 1998), Robert Winer (1994), and Otto Kernberg (1975, 1976, 1995), to name those who have most influenced my thinking. This work aims to augment object relations and other clinical approaches to couple therapy by the addition of a multifaceted view of relationship development that can act as a valuable guide for assessment and treatment.

Through understanding the optimal development and common pitfalls of each relationship pattern, the therapist can more readily identify which pattern(s) is causing difficulty for a couple and at what point in this development the partners have become derailed, either temporarily or more permanently. This assessment is then helpful in determining treatment difficulty, where and how to focus interventions, and the possibility of a certain kind of relationship forming between therapist and couple that may interfere with treatment progress.

Clinical interventions are more or less effective, depending upon as-

sessment of the couple's area(s) of conflict and to what extent the partners' relationship capacities have developed in that area. For example, a
couple that exhibits considerable difficulty in moving beyond romantic
forms of merging, idealizing, and nurturing will respond favorably to an
approach that explores the adaptive and defensive needs to sustain these
modes. However, such a couple will likely not respond to *initial* interventions that promote separateness too rapidly or that assume the partners'
to be more differentiated than they are at the time. This assessment also
predicts that as treatment unfolds, the couple is likely to idealize the therapist as a perfect mother and the therapist may be induced to idealize the
couple in return. Awareness of this likelihood can help the therapist to
use such an enactment productively and forestall a potential stalemate in
treatment.

My criteria for the *optimal* or *normal* development of each pattern
have evolved over thirty years through the study and treatment of hun-
dreds of couples. For certain patterns (nurturing, idealizing, and devaluing), I present a couple with problems in the mild to moderate range of
difficulty, followed by discussion of longer-term treatment with a more seriously disrupted couple. The patterns of controlling and competing are
each illustrated with one case example, reflecting common problems of
moderate treatment difficulty. Although couples are likely to have trouble
in more than a single mode of relating, often one defensive pattern dominates the foreground of their relationship, though others may come into
focus at a later point.

The theoretical concepts are derived from an exploratory form of
study and thus require verification and refinement in subsequent research. From initial observation, the relationship patterns do not seem to
develop in a linear progression as most stage theories hypothesize.
Rather, they appear to develop in the form of a spiral by recapitulating
earlier steps, though at higher levels of organization, many times throughout the life of the relationship. Some of the patterns appear to be more affected (either progressively or regressively) by life events, personal development, and early family experience. Other patterns seem particularly
affected by culture and gender stereotypes. These differences will become
apparent in the varying ways each developmental process is described.
Whether relationship development can be refined into a more consistent
framework remains for future study to determine.

My concepts are also restricted by the kind of couples I have treated
and studied over the years. These couples have been mainly white, heterosexual, and from the middle- to upper-middle-class socioeconomic groups.
It cannot be determined at this point whether these developmental formulations reflect the processes of other couple populations. However, in my

minimal experience of treating gay and lesbian couples, I have found this approach to be applicable and meaningful.[7]

Midstream in the writing process, I realized that if I made the effort to write in clear, nontechnical language, the concepts and treatment illustrations could be helpful to couples having difficulties and to those who were experiencing couple therapy. I hope distressed couples will be comforted by the concept of marriage as a complex, developmental process that in its normal progression is fraught with periods of great difficulty, turmoil, and conflict. Steeped in the ideals of romantic and devoted love, many couples feel they are failing in their relationships if they experience disappointment and conflict. I underscore that much of what feels like painful failure often reflects aspects of a normal developmental process.

The downside of this conception is that we are taken back to my mother's knee and her observation that having a good marriage involves a lot of work—but then again, so does having a bad one. This book tries to make that work less vague, more manageable, and sometimes fun.

Just as couples' relationships are difficult, so too is doing couple therapy. Most therapists who first begin seeing couples, even though experienced in individual therapy, are shocked at how difficult it is and how overwhelmed they feel. Many flee in horror, never to return. These strong reactions reflect the powerful feelings stirred up in therapists by couples' anxiety and openly expressed conflicts. In discussing treatment of difficult couples, I pay particular attention to the therapist's evoked emotional reactions (countertransference feelings). I hope to provide support and comfort to therapists by demonstrating how the understanding of these feelings and their utilization of them in treatment not only significantly enhances the treatment process, but also can make couple therapy feel less like drowning in a swamp of emotions and more like an interesting, if not always easy, therapy experience.

I also hope therapists will benefit from my efforts to illustrate the treatment process and therapy approach with in-depth case examples that not only reveal the couple's interaction but also what I do, say, think, and feel. I have often felt unenlightened when reading case examples that only describe a fragment of treatment or the therapist's activity in summarized terms. The dialogues with couples presented throughout the book to illustrate couple development and treatment have been taken from detailed notes and my memory of sessions. They have been condensed, edited for

---

[7]Several authors have written about women's struggles in lesbian love relationships with respect to many of the same themes and patterns described in this book. In particular, see Peglau, Cochran, Rosh, and Patesky (1978), Lindenbaum (1985), and Burch (1985, 1987).

clarity, and identifying information has been altered to protect confidentiality, though I have tried to preserve the accuracy of the partners' dynamics. At times, I have made myself sound more articulate and to the point than I actually was, in the hope of providing better dialogue.

Many years ago, I was trained to "solve" a couple's problems in twelve sessions. Then, I spent the next decade trying to figure out how really to do couple therapy. Today, I hear of treatment approaches that purport to do the job in six sessions. Troubled partners who need to be in treatment longer than the few sessions specified by their health maintenance organization (HMO) or therapist's approach then feel even more like failures. Likewise therapists who cannot fix a couple in six or twelve sessions begin to wonder what is wrong with their skills.

This book aims to counter these unhelpful attitudes by speaking to the difficulty of both creating a good marriage and doing couple therapy. By offering an assessment process and treatment approach tailored to a couple's needs, I also hope to encourage more enlightened views. Many couples come to therapy with problems stemming from the stresses of a normal developmental process. Often, these couples can benefit from short-term treatment. Many other couples, however, have deeply entrenched difficulties that require a more substantial, longer-term approach. These diagnostic distinctions should be made about couples, just as they are about individuals.

The couples whose treatment I describe in this book not only reveal fascinating, true-life love stories but also demonstrate what it takes to work out of painful patterns and move forward. Each of their stories presents a unique and priceless tapestry of the ways we love.

GENERAL PHASES	PATTERNS OF CONNECTION			PATTERNS OF SEPARATENESS			
	Nurturing	Merging	Idealizing	Devaluing	Controlling	Competing for Superiority	Competing in Love Triangles*
Romantic Love	Romantic nurturing	Global merging: oneness	Romantic idealizing		Controlling to foster connection	Competing as courtship play	Competing *for* the partner
Disappointment and Disillusionment	Integration of disappointment	Deflation: recognition of differences	Deidealizing	Global devaluing Devaluing to create separateness	Controlling as parental domination Controlling to foster autonomy	Competing for admiration and superiority Competing to cope with envy and inadequacy	Competing *with* the partner
Differentiation and Acceptance	Differentiation of needs	Acceptance of needs to be close and separate	Acceptance of the real partner	Acceptance of flaws in partner and self	Differentiation of self-control from partner control	Acceptance of needs to compete	Reworking past competitive triangles
Modulation and Integration	Reciprocal nurturing	Regulation of being together and apart	Modulated idealizing	Devaluing as a distress signal	Acceptance and modulation of wishes to dominate and submit	Modulation of dyadic competing	Regulation and modulation of competitive triangles
Mature Love	Triadic nurturing	Attainment of mutuality	Intermittent romantic idealizing	Respectful criticism	Controlling in service of cooperation	Competing to enhance collaboration	Winning first place with the partner

*Serves both connection and separateness.

FIGURE 1. Development of couple relationship patterns.

PART I

Patterns of Connection

Nurturing

"Someone to Watch Over Me"
—GEORGE GERSHWIN (1926)

CHAPTER 1

The Foundation of Loving

If one pattern of relating could be singled out as the most important and fundamental in love relationships, it would be nurturing. Loving our partner, translated into day-to-day living, includes a commitment to both taking care of and receiving care from that person. Nurturing is one of the most important ways love is expressed and connection is experienced. How well partners can give and receive nurturance is usually a central determinant of their overall well-being as a couple.

The majority of couples who come for therapy suffer from feeling unnurtured in their relationships, even though they may define their difficulties as poor communication, drifting apart, or an unsatisfying sex life. Sooner or later, one or both partners may cry out from this core of their unhappiness: "I do all the giving and get nothing in return!"

Rina and Zack, a bright, engaging couple in their late twenties and married for four years, came for therapy because of increased fighting, a minimal sex life, and growing feelings of estrangement. Although difficulties began within the first year of their marriage, their fighting had gotten more intense and frequent since the birth of their daughter, Eliza, now two years old. Both were concerned about the effect of their conflict on Eliza, who was described as overly fearful. Zack thought Rina's "need to control" was the major problem, and Rina thought Zack's "distance and depression" were ruining the marriage. Their formulation—that the other's unfortunate traits were the cause of their problems—is a familiar presentation. Interrupting their blaming, I asked Rina how Zack's distance and depression affected her.

RINA: I feel deserted and alone. He's just not there . . . not emotionally present. We never talk about our feelings like we used to.

ZACK: We don't talk because we're both too exhausted by the time we're alone together.

RINA: But I would feel so much better if we talked.

ZACK: When do you suggest we talk? We get home late from work. After Eliza goes down, I just want to zone out or go to sleep. I don't have the energy for talking and neither do you.

RINA: That's not true!

I see the lines of strain etched in their young faces and hear the irritable edge in their voices. Rina's attractiveness is marred by a fixed scowl and deep furrows in her brow. With her sculpted face, huge brown eyes, and black hair, she reminds me of Audrey Hepburn playing the waif in *Breakfast at Tiffany's*. Zack looks at me, a plea in his intelligent gray eyes. He has the sensitive features and sickly pallor of a starving poet. He wears his long blond hair pulled back into a ponytail, and Birkenstock sandals wrap around his bare feet. I deduce he's a graduate student or on the faculty at the University. Both are very tall and rail thin, looking like tender saplings that could easily blow over in a high wind. They sit tensely, waiting for the next scrape on raw nerves to send them flaring into open conflict. I feel like offering them a square meal and a good night's sleep. Instead, I ask for a description of their daily lives to expose the most immediate causes of their plight.

Both perk up with this request, perhaps as something to do, other than following their usual groove into a bruising fight. In recounting the details of their less than storybook life together, each one's sense of humor and capacity for insight begins to surface. Zack, an assistant professor of music, has a gift for turning the most mundane events into black comedy. Rina responds to Zack's humor with a sharp wit of her own. Rina, an architect, works for a local firm. The essence of their description of a typical evening together is similar to many I've heard over the years and is indicative of *marital malnourishment*, the most common condition plaguing couples who come for therapy.

Zack arrives home about 6:30 P.M. to their old, fixer-upper of a house in the endless process of being refurbished. He's exhausted from a stressful day at the University and spending forty-five minutes on the freeway in traffic. He's greeted by a dying lawn, a garage door that does not open, every room in total disarray, and nagging reminders of disrepair everywhere.

Rina picks up Eliza at day care and then carries a fussy, hungry child into the house about 6:45 P.M.. Before an exchange of greetings, she announces that Eliza has come down with a cold and has diarrhea. Zack groans. The sequel is predictable to both. One of them will have to jump through a dozen hoops to stay home from work if Eliza gets sicker. A doctor's appointment will need to be arranged. Eliza will be more difficult, and they will both likely catch the cold.

Eliza starts to cry. Rina attempts to soothe her without success and then hands her to Zack. It's her turn to cook dinner. Tired and frustrated, she stomps around the kitchen banging pots and throwing leftovers together, while barking out complaints about the counter littered with dirty dishes that Zack should have cleaned up. Zack tries to defend his lapse, while alternately checking his e-mail and bouncing Eliza on his knee to keep her amused and quiet.

There is no meaningful conversation at dinner. Eliza needs constant tending. She smears food on her face and laughs. Zack scolds her. Rina criticizes Zack for scolding Eliza. In fits and starts, each reports the facts of the day, what needs to be done, and who will take care of it. Zack asks if Rina got the dishwasher fixed. She forgot to call the repair man because she was so busy. Zack is clearly annoyed, because he is this week's dishwasher. They argue about who is more stressed, and who has more to do. Zack suddenly stops the quarrel, because he must prepare two lectures for the next day. Rina tries to get Eliza ready for bed, in between answering the phone and picking up the toys, shoes, and clothes strewn around the bedrooms and down the hall.

After putting Eliza to sleep with three stories and several songs, Rina returns a call from her mother, who is anxious about her upcoming bypass surgery. She listens and soothes her mother's fears for a half an hour. Her mother makes her feel guilty for not calling sooner, not calling her often enough, and not being there with her to provide better support. Rina then shuffles into bed to read her novel for a treasured few minutes before passing out.

On her way to the bathroom, she finds Zack snoring in front of the television. She wonders whether to wake him or just let him sleep. She worries that if she wakes him, he might impinge on her urgent need for time to herself by trying to initiate sex. Awakening briefly, he worries that she might want to talk about their problems, and then he will not get enough sleep to do well in class the next day. He falls back to sleep on the couch. Returning to bed, Rina feels relieved, lonely, and acutely sad. She cries quietly over the day's painful reminders of her inadequacies as a daughter, a mother, and a wife.

CREATING A "HOLDING ENVIRONMENT"

An important early intervention is to help depleted partners recognize their chronic fatigue, stress, and anger about overgiving and feeling unnurtured in return. After hearing their story, I said, "This is a very demanding, stressful life you're describing, and I think each of you is suffering from giving too much and getting too little. A lot of your hurt and anger with each other is coming from the reality of trying to meet too many demands without being replenished in important ways."

The initial identification of a couple's deprived feelings, underscoring their shared experience, helps promote empathy between both the partners and the therapist and the couple. This kind of explanation also helps to allay fears each partner may have about being the cause of problems—the one who is wrong or a failure. Such underlying fears are typically expressed by projecting fault and blaming the partner. Reducing these fears and their defensive expression aids in the creation of an empathic "holding environment," so that deeper exploration of the couple's difficulties can more easily occur.

Donald Winnicott (1965) introduced the term "holding environment" to describe certain aspects of the therapy relationship that were like the mother's care of her infant. The importance of the therapist's creation of a holding environment in providing a safe climate for emotional expression has been particularly emphasized by those clinicians who use object relations and self psychology concepts in the treatment of individuals, couples, and families.[1] In couple therapy, creation of such an environment requires the therapist's initial and ongoing demonstration of empathy, understanding, reliability, maintenance of appropriate boundaries, protection of the partners from injury, and refraining from retaliation.

Provision of this climate is generally desirable, but it is particularly important for people with nurturing deficits. The holding environment provides certain aspects of nurturing that are lacking in the couple relationship and in itself has a healing, growth-promoting effect. A major goal of treatment is to promote the couple's gradual ability to bring into their own relationship the elements of the therapeutic holding environment.

Many conditions affect the therapist's ability to create a good-enough holding environment. Training, experience, and general sense of life satisfaction are important factors in determining the therapist's self-confidence, capacity to give appropriate support, and ability to refrain from unprofessional reactions to partners. Couples who frequently engage in unmodulated expressions of anger and injury certainly test such capacities more strongly than do most individuals in treatment. The kind of role relationship that develops between couple and therapist and between each partner and the therapist are also significant factors in the therapist's ability to sustain a safe environment.

---

[1]See Arnold Modell (1976), the Scharffs (1991), Siegel (1992), and Luepnitz (1988).

Another important consideration is the quality of the couple therapist's relationship with any other therapist who may be involved in the partners' treatment. The therapeutic environment may become difficult or impossible to sustain if one or both of the partners' individual therapist(s) undermines the couple therapist (or vice versa). The confusing and sometimes toxic environment that may develop is akin to the climate created by parents who undermine each other in the care and discipline of their children. (Although this unfortunate, but all to common, difficulty is not examined in this book, the reader is referred to an excellent paper on this subject by Carolyn Maltas, 1998).

ASSESSMENT OF NURTURING PATTERNS AND PROBLEMS

It is important for the therapist to understand how partners nurture each other, since most couples who come for therapy have difficulty in this area. Assessment entails exploring with the couple a number of interrelated factors that are only introduced here but elaborated in the next three chapters. In the course of an evaluation, the therapist seeks to understand (1) the fundamental ways that partners give and receive caring, (2) the severity of their malnourishment, and (3) the causes of their nurturing problems.

The Evaluation

One of the first acts of good caregiving that benefits both the couple and the therapist is the provision of a defined evaluation period. Structuring time to understand a couple's relationship and its unique problems helps the partners feel well cared for, even though many couples will press for immediate solutions. Couples are very complex systems and are not quickly understood. In general, magical expectations of the therapist and therapy may also be reduced by helping couples understand the necessity for an in-depth evaluation. Space and time are given for everyone to consider carefully what constitutes the problem, who feels what and why, and the therapist is restrained from rushing prematurely into a "fix-it," action mode, driven by anxiety or grandiosity (or both). The greater efficacy of understanding before taking action is also modeled.

It is important for the therapist to understand each partner as an individual, the couple and family system, and the interplay between individual and interpersonal dynamics. Since couple relationships consist of two separate, individual personalities and their interaction, it is helpful to have an evaluation format that is congruent with this reality, one that includes both conjoint sessions and individual sessions for each partner.

Partners often relate much differently with the therapist alone than when they are together. The inclusion of individual sessions is of particular help in forming a therapeutic alliance with each partner more rapidly than can usually occur by meeting only conjointly.

I have found six sessions to be a good average number for an in-depth evaluation of a couple. The first session is conjoint, the next four are allocated to two individual sessions with each partner, and the last session is focused on collaboratively summarizing the couple's strengths and difficulties, followed by a discussion of the therapist's recommendations. This is a general and somewhat ideal format that may not always be possible or appropriate. One may only have six sessions to work with a couple who must rely on coverage from their HMO. Some couples cannot tolerate being separated for individual sessions, in which case the evaluation should be done conjointly. Also, if the couple is in an acute crisis, individual sessions may need to wait until the crisis has subsided. It is possible to understand the needs of certain couples in one session, while with others, twelve evaluation sessions would not seem to be enough.

The evaluation does not just involve information gathering that provides little help to the couple. It can be very therapeutic. Sometimes a couple's forward development is restored in the course of a good evaluation, because identification of the "real" problem or causes of problems have been enough to enable the partners to work on their own. A detailed example of conducting an in-depth evaluation that provides considerable therapeutic benefit to the couple is presented in Chapter 9.

The Ways Couples Nurture

While often associated with the giving of food and other forms of basic care, "nurturing" here is meant to encompass all forms of caring that a person *subjectively* experiences as giving and receiving nurture. Feeling nurtured and cared for are usually central aspects of feeling loved. Since being nurtured was our first experience of relating, mutual nurturing between partners is the most fundamental mode of connection. Partners nurture each other in a number of ways that can be organized into three categories: (1) *basic care*, (2) *emotional support*, and (3) *affectionate expression, both sexual and nonsexual.*

Basic care is the most fundamental form of nurturing. It includes the activities of feeding, sheltering, clothing, comforting, protecting, financial support, and nursing care when a family member is ill. A couple is challenged daily by the management of these aspects of giving and receiving. The difficulties of many couples are focused in this area, ranging from mild conflict over chores or finances to major competitive strife over whose needs get met. Other couples, like Rina and Zack, may collaborate fairly well in the daily mechanics of living but experience deficits in emotional support, and affectionate and sexual expression.

Emotional support in all of its various aspects is central to a couple's well-being, including giving and receiving empathy, encouragement, admiration, appreciation, time, companionship, and assistance of all kinds. Particularly important is support of the other's life work, whether it be a career or homemaking. One of Rina and Zack's strengths was their belief in the value of each other's career. Each took an interest in the other's activities, admired the other's achievements, and actively helped the other meet career responsibilities. However, each also felt certain significant deficits in the other's emotional support. Zack felt criticized and unappreciated by Rina for never being good enough in meeting her needs. Rina felt that Zack did not provide the intimate sharing of feelings and empathic listening she required to feel nurtured.

Affectionate and sexual expressions of caring, including verbal as well as physical expressions of love, are needed by most partners on an ongoing basis to feel loved. One of the difficult tasks for couples is being able to sustain the nurturing aspects of their physical and sexual relations. So often, physical affection becomes a dutiful kiss or a hasty hug rather than a spontaneous expression of tenderness. Rina complained that Zack's affectionate expressions only occurred as a prelude to having sex. Zack said he had withdrawn from giving affection because of Rina's frequent sexual rejections. Both felt their sex life lacked intimacy. Rina had lost her desire and withdrew from sexual relations, because the experience too often left her feeling emotionally disconnected and unloved.

Severity of Problems: Temporary or Long-Term Derailment

Although Rina and Zack were in acute pain when they came for therapy, their angry, hurtful interactions were not long entrenched, nor did they characterize the overall quality of their relationship. While the history of each partner revealed certain dependency and control conflicts stemming from their family-of-origin experience, there was no major psychopathology. Much of their conflict appeared to result from overwhelming demands without adequate help, a condition that interfered with the optimal development of their nurturing capacities. In our society, most couples go through very hard times when they are trying to care for young children and manage dual, demanding careers (or even one career). Typically, it is the relationship that suffers, more so than the child or the careers. Couples with this kind of problem can often respond to short-term treatment.

While the problems in nurturing represented by Rina and Zack signify a temporary derailment or stall in the normal development of nurturing capacities, there are many other couples whose nurturing deficits are much more severe, signifying a serious, long-term derailment. Development has not only come to a halt, but also destructive defensive patterns have become entrenched. In the most severe cases, the partners have lost all spontaneous desire to give and end up punitively depriving each other. Prolonged regression to childhood states has occurred. Each partner has come to feel and act like an angry, hungry baby crying out for an unavailable mother. The partners' interactions can become a ferocious competition for crumbs of sustenance—the scarce supplies of basic care. Emotional support, affection and sex are also lacking but feel less crucial to survival. John Cheever (in his *Journals*) captures the essence of marital starvation in describing his parents' attacks on each other at the breakfast table.[2]

> "Leave me alone, just leave me alone is all I ask," says she.
>
> "All I want," he says, "is a boiled egg. Is that too much to ask?"
>
> "Well, boil yourself an egg then," she screams; and this is the full voice of tragedy, the goat cry. "Boil yourself an egg then, but leave me alone."
>
> "But how in hell can I boil an egg," he shouts, "if you won't let me use the pot?"
>
> "I'd let you use the pot," she screams, "but you leave it so filthy. I don't know what it is, but you leave everything you touch covered with filth."
>
> "I bought the pot," he roars, "the soap, the eggs. I pay the water and the gas bills, and here I sit in my own house unable to boil an egg. Starving."
>
> "Here," she screams, "eat my breakfast. I can't eat it. You've ruined my appetite. You've ruined my day." (1991)

The following interchange between Eva and Sid, married for twelve years, also exemplifies a serious derailment in nurturing. The same theme is expressed of the unnurturing mother who withholds food from a starving infant.

SID: I come home after working all day and there's no dinner on the table, and then I find there's nothing in the refrigerator. I have to go out to the store to get something to eat. Driving there, I realize I have

---

[2]I am indebted to Michael Vincent Miller (1995, pp. 34–35) for bringing this wonderful quote to my attention in his book, *Intimate Terrorism*. He uses this interchange to illustrate the kind of "intimacy" in which battles for control permeate every aspect of a couple's relationship. This interaction also illustrates other patterns of relating used defensively: devaluing and competing for love. In this case, love has become equated with food.

to take care of everything in this relationship! I ask myself, what am I getting? Nothing, is the answer!

EVA: What about me? What am I getting? I get nothing but abuse. If I were to be the dutiful little wife you want and make your dinner, you'd say it wasn't fit to eat.

SID: I only say that when you burn the rice. No one can eat burned rice.

EVA: I don't burn the rice. That happened one time when Laurie was shrieking bloody murder. I should have saved the rice I suppose and let our child be beaten to death by the neighborhood bully!

SID: I can't count the times I've come home to the smell of something burning on the stove. Usually I find you napping or taking a bath. Laurie could be murdered or kidnapped for all you'd know.

EVA: I won't be burning your dinner from now on. You can eat your own shitty words and choke.

Unlike Rina and Zack, Eva and Sid were not able to become parents in the sense of forging an adult partnership that could embrace a dependent child. They remained mired for years in an endlessly frustrating parent–child interaction of their own.

Causes of Nurturing Problems

In attempting to understand why a couple's nurturing patterns and problems have developed in the way they have, the therapist should evaluate the possible impact of several important factors including (1) culturally ingrained attitudes about giving and receiving, (2) the stresses of normal development, (3) the partners' nurturing experience in their families of origin, (4) existence of substance abuse, (5) existence of mental or physical illness, (6) depression of one or both partners, (7) gender differences, personality traits, and genetic endowment of the partners. Most often overlooked by therapists are cultural attitudes and their role in couples' failure to thrive. Because our culture provides the context in which development and other marital dramas unfold, cultural myths and marital malnourishment are the first to be discussed in Chapter 2.

The normal development of nurturing, which is closely interrelated with the life cycle of a marriage, is a difficult, stressful process even under the best of conditions. Many couples' nurturing problems are partially or wholly a result of the trials and tribulations of normal development. Different kinds of nurturing are called for at different phases in the life cycle of a marriage. In the early phase of a relationship, romantic kinds of nurturing are often most desired. But when a baby arrives, each partner's ability to support the other while giving constant care to the new baby calls upon a more complex and demanding set of nurturing capacities. Like many couples, Rina and Zack, and Eva and Sid ran into trouble with the birth of their first child. Each new child and each new phase in the children's development impact the couple's relationship and the family's nurturing environment. The onset of middle age, the empty nest, retirement, and old age creates yet other challenges to the partners' abilities to care for each other. Developmental derailment can occur at any point. In Chapter 3, the normal development of nurturing is presented, along with the common pitfalls encountered. The case example of Rina and Zack is used to illustrate the developmental steps, as well as how this knowledge is utilized by the therapist in treatment.

People vary widely in how they demonstrate caring and what makes them feel cared for in a relationship. The kind and quality of a partner's nurturing are strongly shaped by experiences in his or her family of origin. Especially early on in relationships, partners often give and expect certain kinds of care based on their own family experience. In reverse, they frequently want to give or get the opposite kind of care than was experienced. When one's partner does not follow the familiar script (or follows it too well), disappointment can be acute.

In addition to the usual problems caused by the partners' different or similar family-of-origin experience, one or both partners may have experienced inadequate or distorted forms of care. Deficits in nurturing from childhood can cause mild to severe repercussions in adulthood and marriage. In Rina and Zack's case, their experiences led them to create a certain kind of role relationship—*the caretaker and the self-sufficient child*—to protect themselves from reexperiencing the pain of childhood longings for basic care. Because their difficulties were not deeply entrenched, this couple responded relatively quickly to appropriate treatment.

However, when each partner's early deprivations are more serious and become reenacted in the marriage in a pervasive way, treatment can be very difficult and long term. In their enactment of a common collusive relationship—*the caretaker and the needful child*, Eva and Sid were caught in the hopeless attempt to fulfill childhood needs or find satisfaction in revenge. Their in-depth treatment is presented in Chapter 4.

A couple's nurturing environment can also be adversely affected by the individual problems of partners that may stem from unfortunate childhood experience, as well as biological factors. One or both partners' substance abuse and mental or physical illness can dramatically drain or destroy a couple's nurturing supplies. The illness or addiction of one partner may force the other into a caretaking role. This situation usually causes great strain, even with couples whose psychological needs are fulfilled in such a role relationship.

Some degree of depression is the most common disorder affecting one or both partners whom I have seen in consultation.[3] The depression may be a result of their troubled relationship or may be one cause of the problems. While major depression or a bipolar disorder can incapacitate a partner, milder depressions can interfere with sexual interest and satisfaction, spontaneous expression or reception of affection, and the ability to give or receive emotional support. Whether a spouse's depression is caused by cultural, psychological, relational, or biological factors, the potential benefit of antidepressant medication should always be considered. The improved mood and well-being of one partner can revitalize the couple's relationship. Many partners initially refuse to consider medication and need to overcome their perception that taking medication means craziness, weakness, neediness, or some kind of psychological or biological flaw. In the two cases introduced, I recommended that both Zack and Eva be evaluated for antidepressant medication. Neither partner was amenable to this suggestion until the midphase of therapy. When they ultimately followed through and experienced substantial benefit, their relationships were dramatically and positively affected. Deeper work in therapy also became possible.

Gender and personality differences may be important determinants of how each partner gives and receives care. A man who is very self-controlled and intellectual will likely have difficulty with spontaneous expressions of feelings and affection. A woman who experiences the world primarily through her feelings may have great difficulty with certain aspects of basic care, such as organizing the household or keeping track of finances.

Understanding how each partner's unique, inherited temperament affects their interactions and general well-being can also be particularly helpful to couples. At the end of Rina and Zack's evaluation, I made the observation that each shared certain traits—high intelligence and great sensitivity—that were very desirable on the one hand but caused them difficulty on the other. Superior intelligence and sensitivity often go hand in hand with thin, tender skins and greater emotional reactivity. These qualities would make them feel their feelings acutely. On the positive side, good feelings would be heightened but hurt feelings, anxiety, anger, and depression would also be amplified. I suggested that it would help them to keep awareness of these endowments in mind in working with their own

---

[3]See Coyne, Kahn, and Gotlib (1985) for a review of studies on marriage and depression. See also the edited volumes of Jacobson and Gurman (1986, 1995) for many chapters describing treatment of partners suffering from a variety of personality and psychiatric problems that mildly to severely affect their nurturing capacities.

and each other's reactions. Both partners felt supported and enlightened by this understanding.

I also determined that Zack was hypersensitive to sound. He became overwhelmed in situations with a lot of commotion and noise, such as big parties or crowds. In addition to the emotional impact, the sheer noise of loud arguing, crying, or expressions of anger deeply disturbed him. Even the volume of the sound system in movie theaters was hard for him to tolerate. To endure these situations, he would instinctively withdraw like a turtle—behavior that had left Rina feeling deserted on many occasions. When this behavior of Zack's was better understood as an aspect of his hardwiring, Rina could empathize and help protect him. Zack also became better able to protect himself from overstimulation and the need to withdraw.

Modality of Treatment

The best modality of treatment for couples continues to be a hot topic of debate. The strongest disagreement occurs between those clinicians who think couples should be treated only conjointly and those who feel that the inclusion of individual sessions with the partners (a combined modality) is sometimes desirable or even necessary. There are good arguments in favor of each position. I do not here present all aspects of this multifaceted subject, since thorough discussions exist elsewhere (see Nadelson, 1978; Sander & Feldman, 1993; Siegel, 1992; Birk, 1984). In my own view, the modality of treatment selected should be tailored to the couple's goals, developmental needs, ego strengths, and vulnerabilities.

An additional important consideration is the experience and comfort of the therapist in managing the formats of treatment. Because of training or other factors, one therapist may *only* be comfortable working conjointly, while another therapist has become skilled at combining modalities to effect greater depth of treatment. In general, it takes long experience to make good judgments about when and how to combine modalities and to manage the problems that may be stimulated by different formats. For this reason, beginning therapists are likely to be more comfortable sticking with a conjoint modality. There is less chance of making major errors. On the other hand, depth of treatment and potential progress may be sacrificed.

Conjoint therapy should be the first option considered if the couple is coming for improvement of their relationship. Relationship dynamics are best seen and can be more effectively addressed with both partners present. A *consistent* conjoint modality is especially important for those couples, like Rina and Zack, who have major difficulty in forming a strong couple bond and couple identity (discussed in Chapter 3). A conjoint framework in itself addresses this problem, giving time and attention to the relationship.

For the opposite reason, a consistent conjoint modality is often necessary for couples who are enmeshed and use devaluing and blaming as major defenses. These couples, like Eva and Sid, cannot emotionally manage individual treatment with separate therapists or the inclusion of individual sessions by the same therapist (at least, not until they become less merged). Any separation of the partners can lead to overwhelming anxiety. Both fear the loss of their crucial bond and that one partner will form a stronger alliance with the therapist and the other will be identified as the flawed one with the problem. However, the partner who is striving for greater independence may wish for individual appointments to strengthen his or her position with the therapist (viewed as a powerful parent) and may succeed in seducing the therapist into providing individual appointments. This situation occurred in the midphase of treatment with Eva and Sid, and the deleterious effects of not holding firm with the conjoint format are demonstrated in Chapter 12.

However, in many other situations, I have found it to be beneficial and necessary to include individual sessions or to treat each partner in individual therapy for a time (termed "concurrent treatment"). When mixing modalities, the therapist's attunement to potential problems is a major key to success. Ground rules about sharing of information from individual sessions must be clearly defined. The partners' possible fears of feeling left out of an alliance should be thoroughly discussed in advance. The couple should be strongly encouraged to share such feelings when they occur. Since it is impossible always to know how a partner may react, it is advisable to plan in terms of a trial period for mixing modalities that can be quickly altered if too many problems arise (e.g., unyielding suspiciousness, repeated use of the therapist's comments as a weapon with the partner, or the sharing of a secret, such as an affair, that puts the therapist in an untenable position).

From a developmental point of view, some couples are unable to manage a triangular modality or three-person format because it can stimulate strong competitive feelings. Partners' inability to modulate competitive impulses to win the therapist and defeat the other partner may be so great that conjoint treatment becomes destructive to one or both partners (or the therapist!). Provision of a safe holding environment may necessitate temporarily abandoning conjoint therapy until the partners come to understand and manage rivalrous feelings in more modulated ways.

Additionally, some partners are too narcissistically vulnerable to manage the kinds of injuries that inevitably occur in conjoint therapy. One partner may criticize or become angry with the other in way that is destabilizing and destructive to that partner. The couple's angry escalations can become difficult or impossible to control. The therapist might be able to keep destructive episodes to a minimum by discouraging the couple's interaction and doing individual therapy with each partner in a conjoint frame. But sometimes the conjoint format cannot be constructively maintained in spite of skilled therapeutic management, and the partners may require preparatory or adjunctive individual treatment.

Including individual sessions in the therapy plan can also significantly advance treatment. Meeting individually with partners can be of great help in working out of a stalemate in treatment or working through the negative feelings one partner may have developed toward the therapist. Partners who are striving to define and sustain individual identities can often utilize individual sessions for strengthening a sense of self that enables them to use conjoint therapy more constructively. For couples mired in an idealizing mode of relating and mortally afraid of conflict, the use of individual sessions to unearth the partners' angry feelings and explore fears of conflict can much more rapidly effect positive change in the relationship. The importance of including individual sessions for such couples is detailed in Chapter 9.

Group therapy and couples group therapy can also be very beneficial to many couples. Unfortunately, there is a paucity of couples groups available, since so few therapists undertake this form of treatment. The advantages of couples groups used alone and in combination with other modalities are well discussed by Framo (1973), Birk (1984), and Gershenfeld (1985).

I was introduced to couples group therapy about fifteen years ago when I had the unique opportunity of working as a cotherapist (in training) with James Framo. I could see the great benefit couples experienced in the process of sharing their shame, struggles, and attempted solutions. The supportive climate created by the group encouraged understanding and change more rapidly than may often occur in traditional conjoint therapy. In the conjoint format, the therapist is the lone supportive figure, who is also likely to provoke more intense competitive rivalry between the partners because of the triangular constellation. In these respects, the creation of a safe environment may be easier to achieve in a couples group.

A couples group may be the ideal modality for malnourished couples in its provision of a familial kind of caring environment, where support and helpful interventions come from a variety of sources. Such a group would also supply meaningful connections with the outside world to counteract the loneliness and isolation of many couples and families in our current society.

Framo (1976, 1992) adds a potentially powerful additional technique to couples group therapy (also used in conjoint marital and family therapy). In the context of identifying family-of-origin sources of a couple's problems, he encourages both partners to bring in their original families for direct therapeutic work on the unresolved issues that contribute to their marital pain. When used effectively, this technique can achieve the dual important purposes of dramatically improving a couple's relationship while at the same time restoring the partners' original families as sources of love and support, a crucial source of nurturing that is so often missing in the lives of couples today.

CHAPTER 2

Cultural Myths and Marital Malnourishment

Our culture perpetuates certain myths that significantly contribute to marital malnourishment. Cultural influences are often overlooked by therapists, couples, and the psychological literature on marriage relationships. The therapist who is attuned to these influences can help couples understand this aspect of their conflicts. Since partners often share belief in certain cultural myths, their understanding in this area often contributes to an expansion of mutual empathy, a softening of defensiveness, and the creation of a safe holding environment for deeper therapeutic work.

In his remarkable and eloquent book, *Intimate Terrorism: The Deterioration of Erotic Life* (1995), Michael Vincent Miller examines the effects on couples of the myth of romantic love and the myth of the nuclear family as the source of all love. To these I have added the myth of selfless love and the myth of couple self-sufficiency. A combination of belief in these four myths and a young couple in love supplies all the ingredients necessary for marital malnutrition. These myths appear to have their roots in the sociocultural ideals of romantic love, Judeo-Christian morality, the Protestant work ethic, American rugged individualism, and the idealized nuclear family.

THE MYTH OF ROMANTIC LOVE

The ideal of romantic love is still embedded in our culture, however tarnished and faded some of its trappings may be. The knight on a white charger may be a heartthrob of the past, but belief in the power of love to transport, to heal, and to provide everlasting rapture remains. For those romantically in love, giving love and nurture is spontaneous and effortless. Just by virtue of being in love and loving, couples expect that all of their needs will automatically be fulfilled. And if they sustain their love, this abundance and need fulfillment will go on indefinitely. Consequently, the idea that married people need to learn how to nurture each other, that nurturance is not a free commodity and is often in scarce supply, comes as a shock to many couples. Miller describes this painful recognition and its aftermath:

> The discovery of scarcity can sneak up on people in a particularly vindictive way after they marry. It mocks their fondest dreams. For what it tells them is that marriage consists of two people trying to make a go of it on emotional and psychological supplies that are only sufficient for one. As a result, they are liable to lapse into a barbaric competition over whose needs get met. The likelihood of this regression increases as marriages and families in America slip further from their moorings in purposeful connections to the larger society. (p. 93)

In addition, the myth of romantic love has discouraged the development of adequate psychological theories of love relationships. Pervasive attitudes that love either happens and lasts or becomes sick and dies are so embedded in our culture that the idea of love as involving multiple aspects of relating that develop over time, and that a love relationship needs to be nurtured so that it can develop and flourish, are topics that rarely come to mind for investigation.

THE MYTH OF SELFLESS LOVE

The automatic fulfillment of needs promised by romantic love exists in contrast to the hard work and sacrifice demanded by the myth of selfless love. Inculcated in us from Judeo-Christian morality are the beliefs that "it is better to give than to receive . . . cast your bread upon the waters. . . . " Wanting, asking, and receiving are thought of as baser forms of behavior—greedy and selfish—above which one should endeavor to rise. At the core of this myth is the belief that if love is given selflessly, without expectation of reward, it will be returned in abundance. People will get back more than they give and, said Jesus, "The meek shall inherit the earth."

After marriage, partners soon feel the effects of trying to operate according to these notions. The virtue of giving selflessly is not enough for subsistence. Resentment and feelings of exploitation begin to accrue. There are no signs of a just reward on the near or distant horizon. Instead, it seems like the more one gives, the more one is expected to give. The partner and the relationship begin to feel like a bottomless pit of need.

Even though the myths of selfless love and romantic love are contradictory, many partners believe in and operate according to both. The toxic combination of these myths sets up a couple for double-barreled disappointment and resentment. Rina and Zack were most aware of their disappointments in operating according to the myth of selfless love. Both felt they had given greatly to the other without adequate reciprocation and with minimal appreciation. Because both felt they should give selflessly, their great resentment over giving and not getting enough in return was difficult to acknowledge or discuss.

Compounding this resentment was a more unconscious disappointment in the failure of romantic love to deliver the automatic fulfillment of needs. Rina and Zack were angry that giving to the partner had turned out to be such hard work. Giving and receiving were supposed to occur spontaneously. The failure of these deeply rooted beliefs to provide expected rewards leaves a couple feeling betrayed and without anyone to blame except each other.

THE MYTH OF THE NUCLEAR FAMILY AS THE SOURCE OF ALL LOVE

"We are taught that the family is supposed to fill virtually all our early needs for love," says Miller, "romance with an enchanting stranger our middle ones, and a family once again our later ones" (1995, p. 93). Unfortunately, this idealization of the nuclear family resonates with the myth of romantic love to amplify a young couple's disillusionment. Both of these myths lead partners to rely on each other (and their children, when they arrive) for all of their emotional needs. This reliance puts too much strain on a system that was only meant to do part of the job.

It is not surprising, however, that many of us look to the nuclear family as the primary or *only* source of intimacy, love, and nurturance. Because a parent's career was likely to require a move sooner or later, growing up without extended family nearby is a common experience. Unlike preindustrial times, when families were surrounded by their extended family and ties to the community, today's nuclear family members more often live without this kind of support. Rather than bemoan the disadvantages of this change in economics and family life, we tend to rely on the nuclear family to meet all of our needs. In fact, many think of it as liberating to live on one's own, away from the intrusive meddling of parents, inlaws, and other relatives.

Because wishes to make it on their own took them away from their home towns, couples like Rina and Zack began their life together with no extended family nearby, no deep ties to a community or church, no long-term friendships, and no social institutions to support them. This isolation encourages partners to turn to each other to meet all of their needs. When a baby arrives, the problem of scarcity can increase to famine proportions. Having given up on each other, couples may tragically look to the baby as their new hope for everlasting love. In her excellent discussion of the family in history, Deborah Luepnitz (1988) noted this disturbing trend: "Whereas family scholars have sometimes said that the nuclear family replaced the village in modern life, I have said that the child has replaced the village in modern life" (p. 145). When Zack fell asleep on the couch, Rina had the impulse to bring Eliza into bed with her for comfort and cuddling. Concern about damaging her child stopped her from using Eliza as a substitute for Zack.

These unfortunate conditions and their impact on current and future generations have received considerable attention in social history texts but have been very poorly integrated into psychological and therapeutic approaches to marital problems, though Miller's and Lupnitz's books are notable exceptions. This is a surprising oversight, since our developmental theory so strongly underscores the necessity of a nurturing environment for the healthy development of a child. A nurturing environment is also needed for the healthy development of a love relationship, which is just as difficult to raise successfully as is a child. In couple therapy, helping one or both partners to develop a support system outside themselves and their children is often an important aspect of treatment.

THE MYTH OF COUPLE SELF-SUFFICIENCY

Idealizing independence from parents and ties to established institutions (such as the church) feeds into another unhelpful myth—the glorification of couple self-sufficiency. This myth involves the grandiose notion that if couples work hard enough, they can do everything perfectly and should need little or no outside help. This myth seems to derive from rugged individualism applied to couples, combined with the myth that the nuclear family is the source of all nurture.

Rina and Zack are an example of the many couples I have seen who try to live according to this myth. Both came from families on the East Coast and went to college in the East. They moved to the West Coast not only because of the good position Zack was offered at a local university but also because he particularly wanted to live away from their families, fearing the intrusiveness of both sets of parents. So they journeyed west,

leaving families, long-established friends, and lifelong associations behind. They had no ties in their new city, and that seemed romantic and
adventurous to them at the time. They would feel freer to build their own
lives away from the critical eyes of narrow-minded, conservative family influences.

In addition to providing totally for each other's emotional and physical needs, both believed they should also be capable of engaging in successful careers, creating a wonderful home, amassing savings, participating in an active social life, maintaining physical fitness, and raising perfect
children. Couples with these impossible expectations are usually in the
middle and upper-middle socioeconomic classes. Wealthy couples may
more often tend to feel entitled to have everything done for them. Lower
class and poor couples are preoccupied with issues of basic survival and
need to rely on extended family and the outside world for help, even
though they may feel conflicted about such needs.

Rina and Zack were only mildly unrealistic in their expectations compared to another idealistic young couple that came for consultation. I saw
Stella and Chad only briefly, because they were on their way to a third-
world country, where they were going to live in a small village with a family, learn the language, and help to establish a medical clinic. They were
hoping I could put some life back into their marriage in a few sessions before they left. Stella was about four months pregnant and had morning
sickness. The couple's two young children, a two-year-old and a five-year-
old, were going with them. Their marriage was in serious trouble, each
feeling isolated and distant from the other. Stella was so exhausted from
being up with their sick two-year-old for several nights that she could
hardly speak coherently. Chad's boyish face was so strained by fatigue
from too many responsibilities that he looked twice his age.

Although financially comfortable, this couple had a minimum of
household help; a cleaning woman came once per week. They had no extended family living in the area. Although the couple thought their problems had to do with diminishing passion, I thought they were wasting
away and deeply angry from lack of basic care and so had no desire or energy for sex. They were like two malnourished children, who did not even
know they were hungry, hoping to save themselves by saving the world. In
fact, it seemed they were really looking for maternal care and a sense of
connection from a third-world family, and this likely was another reenactment of their histories of trying to get something from an impoverished
nuclear family. Though I prevailed on them to consider carefully their
motivations for making this journey, along with the potential physical and
emotional consequences, they left as planned.

Many months later, after the new baby was born, I heard from Stella
again. They had lasted about two months living in a hot, dirty hut with a

family so poor they could not provide enough food for the ravenous, pregnant Stella. These hardships sent the couple back to civilization, where a new baby and an overwhelmed mother finally impelled them to consider changing their way of living. The first step was to hire adequate help, so that both Stella and Chad could get enough sleep. With enough sleep, they could begin to eat properly. Over time, they became able to address their psychological problems.

While this is an extreme example of physical and emotional malnutrition, the majority of couples with young children I see have similar symptoms: strained faces, irritability, hair-trigger tempers, chronic fatigue, depression—the characteristics I have come to associate with marital malnourishment. Whatever the couple's deeper issues, their physical and emotional depletion from trying to keep up with impossible lives, without adequate help, is their most striking problem.

Repeatedly faced with these issues, couple therapists act, in part, as modern-day substitutes for the extended family. With increasing insistence over the years, I point out that partners' irritability, depression, and feelings of deprivation are a result of chronic depletion from trying to fulfill too many demands without support. Trying to run a marriage without nourishment is like trying to run a car without gas.

Sometimes it is necessary to start with the basics, such as getting enough sleep, a healthful diet, and time for exercise and relaxation. I speak emphatically to couples about getting more help or doing less work. Even affluent partners, who can easily afford to hire more help, resist this solution because of unrealistic or puritanical expectations of themselves. Many prefer to see their marital pain as caused by psychological problems in their partners or themselves. This resistance is bolstered by our culture's worship of superachievers, who, more android than human, seem never to need rest or any other human forms of replenishment. To many partners, finding that they need basic care feels like a narcissistic blow. Recognition of such human limitations threatens their defensively inflated self-image of having no needs.

One can speculate that this lack of need recognition is also a survival mechanism, developed in families in which emotional supplies were scarce. For example, Zack, whose father was rarely present due to his high-powered political career, was the oldest of three children, and his overwhelmed mother needed him to act as a helpmate to her and a coparent to the younger children. He learned very young to deny awareness of his own needs. He could win his mother's love as a helper but not as a needy child, so he buried his childish needs for caretaking and developed a counterdependent defense. His pseudoindependence was built on the false construction of not needing and not wanting nurture.

For those like Zack, raised in a family of emotional scarcity, not to need basic care was less painful than always to feel hungry for love, with no one to respond. It may be a positive step then to develop pride in being self-sufficient and self-sacrificing. However, this defensive structure prevents the possibility of intimacy in a love relationship, especially in being able to receive love and nurture. Unfortunately, without awareness or intervention, the whole syndrome deriving from the scarcity of emotional supplies tends to be perpetuated from generation to generation. The children of emotional scarcity are likely to create families in which nurturing for their children is also in short supply, even though they may give their children much more than they got.

A common occurrence that lends credence to this speculation is the experience reported by many couples of their parents' visits. It used to be in the good old days (or so it's been said), that parents and extended family substantially helped the young couple and family. Mothers, aunts, and cousins came over to help when a new baby arrived, when someone got sick, or whenever there was a need. However, most couples I see today dread the visits of their parents, although this dread is frequently masked as vague anxiety. In the climate of couples' highly demanding lives, parental visits usually mean more work, more giving, and more caretaking without getting anything in return except, perhaps, criticism or silent disapproval of how they live. In a sad reversal of our ideal of the extended family, parents more often seem to be visiting their children to get nurturing rather than to give it.

CHAPTER 3

The Development of Nurturing
Common Treatment Problems

Capacities of partners to nurture in the particular ways each one needs are not usually present at the outset of a relationship; they require development. In an ideal developmental process, couples in love first nurture each other in romantic ways. They focus intensely on each other, creating a cocoon in which each feels at one with the other and of indispensable importance. They share an unconscious expectation that *love means the automatic fulfillment of both partners' needs.* As day-to-day reality intrudes, romantic expectations are disappointed, although these wishes may persist as attainable. Partners who can integrate their disappointments and mourn the loss of romantic ideals are able to accept one another as separate, imperfect persons with differing needs. Once they begin to accept each other's individuality and form a distinct couple identity, they are in a good position to find satisfying ways to meet each other's needs. Ideally, when the partners have learned to nurture reciprocally, they are ready to take on the care of a baby and the demands of a three-way or triadic nurturing pattern. To care for a baby, while also sustaining a strong couple bond, requires the partners to evolve more complex ways of nurturing. These steps in the development of nurturing are summarized as follows:

- Romantic nurturing
- Integration of disappointment
- Differentiation of needs (self, partner, and relationship)
- Reciprocal nurturing
- Triadic nurturing

37

Although this development is presented in sequential steps, the steps overlap to a great extent even under optimal conditions. Often, circumstances and life-cycle events (such as the arrival of a baby at the beginning of the relationship) challenge a couple to develop simultaneously most of the capacities associated with each step. Such pressure can accelerate the partners' maturing but, more often, it causes an array of problems. Even under the least demanding of circumstances, many couples run into difficulty navigating these steps.

A therapist's knowledge of the optimal evolution of nurturing capacities can aid in the assessment of where the partners' development may have stalled, regressed, or derailed altogether. Understanding this developmental progression is also useful as a guide for conducting therapy. Each step incorporates a number of interrelated psychological tasks. Attainment of more complex relational capacities usually requires the prior achievement of other capacities. For example, partners who have not accepted their disappointment in each other cannot easily move on to accepting the other's differing needs. To be most effective, the therapist should first aim to help the partners integrate disappointment before expecting them to work effectively on differentiating their needs or to develop reciprocal nurturing. Figure 2 details the developmental steps with their associated psychological tasks and the common problems encountered.

RECAPITULATION, REGRESSION, AND DEVIANT DEVELOPMENT

Most developmental stage theories hypothesize a linear progression of stages, phases, or steps. However, in my observation the steps in the development of nurturing and other relationship patterns progress in the form of a spiral rather than in a linear sequence that only occurs once. In the spiral form, the steps are repeated, or *recapitulated*, at more mature levels throughout the life of the relationship.[1] Thus, the steps of romantic nurturing, differentiation of needs, and reciprocal and triadic nurturing are reexperienced in new ways by both partners over and over again in a couple's life together. With each repetition, the partners' capacities to give and receive care develop further, becoming more elaborated, flexible,

---

[1]This recapitulation theory of relationship development is a loose adaptation of Jean Piaget's (1950) concept of vertical décalage, a central tenet of his theory of cognitive development, wherein the attainment of each new level of cognition involves a recapitulation of all previous developmental phases but at a higher level of organization. I originally adapted the recapitulation aspect of his theory to the child's development of object relations (Sharpe, 1984).

Steps in Development of Nurturing	Tasks for Couple/Guide for Therapy	Common Problems (Points of Regression and Derailment)
Romantic Nurturing	Experiencing automatic fulfillment of needs Creating a romantic cocoon Forming a secure *couple bond and couple boundary*	Early failure of fantasy Inadequate cocooning Insecure couple bond, weak boundary Clinging to romantic cocoon/idealizing
Integration of Disappointment	Recognizing anger over unmet needs Accepting disillusionment in the partner Mourning the loss of romantic ideals	Regression to cocoon/idealizing to avoid anger Stalled in anger and disillusionment Avoidance of mourning, regression to anger Partial integration, deviant development
Differentiation of Needs (self, partner, relationship)	Recognizing confusion of self with partner Clarifying differences and similarities Identifying partners' internal conflicts, and nurturing collusions Defining *separate identities* and a distinct *couple identity*	Confusion between needs of self and partner Assertion of own needs without listening to partner Enactment of caretaker–child collusions
Reciprocal Nurturing	Identifying problems in accepting neediness, asking, giving, receiving Working through intimacy fears Modifying identifications with parents, siblings, gender stereotypes	Denial of neediness in self or partner Inhibition in asking, giving, or receiving Maintaining global identifications
Triadic Nurturing	Including baby/forming a *parental bond* Sharing attention with baby Expanding nurturing roles *Maintaining* couple bond and identity Reworking past love triangles	Exclusive couple maintained at expense of baby Competition with or withdrawal from baby/partner Romance with baby, with exclusion of partner Couple bond sacrificed for parental bond Past love triangles destructively reenacted

FIGURE 2. The development of nurturing.

39

and effective. However, as is also true of child development, the partners' first time through the developmental sequence is the most important, since it becomes the foundation upon which their capacities to nurture are later reworked.

A couple's development of nurturing is strongly affected by external demands, life-cycle changes, and individual development. Each significant event in their lives, each personal developmental step, each new important person entering their family or social orbit requires a reorganization of existing perceptions and understandings. In returning to the fundamental relational tasks time and time again, a couple reexperiences romantic longings, redefines their separate and couple identities, renegotiates reciprocal agreements, and reworks triadic nurturing patterns.

For example, early in their marriage, Zack needed Rina to help him feel more comfortable socially, and Rina needed Zack to admire her social and professional competence. Later on, when both partners had developed greater personal security, Zack wanted less of a social life in order to devote more of his time to composing music. Rina wanted Zack to spend more time alone with her (no longer needing to be admired for her competence). Thus personal maturing evoked a redefinition of their needs, which then required a reorganization of the kind of care each needed from the other. Likewise, when Zack and Rina had their first baby, their agreements about basic care, emotional support, affection, and sex had to be totally renegotiated. Problems can emerge at any point in the reworking of a formerly established pattern, as well as during the original development of nurturing capacities.

The recapitulation of earlier modes of relating should be distinguished from the process of regression, which also involves a return to an earlier position. Regression, in this context, involves a couple's retreat from forward development because one or both partners feel too threatened by the demands of a new developmental task. For example, one or both partners may begin to differentiate their needs but become anxious about the degree of separateness this process entails, and so they regress back to the romantic cocoon and the safety of oneness. They may stay there briefly to reassure themselves before moving on; they may be stalled there for quite a while, or they may nest there indefinitely, their development permanently derailed.

In contrast, recapitulation involves reexperiencing aspects of the earlier mode in a new way in order to revitalize the relationship and advance development. The couple does not become stalled or derailed in an earlier position as occurs in a regression. Instead, responding to romantic wishes or feeling unhappily distant, the couple will make plans to spend a weekend alone together in order to become closer. In this action, they create a new version of the original romantic cocoon to deepen their connection. By paying attention to their needs in this way, their connection is strengthened and they are better able to support each other's separateness and their children when they return.

Adding another layer of complexity to the assessment of a couple's nurturing capacities is the possibility that the partners, in coping with a number of stressors, have managed to continue their development but in less than optimal ways. The most common deviations are what I would describe as restricted development and pseudodevelopment. When development is restricted, it is uneven and patchy. Partners advance in certain ways but not in others. For example, a couple may develop an emotionally supportive relationship but be unable to evolve physical expressions of caring. Additionally, one or both partners may develop symptoms in order to manage or avoid certain developmental tasks. Certain symptoms may stabilize the relationship but interfere with the development of nurturing in various ways. A depressed or sick partner, for example, may have difficulty giving emotional support or engaging in a sex life.

The pseudodevelopment of nurturing capacities is similar to the development of pseudoindependence in children who have been required by neglectful or overwhelmed parents to become self-sufficient and caregiving (parentified) before they are emotionally ready for such responsibility. Partners who have developed a false maturity in reaction to too many demands are able to look like they nurture collaboratively and may be good parents, but they feel greatly deprived and angry at each other (though these feelings may be kept out of awareness). This prevalent form of relationship development is fostered by the same kinds of cultural myths, social values, and expectations that produce marital malnourishment. Additionally, partners who were parentified as children are likely to be more vulnerable to pseudodevelopment in their marriages.

Rina and Zack's difficulties in nurturing reflected both restricted and pseudodevelopment. Stalled in the anger phase of disappointment, they were still able to partially differentiate their needs and develop reciprocal and triadic nurturing capacities in a limited way. However, built upon the unstable foundation of unresolved disappointment and anger, their apparent achievements collapsed easily under stress, and both partners paid the price of depression with symptoms of chronic fatigue and frequent illness. Since their attainment of complex nurturing capacities resulted from overly accelerated development, their treatment required a reworking of all of the nurturing tasks.

ROMANTIC NURTURING

At the beginning of a relationship, when partners are passionately in love, nurturing is often given spontaneously, extravagantly, and in every conceivable way. Lovers pay attention to each other as though nothing and no one else matters. They listen to, understand, encourage, praise, and appreciate each other. If one is injured, the other rushes to the rescue. Some couples gaze into each other's eyes, radiating mutual love and adoration. Others coo and goo at each other like mothers with their cherished infants. Without holding back, each gives sexual pleasure, fun, joy, and presents to the other. They are often seen hand-feeding each other, taking the food from their own plates.

The Automatic Fulfillment of Needs

The question arises as to why nurturing that is so effortless at the beginning of a relationship so often becomes onerous later on. Being in love and viewing our partner as ideal motivates us to feel connected in all ways, through nurturing, affectionate, and sexual forms of expression. Additionally, the desire to give is supercharged by our lover's concentrated attention. Certain unconscious fantasies also fuel positive displays of caring. These fantasies can be stated in the form of the following irrational beliefs (the first is the usually the closest to consciousness):

- My partner will appreciate what I give, and I will *automatically* get what I need in return.
- My partner will want what I want to give him or her.
- Giving to my partner is giving to myself, since our needs are the same.
- When my partner is fulfilled, I am fulfilled.
- When I am fulfilled, my partner is fulfilled.
- My partner will intuitively know and meet all my needs, and I will intuitively know and meet all of my partner's needs.
- In summary, *love means our needs will automatically be fulfilled.*

These beliefs assume a merged relatedness between partners, sustained by fantasies of oneness. Romantic forms of merger underlie all irrational beliefs that needs will be met automatically and without effort. Thus, a good portion of the high energy for nurturing shown by lovers may be stimulated by fantasies that love means the automatic fulfillment of each partner's needs.

The merger fantasies of lovers and their expectations of total fulfillment stem from cultural portrayals of romantic love (as discussed in the previous chapter) and from our fantasized experience in the mother–infant relationship. We think we remember, or we imagine, that mother was always there to fulfill our needs when we were young. Even for those who know that they had neglectful mothers, the possibility of finding perfect maternal care is strongly embedded. This fantasy of an all-giving mother remains with us as an ideal, and is revived, in full force, in the experience of romantic love.

Creating a Romantic Cocoon

Optimally, in this early romantic phase, each partner experiences a grown-up version of that ideal state of being the one and only cherished baby who receives the total love, attention, and devoted care of the other. With enough time in this cocoon of loving nurture, each feels fulfilled, develops a sense of security in the other's love, and feels safe in the relationship. As in child development, the partners get enough of this kind of sustenance, enough of being the primary focus of attention and care, to be able to move on developmentally. In other words, the partners become able to expand their nurturing patterns to include other people, work, and, later on, a baby of their own, without either partner feeling seriously abandoned, rejected, or deprived. Additionally, each becomes able to see the partner as an imperfect, separate person with needs of his or her own.

Inadequate Cocooning and the Waning of the Honeymoon

There are many reasons couples have trouble moving beyond romantic nurturing, but an inadequate cocooning period is a significant contributor to problems. This common cause of difficulties may be overlooked, because there is little recognition in our society or the literature of the need for a couple to have a long, satisfying period of tending only to each other. While a cocooning period is recognized symbolically with the tradition of the honeymoon, current versions of honeymoons (or at least the ones I hear about) are not usually sufficient for this purpose. Often, they involve one or two weeks of travel to an exotic place. The couple returns jet lagged and sunburned, and immediately resumes an impossibly hectic life.

Rina and Zack spent a week in the Bahamas for their honeymoon, an expense they could not really afford. Rina got so sunburned the first day out snorkeling that she had to stay in the room for the rest of the week, swathed in ointments and numbed by painkillers. She could not be touched. The couple tried to enjoy watching videos and ordering room service together, masking their disappointment with good-humored jokes, but it was more of a strain than a pleasure. Both were anxious for this stressful, expensive honeymoon to be over.

Even if the week had been fun, such a honeymoon is a mere bow to a major developmental need and is bound to leave one or both partners unfulfilled. Many couples simply do not have a honeymoon because they cannot afford one or are unable to leave their jobs. Many spend their "honeymoon" visiting family, which may be less expensive but is a step backward rather than forward in its denial that a new family has formed.

Information about the origin of honeymoons and the term itself is vague. One version from folklore is that the honeymoon took place long before wedding ceremonies existed. A man would abduct his chosen bride and go into hiding with her for one month. A month became traditional because it was long enough for angry relatives to stop looking for the bride and for the moon to go through its phases. The couple would drink mead every night, a special kind of wine made from honey—hence, the term "honeymoon."

Thus, in times past, honeymoons may have lasted longer and involved little expense, the outside world was more definitively shut out, and the partners devoted their attention to each other. Restoring this practice might help get marriages off to a better start by supporting partners' development of a secure *couple bond* and a strong boundary around their relationship. Forming a strong couple bond preserves the partners' sense of being securely attached even during separations.[2] The *couple boundary* is a psychological boundary that surrounds couples and protects their relationship from undue invasion by the outside world. After the honeymoon, the couple boundary and bond are strengthened by the partners' maintaining their primary focus on each other, while other people and their demands are gradually integrated. Ideally, couples need several months, even a year, living together in the real world, concentrating on each other, in order to develop a strong sense of themselves as couples with a sturdy boundary around their relationship.

Unfortunately, these ideal conditions hardly ever hold sway. Couples' undernourished beginnings are more the rule than the exception. While we understand that babies and children need special care to develop optimally, we do not apply this understanding to adults and their love relationships. Thus, people marry without planning for the immediate need to give their full attention to each other, or they allow certain circumstances to interfere. Common circumstances that prevent an adequate romantic nurturing phase are marrying quickly because of a pregnancy, marrying just before a long separation (as occurs in many military marriages), beginning a relationship after a divorce or death that too quickly includes one or both partners' children, beginning a marriage with another person or relative living with the couple, and, the most common occurrence, one or both of the partners immediately taking on advanced

---

[2]A couple's formation of a *secure couple bond* is similar to Mahler et al.'s (1975) concept of the child's development of libidinal object constancy, which signifies his or her ability to sustain a loving representation of mother in spite of frustration, anger, and separations.

schooling or a demanding career that requires most of their time, attention, and energy.

All of these circumstances put too much strain on couples that have not yet developed secure and meaningful patterns of caring for each other. By condoning such beginnings as normal, our society fosters their continuation. Society is not the only culprit. As previously discussed, the limitations of existing developmental theory are partially responsible for the perpetuation of these unhelpful attitudes. Additionally, partners unconsciously collude to prevent adequate time alone together at the outset and later on. Detrimental circumstances are not sufficient to explain why so many couples begin their lives with a minimum of concentrated time alone. Couples' unconscious fears of intimacy may often underlie their creation of unnourishing environments.

When this early nurturing period fails to provide security in the relationship, one or both partners remain anxiously preoccupied with achieving this basic security, much like children who have never felt securely bonded with their mothers and so remain anxiously attached (as described by Ainsworth, Blehar, Waters, & Wall, 1978). Particularly for those couples who have had an inadequate cocooning period, the developmental shift from expectations of romantic fulfillment to acceptance of a less desirable reality causes considerable psychic pain and interpersonal conflict. However, this shift, with its integration of the disappointments involved, is necessary for further development to occur.

INTEGRATION OF DISAPPOINTMENT

The responsibilities of day-to-day living and coming to know the partner in more depth and breadth expose each person's wishes, needs, and capacities to give and receive. Regardless of good intentions, experiences of failure to meet each other's needs as expected begin to accrue. Disappointment of romantic expectations of giving and receiving appear in two related forms: each partner's growing awareness that the other is not really giving what was expected, and the feeling that the other does not seem adequately appreciative of the care one is giving. "He doesn't give me what I need emotionally," said Rina. "She doesn't appreciate all I do for her," said Zack. Usually, one or both partners become more pointedly aware of these feelings in connection with threats to their couple bond and boundary—the intrusion of outside demands such as work, school, family and friends, the occurrence of separations, or the arrival of a baby. With an accumulation of failures in empathic attunement and nurturing between partners, a period of disappointment in the partner and the relationship usually results.

The phase of disappointment that marks the waning of romantic love consists of each partner's experience of four major losses: (1) failure of the fantasy of automatic need fulfillment; (2) loss of the romantic cocoon; (3) erosion of the sense of oneness (romantic merger) with the partner; and (4) loss of the ideal partner, the ideal relationship, and the self as ideal.

There are, of course, people who marry without being in love. There may be an inability of one or both partners to fall in love and this inhibition may be directly connected to fears of intimacy—fears of engulfment (related to loss of identity or loss of autonomy or both) or fears of rejection and abandonment that keep the individual from risking any depth of attachment. Other common factors not necessarily related to attachment fears include the decision to marry someone for practical reasons such as financial security or to raise a child.

While marriages that begin without romantic love may not follow the developmental progression of nurturing, merging, and idealizing in exactly the way I describe, there are similarities in the expectations of such partners, followed by an experience of disappointment. Most people embarking on a new relationship begin with certain hopes, ideals, and expectations, though these may not be as unrealistic or hard to achieve as those perpetrated by romantic love.

In terms of nurturing expectations, one or both partners who are not in love may still expect to have their needs automatically fulfilled and to be the primary focus of the other's attention. These expectations are not stimulated by romantic feelings but are a product of cultural and family teachings, along with transference of the early parent–child nurturing situation in a marriage relationship. I have seen many partners marry without being in love yet describe similar kinds of disappointments in nurturing expectations. A safe, secure, need-fulfilling mother (or father) may still be desired in a mate who is not romantically loved.

Reactions to Disappointment in the Partner and in the Relationship

Partners may have four kinds of reactions to experiencing disappointment in each other and in the relationship in general, especially regarding their nurturing needs. First, the optimal response is the couple's relatively smooth management of a period of disappointment, so that understanding, integration, and advancement of the relationship is achieved. In an ideal scenario, partners acknowledge their feelings of disillusionment and anger in modulated forms. The realization that one's needs are not automatically fulfilled by a perfect partner in a perfect relationship is accompanied by a period of sadness, during which the loss of romantic ideals is mourned. The partners then become able to engage in open discussion of each other's differing needs and adjust their expectations to the realities of who each is, what each wants, and what each can give. This is an ideal working through that probably does not describe the majority of couples' experience but does provide a guide for helping couples through these feelings and their expression in therapy.

Second, partners may experience a taste of being disappointed in their mate but cannot tolerate the associated feelings of anger, sadness, and loss. Very quickly, they repress all such feelings and retreat back to former idealized perceptions of their partner and relationship. These partners can make a satisfying, if fragile, adjustment by mutual agreement to stay in a romantic cocoon. However, such adjustments are precarious because of their vulnerability to destruction by the intrusion of a third party (e.g., a child) or one partner's need to become more independent. These kinds of "idealizing" couples and their treatment (when this defensive adjustment fails) are described in Chapter 9.

A third, less than optimal but common response is seen in couples like Rina and Zack, who have difficulty working through this phase and get caught in a repetitive circle of disillusionment, anger, and alienation. Feeling uncared for, the giving of each partner becomes increasingly grudging, mechanistic, and poisoned by anger. Expressions of appreciation decline and become less genuine. In reviewing Rina and Zack's marital history, it appeared that the disappointment phase was likely first instigated by the premature loss of each other's attention, initially due to their demanding careers and later exacerbated by the arrival of a baby. They had not formed a secure attachment, and their couple boundary seemed easily invaded. These demands had overwhelmed them before they had learned how to nurture each other successfully.

The fourth response is that of couples who seem to end up permanently arrested in disappointment with each other, rather than temporarily stalled. These are the couples, like Eva and Sid, who will endure endless misery rather than accept the reality that their spouses are separate, ordinary people who cannot automatically fulfill their needs. Partners often sustain this fantasy because of nurturing deficits or inappropriate forms of care they experienced in their families of origin. Because of neglect or unattuned mothering, they continually crave to be cared for like an infant. These wishes may be blatant or masked behind a defensive compulsion to give and an inability to receive care. Because these wishes are experienced as realistically attainable, both partners feel acutely and constantly disappointed.

Mourning the Loss of Romantic Nurturing

The couples who have gotten mired midstream in the disappointment phase (Rina and Zack, Eva and Sid), openly express anger, disappointment, and feelings of betrayal but are unable to take the next step of giving up their fantasies of ideal love and nurture. Giving up these cherished wishes means experiencing acute feelings of sadness and loss. Most partners wish to avoid this mourning process. With couples who are temporarily stalled or more permanently derailed in the angry phase of disappointment, the therapist aims to (1) help the partners articulate their disappointed expectations, (2) expose and normalize their wishes to sustain unrealistic expectations of each other, (3) interpret feelings of sadness and loss that underlie anger and blaming, and (4) understand the impact of past disappointments on the present relationship, if appropriate.

A careful review with couples of their history together will often bring each partners' expectations and disappointment into focus. If partners are not too entrenched in their anger, a greater feeling of positive connection can result from sharing their story. Anger and defensiveness may soften as the therapist empathically responds to partners' reliving the highs and the lows of their journey together. Rina and Zack are representative of couples who have not had an adequate period of romantic nurturing. They returned from a deeply disappointing honeymoon to high-pressure careers that demanded the majority of their time and energy, and then a baby arrived.

I underscored the premature loss of each other's full attention and their limited time to form a bond with each other before many responsibilities took over their lives. I suggested that these circumstances would likely leave them feeling deprived and longing for a more meaningful and secure connection. At first Zack denied any such longings, but Rina revealed feelings of shame in wishing for their lost romantic closeness. "We're not really a couple," she said. "I'd describe us as best friends, siblings, parents, and *very* occasional lovers." As the therapeutic environment felt increasingly safe, they responded to encouragement to express their disappointed expectations. Interpreting both partners' injury and anger with the other's failings as a means of protecting themselves from the sadness of lost hopes and dreams enabled these feelings to surface.

Rina said, "I was so surprised and hurt to find out that Zack didn't want to cuddle in the mornings, even on weekends. When he wakes up, he just leaps out of bed to go running. I've sort of adjusted to it now, but I long just to be tenderly held. I feel so sad, at times, that this need of mine will never get fulfilled with Zack."

Zack revealed, "I thought we'd never lose our passion for each other. I thought we were different than other couples—those who sacrifice their relationship to status seeking and materialism. We used to have such wonderful discussions about our ideals—how we'd never compromise our special connection and values. That's all down the toilet now. Literally, that's what we talk about now—what's wrong with the toilet and how to fix it."

With these kinds of expressions of sadness and loss, the couple resumed an aborted grieving process. Each was more aware of feeling sad during this phase of therapy, and their fighting abated considerably. Greater acceptance of each other's limitations enabled them to listen and begin communicating their needs in a more effective way. For a couple to integrate disappointments so that they are able to accept each other as separate people, with differing needs and idiosyncratic ways of giving and receiving, can take a short or very long time, in or out of therapy. With Rina and Zack, this aspect or therapy took a couple of months of weekly conjoint sessions. However, with Eva and Sid, a couple more seriously entrenched in disappointment, it took two years of hard work in therapy for both partners to accept their disappointments in each other and mourn the loss of an ideal love.

Although the first round of disappointment in one's partner and the relationship may be the most profound, there are many more to come. Daniel Wile (1985) states: "The history of relationships is in large measure the history of partners' reactions to disappointments, frustrations, and disillusionments" (p. 53). Consequently, partners' ability to share the disappointment of their expectations and accept losses in an ongoing way is crucial to the healthy development of their relationship.

DIFFERENTIATION OF NEEDS (SELF, PARTNER, AND RELATIONSHIP)

Certain realities become evident as partners express their disappointed feelings in each other: The partner cannot meet all of your needs; the partner's needs are different than your own; it is necessary to give what your partner wants (at least to some extent) in order to get what you want. In these communications, who needs what, how, and why can become clarified, understood, and gradually accepted. The needs of three entities must be recognized: oneself, one's partner, and the relationship. The psychological structures optimally differentiated are the *separate identities* of the partners and a distinct *couple identity*. Also created is a sturdy but permeable *individual boundary* surrounding each partner, so that the separateness of each in relation to the other is protected and can be reliably sustained.

In therapy, promoting couples' differentiation of their needs begins with an exploration of each partner's wishes pertaining to the other, to the relationship, and to personal ambitions and goals. In helping partners clarify their needs in each area, the therapist asks direct questions, encourages partners to state unspoken wishes explicitly, and underscores the similarities and differences that emerge in their interaction. The therapist remains carefully attuned to difficulties on the part of either partner in identifying his or her needs, to resistance in revealing unspoken but known desires, and to each partner's injured or angry reactions to the revelation of the other's different needs and goals.

Most individuals benefit from spending considerable time clarifying their needs for themselves and having them understood by their partners. Therapists, in their desire to be helpful or because of discomfort with conflict, will often push for resolving differences too soon rather than recognizing the importance of supporting each partner's full awareness and expression of needs and goals. In this process, each partner's internal conflicts about giving and receiving, dependence and independence, will be revealed as contradictions between verbalized expressions and behavior become more apparent.

Ideally, the therapist is able to attend to the interpersonal meanings of the couple's interactions while also staying attuned to how each partner's internal conflicts may be expressed. Gradually, in the course of therapy, the therapist and couple gain understanding of how each realm of experience influences the other, thus further enabling each partner's expression of individuality. For the therapist, this is an intellectually and emotionally demanding way to work. Many therapists avoid such a high degree of engagement by focusing only on one domain. In conjoint therapy, it usually seems most supportive of the couple's process to begin in the interpersonal arena, where the couple is most aware of difficulty. When obstacles emerge that interfere with forward movement (either escalating anger or repetitive interactions), the focus is shifted to one or the other partner's internal world.

Rina was able to identify and speak about her needs more freely than Zack, who appeared to keep himself unaware of his needs as much as possible. Thus, Rina tended to initiate and dominate interactions, while Zack reacted to her feelings and requests but did not speak about his own wishes. After pointing out the one-sidedness of their self-expression, I shifted the focus to understanding Zack's difficulties in saying what he wanted. His responses suggested that he felt more comfortable trying to fulfill another person's needs rather than focusing on himself. Exploration revealed that he felt guilty about having needs at all and thought neediness was unmanly. These attitudes derived from identification with his father and the cultural stereotype of the "masculine man" who has no needs. These identifications were clarified at this point and later explored in greater depth. Zack's recognition that continual denial of his wishes was harmful to himself, as well as the relationship, enabled him to begin expressing himself more directly, leading us back to focusing on the couple's interaction.

In the following interchange, I worked with Rina and Zack to forward understanding of their differing needs.

SHARPE: Rina, you're very clear that talking personally with Zack is most important for you to feel loved and cared about. But I'm not sure that talking is what does it for Zack.

ZACK: Right. I don't think of *that* kind of talk as helpful, at least not anymore. What I need these days is a little time to myself to recharge—like listening to music or taking a nap. Besides there's a risk with our talking. We so easily get into terrible fights these days.

SHARPE: So you would feel more comforted when you're tired or stressed if Rina left you alone.

ZACK: Probably, at least for a while. I try to give her that kind of time when she's feeling overburdened. I'll take Eliza out for the afternoon or the day.

SHARPE: That's interesting. I wonder if you're giving her what you want, and she's giving you what she wants.

RINA: (*nodding*) I think that's true. If Zack's upset, I try to get him to talk about it. That's what would help me.

ZACK: But it doesn't usually help me. I want to distract myself from problems, not relive them.

SHARPE: (*to Rina*) And he probably leaves you alone when you're upset, thinking that's what you need.

RINA: That's exactly right, and then I feel abandoned.

ZACK: Abandoned? That sounds so extreme.

RINA: I mean it seems like you don't care about my feelings and just want to get away.

ZACK: That's unfair. I just assume you'd want time alone to decompress.

SHARPE: Well, this is a common problem, you know—confusing what you want with what your partner wants.

RINA: (*looking mildly injured*) But that's so self-centered.

ZACK: Well, people are self-centered. You want me to be like you, isn't that true? . . . And I wish you were a little more like me.

RINA: Only a little more?

ZACK: Yeah. If you were just like me, we'd never get together.

Not surprisingly and with good intentions, Rina and Zack ended up feeling uncared for and inadequate in part because neither was giving what the other wanted. Assuming the other was like the self, each had been giving in an egocentric way (reflective of wishes for merging and automatic need fulfillment). Previously, because of such strong feelings of disappointment and anger, they had not been able to clarify their needs and be heard by each other. Usually, when partners have accepted some degree of separateness, explained their needs in a nonaccusatory fashion, and recognized their egocentric ways of responding, they will work to alter their nurturing styles. However, if one or both partners' wishes for romantic nurture remain too strong, this confusion of partner with self will continue. This reaction alerts the therapist to shift from directly fostering differentiation to focusing on the partners' fears of becoming more separate (as was necessary in therapy with Eva and Sid).

Continuing forward with Rina and Zack, the subject of goals for the future of their relationship came into the foreground. Constructing a shared concept of a love relationship entails the modification and integration of both partners' needs. Partners who do little explicit work in this area tend to sustain a concept of their relationship that only fits their own needs, with the assumption that the same picture of the relationship and how it will evolve through time are shared by the partner. Emotional distance is created between partners by keeping their differences concealed, but differences tend to register even if they are not openly acknowledged. Feelings of anxiety, anger, and alienation are generated by this subliminal awareness that the partner is living in a different relationship and going down a different road.

This subject came up when I noted that Rina continually pressed Zack for a close relationship, but their interaction about this tended to go nowhere. The most obvious obstacle to progress was their preference for an abstract level of discussion. I noted this intellectualizing tendency, and then asked Rina to speak more specifically about what she meant by a close relationship. Many people, especially women, say they want a close relationship, but the meaning of this closeness is never defined, nor is there a clear idea of what needs to be done to achieve this desired state.

Rina said she wanted a relationship in which she and Zack could share their most intimate feelings on a daily basis. There would be more affection and time together doing enjoyable things, such as going to art galleries and concerts. They would recapture the fun they used to have when they first met. Then, it was possible to entertain each other for a whole weekend and be happy. But Rina also indicated that she wanted to be the kind of architect who advanced social causes and created better living environments. She desired to have a very active social life, to live in an elegant house in an upscale neighborhood, and to send their daughter to private schools. Zack looked increasingly depressed as these wishes were clarified. He had been subliminally aware of certain major differences between them but had been unable to face them squarely.

Zack then revealed his wishes for a more private, family-oriented kind of life, with emphasis on companionship and a sharing of interests. These aims were compatible with Rina's wish for more closeness. He feared that her career ambitions for both of them would ruin their lives. He wished to spend little time or money toward material acquisitions, goals he perceived as having destroyed his parents' marriage. His own personal goals were to continue composing and teaching music. These activities were not ever likely to bring in a high income or substantially improve the lot of mankind. He had no desire to live in the kind of neighborhood reminiscent of his childhood, where people talked about their boats and cars, obsessively comparing cost, luxury features, and horsepower. Since Zack had spent his youth in the best private schools and had felt like an outcast, he wanted a public school education for his daughter.

Many heated discussions ensued, during which Rina and Zack declared and fought for the rightness of their respective views and wishes. The issues of what kind of house, neighborhood, school for Eliza, social life, religious involvement, and worthy causes to support were clarified but not resolved. Neither partner was ready to modify his or her position for a compromise solution.

A lot of couples stay stalled at this point, midstream in the differentiation process. They are able to recognize and state their own needs but cannot move on to the next step of listening to one another in order to find ways of meeting each other's needs. They often engage in parallel talking, wherein each stridently states and restates his or her own views and wishes like a broken record. Such partners often fear regressing to their previous, less individualized state and so become single-mindedly self-assertive. These are the couples who come for treatment with battles for control and self assertion in the foreground of their relationship. Being unable to listen and understand one another, the partners cannot develop reciprocal patterns of nurturing.

Rina and Zack tacitly agreed to shelve the areas of most strident disagreement, since there was no immediate pressure for resolution. Since both wished for greater companionship and closeness in the relationship, they agreed to work toward this consciously shared goal, which they defined as improving communication about their feelings, spending more time together, being more affectionate and sexual.

Identifying Individual Conflicts and Couple Collusions

As we began work in these areas, discrepancies between Zack's and Rina's stated wishes for closeness and their behavior strongly suggested that each was conflicted about intimacy, particularly in regard to feeling dependent. Although Zack at first appeared to be the one who most obviously had difficulty with intimacy and receiving nurture, it became evident that Rina shared these conflicts. She wanted an intimate relationship with Zack, but her life goals were incompatible with their spending much time by themselves. Most of her behavior in and out of sessions appeared to discourage close contact with Zack. She made social plans to such an extent that they hardly ever had time alone. If Zack suggested that they do something together, Rina would inevitably invite a third person or couple to come along with them. Zack felt injured by Rina's apparent avoidance of being alone with him, though he could not, at first, express these feelings directly. He protected himself and retaliated by withdrawing emotionally and physically.

Observing their interaction over time, I concluded that both were more comfortable giving than receiving most kinds of care. In sessions, Zack's attempts to comfort Rina or empathize with her feelings were typically dismissed as inadequate. Zack tended to ignore Rina's efforts to give to him, whether it be practical help or emotional support. He repeatedly conveyed the message that he neither needed or deserved support. It was as though they had an underground competition going on about who was more self-sufficient and who could be the most self-sacrificing caretaker. As is so often the case, Rina's and Zack's internal conflicts had similar themes and similar protective purposes.

The Caretaker and the Self-Sufficient Child: A "Nurturing" Collusion

The interaction between Zack and Rina began to take the form of an unconscious agreement or collusion in which both partners were attempting to resolve their shared dependency conflicts—the longing for caretaking disguised by the denial of such "childish" need. Both attributed their own needs for nurture to the other, who was then perceived and treated as a needful child. However, each also induced the other to respond like a good parent by acting in needy, self-destructive ways—overworking, getting sick, forgetting to eat, ignoring nutrition, staying up too late, and so on. When the other would step in to provide caretaking, each reacted like a pseudo-self-sufficient child who rebuffs parental help but still so obviously requires it. This interaction took many forms, with the parent and child roles shifting back and forth, but the underlying theme always remained the same: The one playing the caretaker would say (in effect): "I see you need help. Here, let me help you." And the self-sufficient child would respond: "No, leave me alone. I don't need your help." Also implied was that the offered help was not the right kind, anyway. This collusive role relationship (or mutual projective identification system[3]) I describe as *the caretaker and the self-sufficient child*. The collusion not only supported their mutual efforts to deny their own needs for nurture but also expressed their shared gratification in acting as the martyred caretaker who could be virtuously superior and punish through guilt induction.

Since denial of neediness was one of their defensive aims, this collusion effectively prevented them from developing reciprocal nurturing that would be satisfying. Even though they could collaborate and make reciprocal agreements about basic care of each other and Eliza, both sustained the feeling of giving all the time without receiving anything in return. In order for this couple to progress in being able to feel adequately nurtured, their collusive denial of neediness (with consequent continual feelings of deprivation and wishes for martyrdom) had to be identified and worked through in treatment (to be described shortly).

Complementary Nurturing Collusions

Couples create other kinds of nurturing collusions that are more damaging to their development and can be more difficult to treat. Among the most common in my experience are those collusive relationships I call *the caretaker and the entitled child* and *the caretaker and the needful child*. In contrast to the mirror image, symmetrical form of Rina and Zack's collusion, these relationships are complementary. Only one partner denies neediness and acts as the devoted caretaker of the other partner, who is endlessly needy. In these dovetails, one partner is the caregiver, while the other is the receiver of care. Giving and receiving are divided between the partners. Unlike in Rina and Zack's relationship, there is no swapping of parent and child roles; hence, these dovetails are generally less flexible and the partners are more tightly shackled to each other.

In *the caretaker and the entitled child* relationship, the caretaking partner appears to be subservient and submissive, while the entitled partner is

---

[3]Projective identification can be briefly defined as an intrapsychic and interpersonal method of relating and defense, by which aspects of the self and internal objects are assigned to another person through projection or transference. The recipient (spouse or therapist) is then induced to identify with and enact the projected or transferred role. The induction of assigned roles is achieved through behavior and communication patterns that tend to elicit certain responses. *Mutual projective identification* occurs when two persons, either patient and therapist or both partners of a couple, engage in this activity (see Sharpe, 1997).

demanding and dominating. Judith Nelsen (1995) has described these couples as having "narcissistic–overgiving" relationships. In this collusion, the caretaking submissive partner may sustain the illusion that his or her needs are the same as the partner's, or may be aware of differing needs yet suppress their expression because of great insecurity and longings for acceptance. For these partners, feeling indispensable to the partner and safe from the fear of abandonment are more important than getting any other needs satisfied. The entitled partner is constantly demanding and endlessly needy, often becoming very angry if the caretaking partner fails to meet or anticipate his or her needs. This partner is also driven by great insecurity but has an inflated sense of self-importance and entitlement that defends against deep feelings of worthlessness.

The 1970 movie *Diary of a Mad Housewife* depicts a caretaker–entitled child collusion. Richard Benjamin, playing the boorish husband, incessantly demands care and attention from his downtrodden wife, played by Carrie Snodgress, who madly spends her days shopping, cooking, cleaning, washing, and generally catering to his every whim. Her reward for this slavish devotion is her husband's perpetual ridicule and devaluation, behavior that their snotty son begins to imitate. In this depressing story, the wife never finds her way out of this most thankless of caretaker roles.

In *the caretaker and the needful child* collusion, the receiving partner may appear to be quite childlike, excessively needy, and damaged emotionally and/or physically. In this role relationship, the caretaking partner dominates the childlike partner, who appears to be submissive. Even though the caretaker may appear to run things, most or all of this partner's efforts are geared toward taking care of the needful partner. The relationship of Eva and Sid, whose treatment is described in Chapter 4, takes this form. A famous example from American literature is F. Scott Fitzgerald's portrayal of his own marital dynamics in *Tender Is the Night* (1934), wherein psychiatrist Dick Diver marries his mentally sick patient Nicole and devotes his life to her care and cure.

These collusions prevent differentiation because only one partner's needs are defined. They also prevent reciprocal nurturing, because giving only goes one way. The one who gives cannot be needy, and the one who receives cannot give. The more polarized these roles become, the further the couple is from developing separateness and reciprocity, and the more difficult to treat.

RECIPROCAL NURTURING

Partners who are successful in reciprocally nurturing each other have developed a myriad of understandings and agreements that take each other's needs into account in all areas of their lives. They accept, at least consciously, that each is a separate individual with distinctive needs, that the needs of both partners are equally important, and that each should make a reasonable effort to satisfy the other's needs. Some agreements have been openly negotiated, and others have been worked out nonverbally through a back-and-forth sensing, testing, and balancing of who gives and who receives where, how, and when.

Common examples of such reciprocal agreements are as follows: "I will support us financially, and you will stay home and take care of the children"; "You will support me with my schooling, and I will support you with your career ambitions"; "I will give you extra time and attention when you're in need, and you will do the same for me when I'm in need"; "I will cook, and you will clean up"; "We'll have sex my favorite way this time, and we'll do it your favorite way next time."

Working out ways to fulfill each others needs does not happen automatically. Most partners have to struggle with this essential relational task. Many people are able to make reciprocal agreements in some areas but not in others. For example, many couples cooperate and reciprocate in a mature fashion regarding basic care for each other and their children but cannot reciprocally nurture each other in the areas of physical affection, sex, or emotional support. Also, the quality of a couple's reciprocity is dependent upon how well the partners have differentiated their needs. Thus, if a partner is unclear or conflicted about what he or she wants, then certain "agreements" may not reflect his or her true wishes. For example, Zack had agreed to cook while Rina cleaned up. Later, it emerged that he felt emasculated doing this chore and resented Rina's pressuring him to go along with this division of labor.

For reciprocal nurturing to be optimally satisfying, both partners need to be able to give and receive in all domains—basic care, emotional support, affectionate and sexual expressions. If one or both partners have great difficulty giving in one or more domains, the couple's reciprocity and satisfaction will be restricted accordingly. The partner who gives more will feel unfairly deprived and resentful, while the one who receives more may feel perpetually guilty.

In order to meet each others needs effectively, certain capacities are required of both partners. These include the ability to accept oneself and the partner as being needy human beings, the ability to ask directly for what is wanted, the ability to give in response to direct requests (without feeling like one is "giving in"), and the ability to receive what has been requested. These capacities are necessary for partners to negotiate their needs and compromise in order to create satisfying reciprocal agreements. Many partners have not been able to develop one or more of these abilities for a variety of reasons. The therapist aims to understand each partner's fears and wishes that have inhibited the development of certain capacities and may have led to the defensive formation of nurturing collusions.

Problems in Accepting the Partner as Needy

Often a child-like partner will view the other as a parent who is expected to give everything, while he or she receives care without expectation of reciprocation. Those who have great needs or little impetus for growth have usually selected partners who will fulfill the caretaking parent role, in the kind of complementary parent–child nurturing collusions described earlier. In these cases, the task of helping the child-like partner grow to the point of being able to accept the caretaking partner as having needs becomes a major focus of treatment (along with helping the caretaker to accept his or her own neediness). Accepting the partner as needy also involves an acceptance of the partner's separateness and vulnerability, which may be very frightening and profoundly resisted.

Rina and Zack's problems with accepting the other's neediness were more concealed. While each wished to view the other as the needy one and accepted the other as separate and having needs in the abstract sense, each had difficulty in responding in a giving way when the partner's needs were different from his or her own. Rina, in particular, had difficulty hearing Zack's differing wishes, and Zack had difficulty responding to Rina's direct requests (to be illustrated later on). Both partners' wishes to be a needy child who just received and never had to give were deeply hidden behind their caretaker identities.

Problems in Accepting Oneself as Needy

In order to bring Rina and Zack's denial of their own neediness into awareness, I began by confronting both partners' rejection of any form of care when it occurred. This approach brought little enlightenment. When I gently confronted Rina with her rejection of Zack's efforts on her behalf, she would say he gave her the wrong kind of care. If only he would give the right kind of love—tenderness, affection, understanding—she would welcome it gladly. When I confronted Zack with his dismissal of Rina's care of him, he would say she was not really doing whatever it was for him but was taking care of her own needs in some way. This response often occurred when Rina tried to empathize with his concerns, which Zack would interpret as really motivated by her wish to talk about herself (a partially accurate interpretation). Furthermore, she wasn't giving him what he really needed, which was appreciation of what he did for her. There was enough truth in their defensive justifications to keep the question of who was giving and who was receiving nurture endlessly confusing.

This approach seemed to aggravate their defensiveness, possibly because they experienced me as critical and out of tune with their feelings. Upon reflection, I could understand their desire to keep out the kind of awareness I was fostering. By resisting care, they protected themselves from experiencing neediness. Recalling that Rina and Zack were parentified children who had grown up taking care of younger siblings, I understood that feeling needy might provoke an array of intolerable feelings for both.

The following interaction provided me with an opportunity to expose Rina's fears of being nurtured, which also opened the way to address Zack's fears. Because of an incident over the weekend, Zack brought up his frustration in trying to help Rina with her migraine headaches, a recurrent problem for her. They were out hiking in the desert near where they were staying for the weekend. Zack said Rina had momentarily become dizzy walking in the heat without a hat.

ZACK: I know by now some of the circumstances and warning signs of her getting a migraine. Exerting herself in the heat is one of the triggers, and getting dizzy is a warning sign. I suggested we return. She refused and got irritated with me.

RINA: It's true, I thought you were overreacting. I just had a momentary dizzy feeling, and I thought I'd be all right. We were having fun, and it was so beautiful.

ZACK: Yes, I know. But I didn't think it was worth taking the chance. You get one of those headaches, and you could be in terrible pain and out of commission for the whole weekend.

RINA: I brought my Imitrex. If I got a headache, I'd be okay if I took it right away.

ZACK: Your medication was back at the hotel. You've told me you have to take it immediately, as soon as you have one of those symptoms, for it to work. (*turning to me*) I offered to go back and get it, while she sat in the shade. She wouldn't listen. Said she'd be fine. (*turning back to Rina*) We kept walking, and sure enough, by the time we got back an hour or so later, you had a full-blown migraine.

RINA: And you weren't very nice about it.

ZACK: No, I wasn't. I was mad at you for ignoring my advice and being stupid.

RINA: Well, you don't listen to me either. Just last night, I was trying to get you off the computer to come to bed. It was midnight, and I could hear you coughing. You know your cold will just get worse if you don't get enough sleep.

SHARPE: These complaints you make about each other sound very similar.

ZACK: (*grinning*) Yeah. But Rina's a worse martyr than I am.

RINA: (*sounding like a bickering sibling*) Am not. You're worse.

I managed an insincere smile and felt outwitted. They had turned my previous interpretation of their competition for martyrdom into a joke, rendering me powerless to effect insight. I scrambled to think of another way into the problem. Confrontation of their behavior did not work, nor did interpretation, which they either superficially agreed with, ignored, or worked into a comedy routine. I speculated that these kinds of interventions might make them feel put down by an authority figure and competitive. Or perhaps my "caretaking" made them feel child-like, and thus they needed to reject it.[4]

I thought an exploratory approach in which we interacted on the same level (and I did not appear to have all the answers) might have a better chance of success. Thus, I aimed to include Rina at every step in trying to understand the meaning of her behavior.

SHARPE: Rina, going back to your migraine, how would you have felt if you had let Zack go back to the hotel to get your medication while you rested?

RINA: (*brightening up; I've gotten her interest*) Uncomfortable. Very uncomfortable. I couldn't have let him do that.

SHARPE: Why not?

RINA: I would feel guilty to put him out like that . . . and, I don't know, inadequate somehow, like I should have thought to bring the medication myself.

SHARPE: So if you let Zack take care of you, you would feel guilty and inadequate.

RINA: Yeah, and . . . a little helpless.

SHARPE: Yes, I see that. Helpless and out of control. (*I pause to assess her receptiveness.*) How about needy?

RINA: (*making a disgusted face*). I guess that's there too.

---

[4]The couple's reaction to me as a controlling parent blossomed more fully later in treatment and is discussed in Chapter 14.

SHARPE: That's bad is it? Being needy?

RINA: Just the word needy makes me want to gag.

SHARPE: That's a strong reaction. (*Rina nods emphatically.*) I wonder if you
would let yourself feel needy just for a moment, so we might get an
idea of why you feel this so strongly?

RINA: Okay, but it's really difficult. I can feel myself blocking. (*Rina hesitates and groans.*) I think the feeling is vulnerable . . . and pathetic. Believe me, it's not a place I want to go.

When I asked Zack about feeling needy, his antipathy was equal to
Rina's. They worked together on understanding this shared aversion.
Both associated neediness with being vulnerable, unlovable, and useless.
They both imagined being rejected if they allowed themselves to be
openly dependent. Couples who have such conflicts about accepting nurture also usually sustain hidden wishes for a mother to take care of them
unconditionally. This wish can be difficult to access because of the defensive layers developed to conceal such a shameful longing.

Problems in Asking

Partners cannot ask to have their needs met unless they have been able to
accept their neediness and identify to some extent what they want. Even
then, asking is often greatly resisted and feared. Most therapists encourage partners to ask for what they want, rather than to rely on the hopeless
fantasy of getting their needs met automatically. Both Rina and Zack had
great difficulties with asking. Like many couples, they wished to have
their minds read, so that asking would not be necessary. Many of us are
aware of certain irrational beliefs that discourage asking. These include "I
shouldn't have to ask for what I need. If my partner really loved me, he or
she would know what I need and give it willingly"; "If you have to ask for
what you want, it doesn't feel like you really get anything"; "Love means
you shouldn't have to ask."

Asking also goes against desires to be self-sufficient, selfless, or self-
sacrificing, those ideal self-images supported by our society. Fears of making oneself vulnerable and then being disappointed or humiliated also
inhibit partners from asking for what they want. Many seem to find it pref-
erable to suffer in silence for long periods of time without getting their
needs met, and then one day explode. In the act of exploding, it then becomes possible to say what is needed and how the partner has failed. This
was Rina's pattern. In this reaction, the partner does not really take the
vulnerable position of asking, but angrily complains, demands, threatens,
or accuses the partner of failing to meet needs of which he or she should

have been aware. These indirect, angry, and ineffective ways of expressing needs should not be confused with the simple, powerful art of asking.

Other partners suffer along in silence and never explode or get openly angry. Rarely clarifying their needs or directly revealing disappointment when their needs are not met, they hardly ever ask for anything. They manage hurt feelings and anger by withholding and distancing from the partner, and may also get depressed or develop other physical or psychological symptoms, including substance abuse. This was Zack's pattern. Not only was he mildly depressed, but also he smoked heavily and was in danger of developing a drinking problem.

In continuing to explore Rina's resistances to feeling needy and asking, she revealed certain of her difficulties in the following exchange:

RINA: It feels scary to say what I want out loud. It makes me feel naked. (*pausing trying to clarify her feelings*) The first thought I have is that I'm going to be bawled out for saying I want something.

SHARPE: So you shouldn't want anything for yourself?

RINA: I think not. It's selfish.

SHARPE: Says who?

RINA: My mother, of course, and the Church. My mother constantly met everyone's needs without paying any attention to her own. She wouldn't sit down, at the dinner table until everyone else was served. And then she would spend the meal jumping up and down trying to anticipate everyone's needs. I'm not sure I ever really saw her eating her own dinner.

ZACK: (*joking*) She probably ate her food cold in the kitchen while washing the dishes.

RINA: It's no joke. She did exactly that. I don't want to be a martyr like she was. She never got any reward for being the way she was.

SHARPE: Are you sure? How about the rewards of feeling more virtuous and than anyone, and the power of making others feel guilty? [I underscored these gratifications, because Rina had unconsciously identified with these aspects of her mother.]

RINA: (*looking to both of us for reassurance*) God, I hope I'm not like that!

ZACK: Let's just say you're not as bad as your mother.

RINA: (*scowling, her long, elegant nose quivering as though she might be on the verge of tears*) Well, that's not saying a whole lot. I suppose it's true, though I hate to see myself like her in those ways. She made me feel so guilty and mad a lot of the time.

SHARPE: You're mad about. . . .

RINA: She was just so good, so virtuous. She cooked and sewed and cleaned. She would drop everything to make me a costume for Halloween or drive me wherever I wanted to go. There's nothing to be mad about, but I am.

SHARPE: Maybe the things she gave weren't what you needed to feel loved.

RINA: (*reassuring herself*) I *know* she loved me. It's like with Zack. He does so much to help me . . . and I appreciate all he does, I really do. But he doesn't hug me, or hold me, or talk to me. (*Her eyes begin to tear up.*)

SHARPE: These are the things that would make you feel loved. But I guess it's scary to ask for them directly.

RINA: (*nodding*) In one way it feels greedy, like I'd be asking too much. Why can't I just be satisfied with what I do get? That's what my mother would say. (*She pauses, deep in thought.*) There's something else. If I ask for what I really want and don't get it, I'll be more hurt than if I never said anything in the first place.

Rina echoes fears shared by many people. Women in particular tend to feel selfish and greedy about wanting and asking. Many women's mothers are also a lot like Rina's—giving, self-sacrificing, self-effacing. These traits used to be considered an ideal of femininity, ideals of the good wife and mother. Although this ideal is undergoing revision, it still has considerable power, passed down from mother to daughter like a hereditary malady.

Zack's fears about asking were also gender-related and tied to an identification with his father. Wanting something was acceptable, but asking did not fit with his ideal of masculinity. The manly man did not whine, complain, or ask for help. The man made do with what he got. His father never spoke about his own needs. Instead, he had affairs and drank whiskey.

When these impediments to asking are brought to light and explored, partners usually feel freer to make their wishes known to each other. In recognizing their likeness to parents, partners become able to modify those aspects of their identifications that are personally unrewarding and harmful to the relationship (such as denial of needs and overly self-sacrificing behavior). However, much practice in asking and positive reinforcement from the partner are necessary before such a change can be fully integrated into the relationship. Unfortunately, many partners have difficulty responding favorably to direct requests, which can be very discouraging to spouses who finally become able to ask for what they want.

Problems in Responding to Direct Requests

A partner's failure to respond to a direct request may reveal a problem with giving in general to his or her partner, or a more specific problem with giving in response to that particular request, or perhaps any direct request. Zack had all of these problems to some degree. As Rina became more straightforward in expressing her needs, Zack was unable to respond positively (even though he had encouraged her to be direct). His unresponsiveness was not immediately apparent, because he would appear very agreeable about doing what was asked. Rina would think they had an agreement about something, but then Zack would not do what was asked of him. When confronted with this, he would apologize and say he had gotten too preoccupied with other things, such as composing music.

Zack's behavior was very wounding to Rina, who felt her fears were being verified: Ask and you'll be ignored. Zack's repeated forgetting made her feel unloved. He tried to reassure her on this point, asserting that his forgetting had nothing to do with her.

This interaction is commonly seen between partners in couple therapy, particularly when attention is focused on working out reciprocal agreements. It is necessary to explore thoroughly the reluctant partner's resistance to responding, or this passive–aggressive behavior will simply continue, and the couple's capacities to nurture each other will regress, become constricted, or stop altogether.

A few repetitions of Zack's reaction needed to occur before he could be effectively confronted. Since Zack's underlying motives for forgetting were unconscious, he needed to see repetitions of this behavior to believe the problem was anything more than his feeling fatigued and preoccupied. Rina had told Zack how important to her it was to have an affectionate exchange before having intercourse and a time of holding each other afterwards. Zack had agreed, saying he had no problem with this request. In the context of this discussion, he had expressed his wish for Rina to initiate sex more of the time. Rina pointed out that she had initiated sex several times (as he had requested), but he had gone about sex as usual—just focusing on stimulating erogenous zones, having intercourse, and then rolling over to fall asleep.

RINA: The last time we had sex, you rolled over and went to sleep right after. I've told you how much that hurts me. Once in awhile it's okay for that to happen when we're tired. But you always do that. I wouldn't even mind the going to sleep part, if we were holding each other.

ZACK: I thought I was holding you.

RINA: Oh, come on, Zack, you rolled over. You were not holding me.

ZACK: You go to sleep, too. You've fallen asleep before, when it's late.

RINA: (*Does not reply. She just glares. Her whole body radiates frustration and anger.*)

ZACK: (*with resignation*) All right. I didn't do what you wanted. I'm sorry.

RINA: Sorry just doesn't cut it, Zack. I need to understand why. Otherwise I'll just go on having these awful feelings about myself, and I'll start to hate you. It makes me want to pull away and not have sex with you. . . not have any physical relationship.

ZACK: I don't know why. That's the truth. I don't think I should have a problem with what you're asking. It's not unreasonable. I even understand the appeal.

SHARPE: But there's something that gets in the way of your being closer to Rina in this way.

ZACK: I really don't know. I think it must be fatigue.

SHARPE: (*quelling the urge to argue with him*) Can you picture yourself closer, holding each other?

ZACK: (*agreeably*) Sure.

SHARPE: Any images or feelings come up?

ZACK: (*replying quickly*) No . . . no images.

SHARPE: (*pressing*) How about feelings?

ZACK: I feel . . . uh . . . well . . .

SHARPE: Yes?

ZACK: (*grinning boyishly*) I feel like changing the subject.

RINA: Is this making you nervous?

ZACK: Uh, yeah.

SHARPE: Can you say why?

ZACK: I feel like I'm being cornered . . . trapped.

SHARPE: (*hoping he would elaborate*) Trapped?

ZACK: And like I can't think. I feel confused.

SHARPE: That sounds like anxiety.

ZACK: (*looking pushed into agreement*) Maybe so.

RINA: That's awful. I don't want to make you feel that way.

I saw Zack's fears of intimacy being enacted at that moment in the therapy. I sensed that he felt overwhelmed and angered by two women probing and pushing at him. His anxiety also provoked a regression in his sense of self. He described a loss of boundaries and mental confusion. His usual method of coping with his fear of being engulfed and controlled was to agree on the surface but become more distant interpersonally (which was how he behaved in their sexual relationship).

SHARPE: I sense that you might feel irritated and pushed into responding a certain way by my probing into this very private area.

ZACK: (*shrugging*) Well, that's your job . . . to push us farther than we would go on our own.

SHARPE: Say more, if you can, about feeling pushed.

ZACK: I don't want to let Rina run everything. . . . That's my first thought.

SHARPE: You fear being controlled by her . . . maybe by me, too?

ZACK: I don't know if I'd call it fear exactly.

SHARPE: Maybe if you do as Rina asks about lovemaking, you may feel like you're letting her take over.

ZACK: It's true, I don't like being bossed.

RINA: But I don't mean to be bossing you.

ZACK: It's not just what you do. It's my reaction we're talking about.

Zack's reaction to Rina's request for increased intimacy is very common among men: passive–aggressive responses—such as forgetting, not quite hearing, avoiding, half-baked efforts, doing it his way—to ward off feeling controlled. In subsequent sessions, Zack's feelings of being controlled by Rina were explored, along with the impact of his relationship with his mother. We found that he feared being taken over by a woman and had to struggle to maintain his autonomy and masculinity with both his wife and mother. The psychological literature has extensively described men's difficulties separating from their mothers—staying separate, grown-up, and masculine—and their fears of being engulfed by a woman. A particularly cogent examination of this subject is presented by John Munder Ross in *The Male Paradox* (1992).

Women also have engulfment fears, though loss of femininity is usually not a central concern. They more often fear loss of power, control, and assertiveness. In therapy, these fears are brought into the open by a focus on reciprocal nurturing and following up with how each partner carries through with agreements.

Problems in Receiving (What You Ask For)

A partner may become able to ask for what he or she wants, but then cannot receive whatever it is—the hug, the gift, the praise—when it is given. Rina, for example, had a predictable response to Zack's new efforts to give her more cuddling and affection.

ZACK: I tried to hold you last night, and you went stiff as a board. I thought I was embracing the bedpost. When I asked what was wrong, you said you had a headache. Then you got up to get some Excedrin. (*turning to me*) While she was up, the phone rang. She talked to whoever it was for about an hour.

RINA: It was only half an hour. It was my mother. She was hysterical about the side effects of her medication.

ZACK: You didn't have to take the call. We have an answering machine.

RINA: I knew it was her. If I hadn't picked it up, I would've just felt guilty. I couldn't relax thinking she was the one calling. (*turning to me*) My mother is having all these problems since her surgery. She . . .

ZACK: Rina . . . You're avoiding the subject I raised by talking about your mother.

RINA: (*defensively*) What can I say? I don't know why I reacted the way I did. I must have felt anxious about something.

ZACK: Very anxious.

RINA: (*looking pained*) Please don't gloat.

SHARPE: It's no crime to feel anxious.

RINA: But I'm the one who wants to be close. He's the one who's afraid.

SHARPE: (*again aiming to alleviate her feeling exposed and flawed*) Everyone's afraid of closeness.

RINA: (*tense*) Really? I'm not aware of being afraid.

Rina's responses were unusually defensive. She was often willing to examine her reactions. I assumed she must feel very vulnerable and out of control, since her fears of intimacy were being exposed. Providing empathy seemed to make her feel more vulnerable, so I thought it might be a better idea to put her back to work on herself.

SHARPE: How were you feeling when Zack was holding you?

RINA: I liked it . . . at first. But then I started to worry that he didn't really like holding me. He was just doing it out of a sense of obligation.

ZACK: That's not true. I liked holding you.

RINA: I guess I don't believe that.

ZACK: (*with conviction*) It's true.

SHARPE: What if you could believe him. Can you imagine that?

RINA: (*pausing*) It would feel wonderful. But I'm still not comfortable. I'm afraid I'd like it too much . . . and just when I started to relax . . . he'd pull away. He'd jump up and start doing calisthenics or something.

SHARPE: He'd abandon you.

RINA: Yes.

SHARPE: Just when you started to let down your guard and depend on him.

ZACK: (*protesting*) But I wouldn't do that!

SHARPE: This isn't just about you, Zack.

RINA: No . . . it's probably more about my mother. I couldn't depend on her . . . about my feelings. I've always had to take care of her emotionally.

SHARPE: Yes. That does show up in your reaction to the phone call. Her needs come before yours. You couldn't let her wait.

Zack also had problems in getting what he requested. When Rina expressed gratitude for his general thoughtfulness and admiration for his clever planning of their upcoming vacation, he could not accept it. He trivialized his contribution, made a joke of it, or deflected the attention away from himself. It was now possible to link his feeling uncared for with his rejection of emotional support. Not only would he feel unmanly and undesirable if he became needy, he would also end up, like Rina, abandoned and alone.

Difficulties in giving and receiving tap into fundamental attachment needs and fears. This is not surprising, since these are the most basic transactions that go on between people. A treatment focus on the specific problems impeding a couple's development of satisfying reciprocal nurturing—problems in accepting one's own or the partner's neediness, problems in asking, responding to direct requests, and receiving what is asked for—will soon bring partners' troublesome identifications and intimacy fears into the foreground. If they are not rigidly defended, working with these identifications and fears clears the way for partners to nurture each other in more satisfying ways.

TRIADIC NURTURING

If I had the power to influence couples' choices, I would advise them to wait until they developed all of the aforementioned nurturing capacities before having a baby. However, when it comes to love and having babies, no one listens to sensible advice. If couples needed to develop mature patterns of nurturing before having children, we would probably risk extinction.

Ideally, it would be desirable for both partners to feel sufficiently nurtured and secure in their relationship before taking on the challenges of caring for an infant and including a dependent third person in their relationship. The shift from a one-to-one (or dyadic) mode of nurturing to a triadic, three-way pattern requires the couple to grow in a number of ways.

To manage a three-person nurturing system *optimally*, the partners are required to (1) put their own needs on hold for substantial periods of time, in order to take care of an infant's constant needs; (2) share time and attention with the baby; (3) reexperience and manage fears of alliances forming and being left out, and wishes to form an alliance with the partner or baby, leaving the other out; (4) shift and expand their accustomed nurturing roles; (5) work out a balance between caring for the baby (and other children), meeting their own personal needs, and maintaining the couple relationship.

These abilities do not suddenly spring into existence with the arrival of the baby. Couples with satisfying relationships often have difficulty stretching themselves to develop these capacities. Their bond must be strong enough so that the baby does not threaten the relationship but is perceived, for the most part, as a welcome addition rather than as a rival for care and attention. The partners are able to maintain themselves emotionally as an adult couple who develop a parental bond in relation to the baby. No alliances form in which one partner (or the baby) is left out.

However, many partners are deeply threatened by sharing love and care with a baby (or any third party). They unconsciously believe that love and care can only securely exist between two people. Thus, if any love goes to a third person, then one partner will be left with less or without any love. When these fears are intense, a triadic conception can be difficult to access or develop. Any third person, especially a dependent baby, can be perceived as a rival who will take all or too much of the love and attention of the partner.

A triadic mode of relating (in comparison with a dyadic mode) means that partners are able to feel secure in each other's love when a baby (or other third person) becomes included or close to the family. The quantity of love available is not felt to diminish when a third person is added to the relationship. Additionally, the partners understand that there is more than one kind of love, and that the quality of love will vary with different people in different roles. Thus, a wife both loves her husband and child very much, but differently. Ideally, a wife's love for her husband is distinguished by romantic and erotic elements. A mother's love for her child is protective and nurturing. Even though partners must put their needs on hold for periods of time while caring for the baby, they do not confuse this loss of time and attention with the loss of the other's love. However, there is some pain involved in losing the "only child" position in relation to the spouse and in losing the partner's full attention. Optimally, these losses are accepted and compensated for by the gains of becoming the one and only grown-up partner and coparent with the spouse.

Partners who have difficulty developing these aspects of mature love usually have intense fears of sharing love. These fears often stem from feelings of having been deprived and left out when growing up. Either a sibling was experienced as taking mother's or father's love away, or the parents' relationship seemed too close or too fragile to embrace a child. The opposite experience of winning the total love of one parent away from the other parent (or other siblings) also interferes with a person's developing the capacity to feel safely cared for in a three- (or more) person family. Thus, the arrival of a baby can reactivate very strong rivalrous feelings that may be acted out in destructive ways. Since the security of love and care may not seem attainable in a three-person system, partners will automatically strive to maintain the safety of a two-person love relationship.

A couple may take three deviant paths in order to maintain a dyadic love relationship and avoid the more complex demands of a triadic system. The most destructive to the child is the emotional exclusion of the baby by both partners in order to maintain the gratifications of their twosome with each other. Children of such parents are emotionally, and sometimes even physically, neglected. Since these couples are not aware of suffering in their relationship, they do not tend to come for couple therapy. However, they may become involved in some kind of treatment (often family therapy) later on, when their child develops symptoms.

Another common outcome is when the mother shifts her primary love almost exclusively to the baby. Mother and child become the most strongly bonded couple in the family, while the husband is relegated to the periphery. (If the husband is the major caretaker, this kind of alliance could form between baby and father.) Unable to tolerate the loss of his wife's attention, the husband may feel impelled to have an affair in order to compensate for feeling neglected, or he may become wedded to his work (thus finding substitute forms of nurture outside the family). The husband may also regress more obviously, becoming excessively needy and openly rivalrous with the baby for his wife's attention. Both kinds of response from husbands tend to reinforce the wife's exclusive romance with the baby.

A third, increasingly common outcome, particularly seen in equal partnership marriages, is that the baby becomes the primary love object of both parents, who participate equally in child care. In contrast to the previous scenarios, this couple succeeds in forming a parental bond, but at the expense of their couple bond. Both partners' bond with the baby becomes stronger and more romantic than their tie to each other. Rina and Zack's relationship took this route. In responsibly caring for their child, they neglected their relationship, as well as their own personal needs.

One of the reasons for this outcome was the undernourished condition of the couple relationship before their baby arrived. Additionally, the couple had little help in the early weeks and months. Without adequate practical help and emotional support, Rina's anger about the baby's constant needs turned into depression and was also displaced onto Zack. Thus, the baby was wonderful, but Zack was a profound disappointment. Zack also displaced his anger toward the baby onto his wife. Hence, both partners ended up feeling more deprived and angry with each other, which reinforced shifting the romantic, idealizing aspects of their love to the baby.

Couple relationships are unnecessarily damaged because of partners' overwhelming focus on tending their baby, while letting their relationship wither and die. The partners are then bewildered as to why they feel so distant and disconnected from each other. Unfortunately, this pattern is supported by our society. Traditionally, provisions are made for the baby's care (and the mother's care to a minimal extent), but there is no tradition of considering care of the couple. Thus couples are more likely to sacrifice their relationship and personal needs to care for their children. (In Southern California, many people put their physical fitness programs before their relationships.)

With couples who are experiencing the normal range of difficulties in managing this multifaceted developmental step, identification and discussion of the points of stress often result in rapid improvement. An important therapy intervention is to help partners reveal and share their *negative* as well as positive feelings about having a child. Most people feel that having angry, hostile, envious, or competitive feelings about their baby (or children) are not acceptable, so they repress them. This repression then fosters the maintenance of a dyadic system, such as those described earlier, impeding development of triadic nurturing.

When partners share the gamut of feelings that having a baby has provoked, they become less angry and closer to each other. For example, a wife can more easily recognize that she has abandoned her husband too much for the baby (or children). Her husband realizes that he has felt deserted and retaliated by providing little emotional support to his wife. Couples come to recognize that they have ignored their relationship, and the partners will take action to correct this state of affairs.

When identification of the stressors and the sharing of underlying feelings bring about little change, then the couple is likely caught in reenacting triangular relationships from their families of origin. The complex subject of competing in love triangles is only introduced here. Chapters 18 and 19 are devoted to the development of love triangles and treating couples with competitive problems. Although in working with Rina and Zack, it was necessary to explore their past struggles in love to enable them to fully develop a three-person nurturing system, this aspect of their treatment was quite straightforward given the progress made in other areas.

When Rina recognized that her bond with Eliza was stronger than her bond with Zack, she was able to see herself repeating her original family pattern. Rina's mother was most strongly allied with her, the oldest daughter, in caring for the rest of the family. Although Rina's father had been unavailable and working much of the time, Rina realized that her mother also treated him like a less important child (or so she remembered). She won too much of her mother's love, which also entailed too much responsibility and a legacy of anger toward both parents for not allowing her be a child. In recognizing the transference of her relationship with her mother to her relationship with Eliza, while also viewing Zack as the inadequate father of her childhood, she became highly motivated to rework the quality of her attachments to both husband and daughter.

Zack's bond with his mother was similarly the strongest in his family, and they, too operated as the parental couple of two younger sisters and a father who erratically dropped in and out like an irresponsible teenager. When Zack understood the repetition of these patterns in his current family, his fear of reliving the unfortunate history of his parents' marriage provided strong motivation for him to find his way to a closer, romantic relationship with Rina. As we see in the next chapter, these outcomes are not so easily achieved with a couple who is more deeply entrenched in a nurturing collusion.

CHAPTER 4

The Caretaker and the Needful Child

A Nurturing Collusion

"He was right in my face, yelling insults," Eva said in a dramatically injured tone, "and then he pushed me. He shoved me really hard. I just saw red. He's so much bigger than me, and I was forced to defend myself."

Eva's husband, Sid, was certainly larger than she. She was tiny, and he was about six feet tall and muscular. At thirty-four, Eva looked much younger than her years, while Sid looked older than his thirty-eight years. Sid was dark-skinned, with a strong-featured face and black hair. He could easily be cast in tough guy roles (as his wife was successfully doing). Eva was his opposite in every respect. She looked like an angel, with a halo of curly blonde hair and innocent, blue eyes. I could feel her baby blues working on me—drawing me into her orbit of injured innocence.

SID: It was just a little shove. I didn't hurt her. (*He raises his arm protectively, as though a judgment were coming down from above.*) I know, I know. . . . I'm not saying it was an okay thing to do! But she slugged me in the arm, and that did hurt. She may be small, but she sure packs a wallop. (*He sounds proud of her spunk.*)

EVA: (*lifting her hand like a small child with an "owie"*) I'm the one who had to put ice on my hand and take Advil. It's still swollen.

SID: (*in a denigrating tone*) You want I should play the violin? This whole thing started because of your off-the-wall reaction about dinner.

In this first session, Eva and Sid were describing the fight that had brought them to therapy. Screaming at high decibels and throwing things had been allowed in their relationship, but crossing over the line and hitting each other had frightened them. This fight had occurred the night of Sid's return from a ten-day business trip, during which Eva and their six-year-old daughter, Laurie, had been sick with the flu.

SID: *(turning to me)* You won't believe this. I offered to make dinner—I do most of the cooking by the way . . . and she went ballistic.

EVA: *(shrieking)* That's a lie! That's not how it was at all, and you know it. He made me feel inadequate. He . . .

SID: That's not true!

SHARPE: Let's stop here! You're both getting hurt and angry all over again by reliving this event.

CREATING A CLIMATE OF SAFETY

In order to create a safe environment for the couple and the therapy, the therapist needs to stop *destructive* escalation of anger as quickly as possible, especially in the opening phase. (Anger may not be destructive if partners neither attack nor react as though injured.) The more hurtful a couple's fighting becomes, the harder it is for the therapist to intervene effectively. It helps to know what an angry, blaming presentation usually means. This is the gist of what I said:

"I think you both feel bad about having lost control in this way. Losing it like that makes most of us feel ashamed." Eva nodded. "But consider the fact that you stopped yourselves from going any further. That's hard to do. You then recognized you have problem and were willing to come here and expose yourselves to a stranger. That takes a lot of courage."

They were both taken by surprise by my response, and there was a palpable lowering of tension in the atmosphere, at least for the moment. Acknowledging partners' underlying feelings of shame and failure is a good way to defuse escalating attacks and help them feel understood and accepted. In addition, it is important to find and state the partners' strengths in order to reduce their sense of failure. Courage can always be found in a couple's willingness to come to therapy together. The therapist's consistent repetition of these three interventions—(1) containing hurtful interaction, (2) empathic acknowledgment of underlying feelings, and (3) positive reframing of shameful behavior—begins to defuse anger, soften defensiveness, and to create a climate of safety. While empathy and understanding provided a sufficient holding environment for Rina and Zack (from the previous chapter), the therapist is required to ensure safety more actively with vulnerable couples like Eva and Sid.

When a couple's interaction repetitively leads to escalation of hurt and anger, additional interventions are required. Working with each partner individually within the conjoint frame is another effective way to protect the partners and discourage wounding interchanges. Each partner is more likely to feel heard and understood with this approach. Conducting individual therapy within a conjoint context may need to be the predominant way of working with volatile couples until the partners become able to modulate their reactions. Mel Lansky (1986) also recommends this individualizing approach in the treatment of narcissistically vulnerable couples so that the partners can be helped to develop capacities to listen and empathize with each other. Eva and Sid required this approach intermittently in the early and middle phases of therapy.

Additionally, in sessions, the therapist needs actively to discourage partners' disrespectful treatment of each other, both verbal and nonverbal. Eva and Sid engaged in much destructive devaluing of each other. Understanding and managing devaluing between partners is only touched on here, but this subject is discussed in depth in Chapters 11 and 12. Blaming and expressions of contempt—eye-rolling, condescension, mocking, and sarcastic tones of voice[1]—cause great injury and promote angry retaliation.

A therapeutic environment that accepts these kinds of expression cannot really be experienced as safe. A therapist who ignores repeated devaluing is indirectly condoning its use, like the parent who gives tacit permission for drug use by ignoring the odor of marijuana emanating from a teenager's bedroom. Even though it can take a long time for some partners to eliminate this destructive behavior, it is important for the therapist to identify devaluing as harmful to the relationship and engage the couple's agreement to work toward respectful methods of expression. If possible, it is a good idea to address this problem early in treatment, since a therapist can easily be sucked into a couple's system and become immune, especially to the more subtle aspects of their wounding interactions.

During the interval of calm, I asked Eva and Sid about their experience of events that preceded this fight. When they reunited after Sid's absence, each felt acutely injured by the other's failure to provide a warm reception and needed support. Sid described Eva as greeting him coldly.

---

[1] The recent studies of John Gottman (Gottman & Silver, 1999) have shown that partners' frequent expressions of contempt are among the top four behaviors (along with criticism, defensiveness, and stonewalling) that cause marriages to fail.

According to Eva, Sid greeted her with a rash of criticism for forgetting to take care of certain household chores. Eva then blamed Sid for being an insensitive brute and caring more about the dry cleaning than the health of his wife and child. The fight got out of control over the issue of who would prepare dinner—who would act as the caretaker.

Both Eva and Sid were reacting to disappointment in each other for failing to fulfill unexpressed needs for nurturing. Such disappointment can easily ignite outbreaks of injury and anger in couples with major nurturing deficits (or in anyone if depletion and stresses are too great). In this instance, I also noted that the separation and each partner's feelings of inadequacy contributed to the intensity of the fight. Eva felt overwhelmed and inadequate to take care of a sick child when she was also ill. Unable to acknowledge these feelings to herself or Sid, she found fault with Sid. Likewise, Sid had felt extremely anxious about the success of his travels to buy and sell jewels. He was attempting to expand his small jewelry business. Unable to acknowledge his fears of failure, he found fault with Eva.

Eva and Sid had been married for twelve years. In reviewing their experience together, both agreed that the first few years had been very satisfying even though Eva had extensive personal problems. But the feelings of togetherness, of "us against a hostile world," had been lost with the birth of Laurie and Eva's move toward greater self-assertion, fostered by three years of individual therapy and developing her artistic abilities. Although Eva functioned primarily as a homemaker, she also made pottery to sell. Eva, who had originally been sweet tempered and compliant, was now bitter and angry, describing their marriage as a "total disaster." Sid rolled his eyes and said that things were bad, but not that bad. "Eva," he explained, "always exaggerates."

In their role relationship, Sid emerged as the dominant parental partner and Eva as the child no longer as submissive as she once was. Over time, Sid had become a less powerful, angry caretaker, while Eva became a disillusioned, though still needful, child. Eva continued to suffer from colitis, fibromyalgia, bulimia, and bouts of depression, though all of these conditions were improved by individual therapy. As noted in the previous chapter, this couple had been seriously mired in the disappointment phase of nurturing development for many years.

Their mutual disappointment, devaluing, and parent–child role relationship are illustrated in a session from the early phase of treatment (which is reported here). In this session, I attempted to create a safe climate for self-exposure by limiting the partners' devaluing, containing angry escalation, and interpreting their underlying needs and fears. In the early part of the session, I struggled to avoid being absorbed into the couple's collusive system, poor boundaries, and lack of differentiation. In the struggle to maintain my role and sense of self, I experienced typical symptoms of regression and boundary loss—losing focus, becoming confused and uncertain about how to intervene, feeling turned off and overwhelmed by the partners, wanting to withdraw. I worked out of this regressed state by using my reactions to understand the couple's deeper feelings and needs. I then attempted to translate my experience into a meaningful interpretation for them. Sharing humor among the three of us contributed to the partners' integration of the interpretation.

The Pancake Incident: Food for Thought

SID: We had a bad fight. Eva got hysterical!

EVA: I did not get hysterical. I got angry.

SID: Would you believe, she got hysterical . . . pardon me, angry . . . about a pancake?

EVA: You were sabotaging me by waving that pancake under my nose. You know I'm trying to lose weight, and the last thing I should have is a pancake.

SID: I did not know you were on another diet. I can't keep up with your diets. (*rolling his eyes*) She's always going on and off diets. Besides, why didn't you just say, "No thank you"? (*scoffing*) Really, I would not have forced you to eat the pancake.

EVA: Do you hear how he sounds? He makes me look like a demented idiot. I'm a figure of fun and ridicule around our house.

SID: That's not true! You just have no sense of humor. [I was aware of Sid's denigration of Eva. To avoid Sid's feeling ganged up on, I reminded him of our previous discussion of hurtful expressions.]

SHARPE: Sid, your manner does seem disrespectful. She's reacting to that. I understand that you still feel hurt and angry about this fight, but Eva can't listen to you when you roll your eyes and sound superior.

SID: Yeah, okay, I hear you . . . but what about what she does?

SHARPE: The same applies to Eva. If she sounds disrespectful, you need to object, if she doesn't correct herself first.

EVA: (*vindicated for the moment, pressing on*) There's a long history of his sabotaging my diets, and I really, really resent it. It's like he wants me to be overweight and unattractive. (*She begins to sniffle.*)

SID: How do I respond to that? She looks fine to me. You don't look any different to me.

EVA: (*sounding unspeakably pained*) You don't see, and you don't hear.

Eva's attractiveness made it difficult to take her fears seriously. By some standards, she was slightly overweight but the plumpness seemed to enhance her cherubic appeal (a description she would no doubt abhor). Although I liked both partners, Eva's dramatic displays of great injury were difficult to empathize with, and Sid's scornful tone and gestures made him an unsympathetic character. I was also bemused by the turn-around of the usual weight control issue, wherein the husband tries to control his wife's eating to keep her thin.

Their tattle-tale manner of opening a session was typical. Sid played the martyred parent trying to take care of ungrateful Eva. And she played the poor, innocent child, victimized by a domineering bully. I already felt discouraged and drained, like an exhausted mother who no longer had the energy to deal with quarreling siblings. I was worried that my irritation would show.

SID: Food is a really loaded subject in our relationship. I can't say anything about food. How was I supposed to know about the damn pancake the other morning?

EVA: You don't listen. I told you the night before that I was upset about the weight I'd gained. And then, the next morning, you shove this giant pancake under my nose. You just won't support my efforts . . .

SID: Look, I was just trying to do something nice for the family . . . make a special breakfast, and this is the thanks I get. I thought I was being a good guy, feeding Laurie and letting you sleep in. But you always find a way to turn me into the villain.

EVA: (*mocking*) Aren't you the noble one, and sooo blameless.

SHARPE: Eva, I think you felt blamed by what Sid just said, but your hurt is coming out in a mocking tone of voice. I know the urge to retaliate is strong, but Sid will hear you better if you find a less hurtful way of expressing yourself.

EVA: (*sighing and looking put-upon, then assuming a more neutral tone*) I'm reacting to an old issue in our relationship. If you just look at this one instance, he can make me look crazy . . . and like a lazy, ungrateful wife.

The apparent catalyst for this fight was Eva's feelings of defectiveness about herself (feeling fat) and her poor communication about her needs. She expected her mind to be read by Sid and then felt disappointed, imagining that he deliberately thwarted her wishes. What she wanted was not yet clear. Likewise, Sid's needs seemed to involve unstated wishes for her appreciation. I decided to try a simple intervention aimed at identifying their feelings of not having their wishes understood.

SHARPE: Eva, it seems as though you feel very disappointed that Sid does-n't understand your concerns about your weight and how much you need his support.

EVA: Well, yes, . . . but he doesn't even try.

SID: I do so try.

SHARPE: And Sid, I'm hearing your wish for Eva to appreciate your good intentions, even if you don't always understand her needs correctly.

SID: That's right! That's exactly right, but she won't give me that kind of credit.

EVA: How can I, when you try to control my eating all the time?

SID: (*mocking*) Oh, right. And how do I do that?

I intervened to curb further escalation, but Eva talked over me, com-pelled to describe Sid's insensitivity in excruciating detail. I withdrew for awhile, trying to figure out why my intervention not only misfired but fanned the flames. I wondered if Eva felt I had taken Sid's side and so needed to reemphasize his badness. I was aware of becoming increasingly disoriented and unable to think clearly as the sound of their relentless bickering drove me further into a state of numb detachment.

EVA: At dinner, you demand that I continue eating as long as you do.

SID: That's ridiculous. It's the kids I try to get to clean their plates. They need the nourishment.

EVA: If I tell you I need to diet, you press me to eat more, saying it's not healthy to eat so little. You just keep badgering me until I eat more.

SID: (*sarcastically*) Asking if you want a pancake is badgering?

EVA: I got angry this time before you could get into harassment.

SID: (*flushing with anger*) Oh, give me a break! You really are crazy. It's true. . . . I don't support those crash diets. You get weak and de-pressed when you do that. More weight just comes back on in the end.

EVA: (*turning to me for support*) See what he does? It sounds like he's just trying to take care of me, and I'm nuts. Well, maybe I am crazy, and I should just go check into a mental institution.

SID: (*rolling his eyes in disgust*) If you get into that breast-beating thing, there's no point in talking. We should just end the session right now! (*He stands.*)

SHARPE: (*firmly*) Sit down, Sid. We need to try and understand what's happening. We need you here to figure this out.

I was forced to intervene, but it was not clear to me what would be most useful. I knew I should resist their pulls to get me into the content issues—pursuing Eva's complaint that Sid sabotages her diets to keep her unattractive, or Sid's complaint that Eva is paranoid and out to prove he's an insensitive brute. I'd gotten nowhere going down those trails before.

I thought both, but especially Eva, would feel too criticized by any more discussion of their devaluing (which may have already occurred). I needed to find a meaningful statement of their underlying feelings. I tried to examine the reactions they evoked in me, the feelings of an exhausted mother, desperately needed by two rivalrous siblings. Obviously, they both felt starved for some kind of care. Each viewed the other as withholding the right food, and each simultaneously viewed the other as the competitor for mother's care. The main content of the interaction was about the pancake, about feeding and not being fed in return (Sid), or being fed the wrong thing at the wrong time (Eva).

I thought my earlier intervention did not get to their basic needs for nurturing and their repetitive disappointment. It also seemed that my attempt to distinguish their separate feelings and switch from one to the other so quickly was not helpful. I realized that fostering differentiation of their needs was likely premature and threatening. They were still too deeply mired in merger and feelings of disappointment to be ready for this kind of work. It would be better to focus on one of them at a time, or their shared feelings. I tried to speak to their shared pain using what I had learned from my reactions.

SHARPE: It seems to me this argument is about not getting what you need—not getting enough food and feeling like you're starving. (*I paused to let that sink in.*) I think you get into these complicated fights so that anger can distract you from the painful disappointment of needing something and not getting it.

EVA: (*looking confused*) Would you repeat what you just said? I'm not sure I got it.

SHARPE: Getting into these fights is a distraction—so you won't notice how really hurt you feel.

SID: So, you think that's what we're doing?

SHARPE: Yes. A lot of people prefer fighting to feeling in need and disappointed.

SID: It's an interesting thought. (*pausing*) Food for thought. (*He flashes a boyish grin.*)

SHARPE: (*chuckling*) Good one, Sid.

EVA: (*smiling*) It's hard to swallow. (*She makes a show of trying to swallow.*) [This was the first joke I'd ever heard her make.]

SHARPE: (*laughing*) Right. Most interpretations are.

SID: So . . . doctor, what do we do about it? (*He sounds impatient, as though we've played enough.*)

SHARPE: I guess you want to go back to work.

SID: (*Shrugs*).

EVA: (*shaking her head*) We'll just go back to fighting.

SHARPE: We can try this a different way. To start with, I'd like you each to consider why you have so much trouble getting what you need. Sid, would you try just talking about your needs without casting any blame on yourself or Eva. Just stick with you and your feelings. No judgments.

After a faltering opening, Sid gradually worked into the longest series of statements he'd ever made about his feelings (other than his anger). He spoke of feeling "in the dark" "at sea," "at a loss" to know what to do to make Eva happy. He was hurt that what he did do never seemed to count. He felt afraid to expect anything, afraid of the terrible letdown of expecting something from Eva, then being disappointed. He couldn't tolerate feeling helpless. It was humiliating.

Eva revealed some of her own feelings of shame about feeling needy. She also feared that if she asked directly for what she needed, Sid would not respond and might even ridicule her. Uncomfortable with this discussion of feelings, Sid said, "Okay, let's move on to how we solve the problem." I suggested we try understanding the source of their feelings by looking at their life together and in original family experience.

Couples who are struggling with nurturing deficits and conflicted wishes to be merged and separate are helped by some structure and direction. I have found that a more passive, open-ended, "Let's see where they go and I'll follow" approach is particularly unhelpful to couples with these problems. With a more passive approach, such couples often feel unsafe, uncared for, and abandoned, possibly because they felt so neglected and without guidance as children. Particularly with angry, devaluing couples who inflict great injury on each other, it is necessary to set limits. The specifics of the therapy structure provided may not be as important as its predictability and reliability, the same qualities required of the good mother of infancy.

Historical Revelations and Connections

At this point, we spent considerable time reviewing their childhood experience as it pertained to their present reactions to each other. Sid described perceiving his mother as fragile and overwhelmed, needing him to help her organize the household and care for the children. He was the oldest of five children and at a very young age acted as a coparent with his mother in caring for the younger siblings, since his father was frequently away on business trips. He also saw her as a saint who stoically endured chronic pain, unstable finances, and an absent husband. Throughout childhood, he was focused on meeting his mother's needs, not his own.

While he could not yet acknowledge feelings of anger and sadness about this role reversal, he recalled feeling agitated if he did not know what was expected of him, especially when his mother seemed sad or tense. As with Eva, he felt he was supposed to intuit what was wrong and know what to do about it. He recognized that he became similarly tense with Eva when she was upset, and he didn't know what to do to fix it. Consequently, he would either try to block out the problem (which made him seem insensitive) or take over (which made him seem controlling). Either of his solutions left Eva feeling enraged, whereas his mother had seemed to appreciate his take-charge efforts (as had Eva earlier in their marriage).

Sid felt chronically anxious around his father, as was the whole family, because of his father's erratic disposition. Sometimes he would explode if dinner was late or the table was not set perfectly. However well Sid tried to perform, his father responded with either indifference or criticism. Sid maintained that he no longer cared about approval from his father and felt lucky to have had such a wonderful mother.

In contrast, Eva was very aware of feeling neglected while growing up. Her mother had been seriously depressed for long periods during Eva's childhood. She had been hospitalized for depression on three occasions. As far back as she could remember, Eva and her older sister were mainly responsible for running the household, though her sister bore the brunt of the responsibility. Eva's father was a minister who was rarely home, preferring to devote himself to the needs of his flock.

Eva felt frightened throughout her childhood. She feared that her mother would fall apart and her father would abandon them. Her parents' marriage was a disaster that was made to appear perfect for the outside world. The public facade began to crumble in later years as Eva's mother became increasingly unable to function. She also feared losing the scraps of approval she got from her mother for being compliant and pretty. Eva now suspected that her mother took diet pills to remain thin and beautiful.

Eva's preoccupation with her weight and dramatic reaction to being offered a pancake now became more understandable. Eating the pancake was equated with the risk of losing her mother's precarious love. Sid was identified with her caretaking but competitive sister who tried to get her to overeat because she wanted Eva to be fat and ugly. As long as Eva stayed in an inferior role, acted needy and incompetent, she got her sister's care and guidance. Her rage at being used by her parents and dominated by her sister was primarily expressed in occasional abusive fights with her sister, and, in adolescence, by conducting a secret life of promiscuity, drug use, and bulimia.

Midway through college, Eva met Sid, who rescued her from the downward spiral of a self-destructive life. She was attracted to Sid's strength and independence. He always knew what to do. With the support of Sid and individual psychotherapy, Eva was able to pull herself together and for the first time begin to perform quite well academically. She also began to develop her arts and crafts abilities. As long as she stayed in the role of a dependent child who admired the caretaking Sid, their relationship was stable and fulfilling.

Eva and Sid naturally glided into a certain kind of role relationship—the caretaker and the needful child—that seemed to provide a solution to their profound but also conflictual needs for nurture. In this relationship, one partner acts out the deprived child of both and the other partner acts out the role of nurturing parent who is needed by both. The overriding aim of this role relationship is the re-creation of the longed for mother–infant bond.

Histories of partners in these kinds of role relationship usually reveal that they have suffered in childhood from parental neglect (as in Eva's case), marked parent–child role reversal (as in Sid's case), or were otherwise treated as the narcissistic extension of a parent (as were both Eva and Sid). The inability to move beyond disappointment in a formerly idealized spouse is caused by the tenacious wish for an ideal mother, fears of separateness and losing a familiar connection, and the desire to take revenge on the disappointing spouse (who also represents the parent or sibling from childhood).

In the course of this exploration, Eva became aware that she was reacting to Sid as if she were an incompetent little girl in order to ensure care, just as she had with her sister. But she also resented Sid's and her sister's power and wanted to rebel against their control. The painful repetition of the past for Sid was not so straightforward, because of his massive repression of the needy side of himself. He denied his own needs for nurture and projected them onto Eva, so that she was perceived as the needy one. Through caring for Eva, Sid could vicariously take care of his own needs. He could win his mother's love and approval by acting as a competent caretaker, but, at the same time, unconsciously take revenge on his disappointing mother and father by punishing Eva.

REENACTMENT OF DISAPPOINTMENT IN TREATMENT

As discussed in the previous chapter, partners need to recognize and mourn the loss of their romantic wishes and ideals in order to give up nurturing collusions and become able to give and receive in a reciprocal way. However, in order to relinquish unrealistic expectations, understanding the sources of anger and disappointment needs to occur. For many couples (as with Rina and Zack), these feelings primarily stem both from the disappointments that have accrued from the partners' history together and from the normal course of nurturing development. When these feelings are understood, impossible expectations are given up (to some extent) and mourning occurs. However, when partners' anger is also significantly tied to past disappointments with parents and siblings, these feelings must be recognized and distinguished from angry reactions to the partner. A key process in distinguishing past from present is the partners' awareness of seeking revenge for past disappointments by punishing each other.

Although Eva and Sid gained some understanding of how their historical experience with each other and their families of origin affected their relationship, they continued to stay rooted in a parent–child role relationship, even though their reactions to injury had become less intense and more modulated. I thought their resistance to further growth had a lot to do with avoiding recognition of their need to make each other suffer for past, as well as present, wounds. I made no headway on this front until they acted out with me their disappointment and vengefulness. The flowering of their anger toward me corresponded with the flowering of my need to become their perfect caretaker. This caretaking reaction to the couple can create another major obstacle to progress in therapy. However, if this countertransference is recognized by the therapist, it can be used to help the couple connect past feelings of anger and disappointment with both the therapeutic and couple relationship.

Therapist Identification with the Role of Caretaker

In working with couples like Eva and Sid, a therapist is highly susceptible to having his or her own nurturing and merging fantasies activated. Since the therapist is already in a caretaking role, he or she is particularly vulnerable to identifying with the couple's wished-for all-giving parent. The role relationship that may then evolve between therapist and couple mirrors the partners' role relationships with each other. The therapist views the couple as his or her "child" who is in need of rescuing and caretaking. This kind of countertransference is not usually activated with couples like Rina and Zack (previous chapter), who also have nurturing deficits but not to the same profound degree.

In the opening phase of treatment, partners with serious nurturing deficits characteristically transfer to the therapist their shared yearning for the ideal mother of infancy and early childhood. The couple induces the therapist to act out the role of their ideal of mother—the all-giving, constantly available mother who is able to magically fulfill all needs. As a corollary to this shared transference, each partner expects the therapist to act as a narcissistic extension and magically fix the other partner who is, of course, the real problem. Falling for the idealized "you are the one and only" role is very tempting, yet leads to endless quagmires and problems in treatment.

The desperate neediness of this kind of couple, combined with their initial idealized transference, can activate the therapist's own grandiose wishes to be an ideal mother. On the other hand, wishes to flee may also be engendered by the burden of these couples' great demands. This wish may evoke guilt feelings and a resultant reaction formation, particularly in female therapists for whom the role of "bad" deserting mother may be especially guilt inducing.

Assuming the role of maternal savior, however, is not a pleasant experience, particularly with devaluing couples. When heroic efforts to "be there" for the couple are not appreciated and instead promote regressive escalation of inappropriate demands, the therapist experiences disappointment and a deflation of grandiosity. In these instances, one can feel like a transitional object, the baby's special blanket that is cherished when needed and then cast aside when the need passes, as when the couple makes up from one of their horrendous fights. I am reminded of one of my disturbed vacations during the saga of my efforts to treat/save Eva and Sid.

Taking a two-week vacation at home during the Christmas holidays, late in the evening on the day after Christmas, I had a call from the therapist covering for me. She said she'd had an urgent call from Sid, who demanded to speak with me, insisting that it was an emergency. He refused to speak with her. Only I could help. Falling for the "You are the one and only," I called Sid.

He was very agitated and reported that during a fight with Eva, she had run out of the house screaming that she was never coming back. The fight had awakened Laurie, who had heard Eva's threat and was now very upset. Sid was frightened. I reminded him that I had suggested one of them leave for a short time, if a fight seemed to be escalating out of control. He was momentarily reassured.

A few minutes later, Eva called me from her car phone. She had been driving around crying since the fight. According to her, Sid had gotten angry because she had spent the day preparing for her pottery show instead of cleaning the house. I encouraged her to call home and speak to Laurie, since the child was very frightened.

Both partners continued to call me. It seemed that nothing I said would calm the hysteria, until I suggested that they come in to the office the next day for an emergency session. Trudging in to the office the next morning, I wondered why I was letting this couple's fight ruin my holiday. I had the sinking feeling that rushing to their rescue was a big mistake.

When I got to the office, there was a message from Eva on my answering machine. With apologetic cheer, she said they didn't need to come in after all. They could wait for their next scheduled time. Sid was helping her prepare for her exhibition, and later, they were taking the children to the beach.

As I sat in my office feeling sandbagged, I recognized that I had let myself be seduced into their wish for me to act as an ever-available, "savior" mother, who could take any amount of childish mistreatment. I realized I had felt compelled to respond to their pleas, as though they were needy, desperate little children whom only I could save and comfort.

However, I also recognized that my acting out this role did nothing to heal their wounds or foster insight and development. Mother, in their view, was not a separate being with needs, feelings, and a life of her own. Though I felt drained and angry, I reminded myself that I was the one who accepted the phone calls and suggested meeting during my vacation. When the therapist's own wishes to be the couple's "ideal" mother (and so be rewarded with everlasting love and gratitude) fail to be fulfilled, he or she can become angry and punitively retaliate by rejecting the couple or becoming avoidant and unreliable. Awareness of the likelihood of this transference–countertransference interaction helps the therapist refrain from continued acting out and make use of the events and evoked feelings for understanding the couple.

This fight and their call to me signified a regression, since the couple had been stabilized for some time without destructive fighting. Contributing factors were the holidays (a universal cause of regression) and Eva's move toward greater independence. She was having her first solo pottery show. Sid's heightened belligerence reflected the activation of his abandonment fears. My unavailability was also a big factor. I realized that we all had avoided dealing sufficiently with feelings about my then-pending absence. I attributed this oversight to their resistance and my own guilt about leaving my "babies" at Christmastime. Guilty about abandoning them, I was more susceptible to acting out countertransference feelings. They were showing me their anxiety and anger in this incident—and, in the last scene, how it felt to be casually discarded by leaving me behind in my office, while they went off to the beach.

In the next session, I asked Eva and Sid how they felt about this episode. Sid apologized for bothering me on my vacation and said things were a little better between them. Eva looked troubled. She said she felt afraid to come to the session, fearing I might be angry and not want to see them anymore. She thought I must view them as an impossible burden. She spent some time blaming Sid for their fight. I asked how she felt about my arranging to see them and then her canceling the appointment.

EVA: (*covering her mouth with her hand*) Oh, we didn't mean to inconvenience you. [I detected the signs of a smile poking out from behind her hand. Sid's expression went blank, and he avoided making eye contact.]

SHARPE: Well, I wondered about that while I was sitting in my office listening to your message. [I watched Eva's eyes widen and all traces of her guilty smile disappear.] I had the feeling of being suddenly left—abandoned. It made me think how you might have felt about my leaving you for the holidays. Maybe you felt deserted by me.

EVA: (*the words tumbling out in a rush*) Oh, I don't know. Maybe a little bit. But you deserve a holiday. I'm just sorry that we dragged you into our troubles. Sid was the one who did that.

Sid was about to defend himself, but I asked him to hold onto his response. I reassured both of them that my point in pursuing this event was not to induce guilt or cast blame, but to understand the meaning of what happened. I asked Sid for his thoughts.

SID: I think we were so caught up in our own problems, we didn't think about you. I guess you think we were paying you back by not showing up.

SHARPE: Possibly, though I don't think it was a conscious action. [Eva quickly asserted she had no awareness of being angry with me, though she had been very angry at Sid.] Let me describe what I think may have gotten triggered. First of all, I think holidays tend to remind people of their experience as children. Disappointed feelings can be aroused.

EVA: (*nodding*) I always feel depressed around Christmas. I remember how empty and lonely our Christmases used to be.

SHARPE: I think my not being available at Christmastime might have felt particularly painful and contributed to your feeling lonely and empty.

SID: Maybe for her but not for me. I was just glad we didn't have any appointments, because I had too much to do.

SHARPE: What about your experience of Christmas in childhood?

SID: (*frowning*) It wasn't a good time. I mainly remember my mother being angry that my father wasn't there. She would often be sick, and I had to take care of the younger kids and the dinner.

SHARPE: So you were left to take care of things.

SID: (*sighing*) I see what you're getting at, but I wasn't angry at you.

SHARPE: Well, maybe not at me personally, but at the mother and father who leave you alone with all the work. [Sid didn't reply, but I could see his face contract in pain. Eva reached over and tenderly touched his leg, the first empathic gesture I'd seen her make. Tears welled up in his eyes. As he allowed himself to feel sadness, his usual driven expression softened for a few moments. But then his mask of tough impatience snapped back into place, and his voice sounded gruff.]

SID: (*irritably*) I think we should talk about what's going on *now*. There's a lot we need to work on.

Even though there was no further discussion of the Christmas episode, Eva and Sid became much less angry with each other. It was as though some of their anger and disappointment had been channeled back to the original sources through me as the conduit. They were much more accepting of each other's failings and solicitous of each other's needs. It began to seem possible to work more directly on their nurturing collusion.

WORKING WITH THE CARETAKER–NEEDFUL CHILD COLLUSION

In order for Eva and Sid to develop reciprocal nurturing, their parent–child role relationship had to be liberated from its one-way giving and receiving form. Changing this relationship usually meets strong resistance, since it is so deeply rooted in each partner's self-image, concept of relating, and security. The following facets of this role relationship must be explored with the couple for meaningful change to occur: (1) recognition of each partner's role and how they dovetail; (2) the adaptive and defensive aspects of each partner's role, present and past; and (3) the fears each partner has about changing his or her role and the nature of this relationship. This exploration can only proceed incrementally as each aspect becomes available in the course of treatment. Knowledge of the typical dynamic structure of these kinds of relationships, as described here, can be a useful guide in working with this material.

The caretaker–needful child collusion can work reasonably well as long as there is a steady supply of appreciation given to the caretaker in return for acting as the responsible parent. These supplies also serve to keep at bay the caretaker's underlying longings for nurture and anger about deprivation. Many partners can find satisfaction in this mode as long as the child partner is gratified in this position and the caretaker remains out of touch with his or her needs. However, when the child begins to try and grow up, he or she requires a different kind of sustenance than what the caretaker has been providing, for the caretaker has inevitably been providing the kind of nurture he or she unconsciously needs and not necessarily what a "growing" child needs. In the earlier interchange, Sid wanted to feed Eva the pancake because he wanted to be cared for in this way. The pancake was not the right kind of care for Eva.

The growing child (or developing partner in a marriage) begins to need acknowledgment and support of individuality and becomes hurt and angry when this growth is discouraged. This developmental need to become a separate individual is exactly where parental support and encouragement was usually missing in both partners' childhoods. The child partner in a marriage, then, withholds the supplies necessary for the caretaker to maintain his or her defensive adjustment as a caretaker, that is, compliance and appreciation. Instead the child becomes angry and rebellious. In response, the caretaker begins more actively to suffer rage and anguish about unmet dependency needs in the guise of martyred cries: "I do everything, and I'm not appreciated! I do everything, and I get nothing in return."

However, the caretaker's aims are usually not so straightforward, for the caretaker also becomes disappointed in the old system. The rewards are not as great as he or she thought they would be. It is exhausting and unfulfilling to be just the caretaker. Envy of the child's position may start to invade consciousness. Hence, often both partners are stalled in the conflict between wanting the security of the old relationship versus wanting another, more liberated system in which all aspects of themselves can be expressed and accepted. Because moving backward and moving forward are equally threatening, the partners stay stalled in a caretaker–child role relationship that has become polluted by anger and disappointment.

Mutual blaming protects them from a backward slide into merging and feared engulfment, and from a forward move into the unknown and the threat of abandonment.[2]

One of the best openings for direct work with this collusion occurs when one of the partners begins to complain actively about his or her role. For example, as Sid became less defended against recognition of his needs, he began openly complaining about his role—"It's like I'm the parent. I have to take care of everyone. I just can't do it all, now that we have a child, and I'm trying to develop my business. Our relationship worked fine before we had a child. I had lots of energy, and I could take care of Eva and everything else with no problem." I seized this opening with Sid to begin exploration of how each of them felt in their roles, present and past.

Eva felt Sid's characterization of their relationship only applied to the past. She agreed that Sid had done most of the work, such as care of the household and providing, because she was depressed or sick so much of the time. But in recent years, she had tried very hard to be a good mother and wife, and felt unfairly criticized by Sid. Sid found it difficult to appreciate her contribution because he felt more burdened by ever-expanding responsibilities. Continued exploration of their complaints and wishes for change exposed both partners' conflictual needs to maintain their roles and their fears of change.

The focus of therapy moved naturally toward the clarification and reworking of roles between the partners. The partners wished to construct a more satisfying division of responsibilities. Sid wanted more help, and Eva wanted more respect. In the midst of attempting to develop reciprocal nurturing, Eva and Sid made agreements about who would take responsibility for which tasks. As with Rina and Zack, the failure of these agreements brought each partner's fears and resistance to change into focus. The collusive pattern of Sid taking over Eva's responsibilities, and Eva's inducements for him to take over were revealed in the following midphase therapy session. Sid began by berating Eva.

SID: You were supposed to have dinner ready for the guests Friday night by the time I got home. We agreed on that, remember?

EVA: Yes, but something happened, I . . .

SID: I don't care what happened. Nothing was ready. The lamb chops we decided to have weren't even in the refrigerator.

EVA: I'd decided it was better to have a roast chicken.

---

[2]See Chapter 12 for a more detailed discussion of the protective functions of blaming.

SID: But there was no chicken there, either. You were in the shower. I had to rush to the supermarket, buy the lamb chops, rush home, and cook the dinner. I always end up having to do everything.

EVA: I told you when we talked on the phone, I was a little behind schedule. You didn't listen to what I was saying. I had everything under control.

SID: How could that be? The guests were due to arrive forty-five minutes after I got home. Nothing was prepared.

EVA: I had a plan. You just interfered and took over. I was going to get a precooked chicken from Whole Foods. There was plenty of time.

SID: There was not plenty of time. Besides you never told me about a change in plans.

SHARPE: Sid, I realize you're angry about what happened, and I can see why. You felt Eva had dumped everything on you. But going back to your agreement, making the dinner was supposed to be Eva's job. Why did you take over? Why did you not let her take care of it, however she was going to do it?

SID: She was in the shower. There wasn't enough time for her to take care of things.

EVA: That's not true. I was aware of the time. I had it planned.

SID: I saw no signs of any plan.

EVA: You could have asked me, instead of just assuming I screwed up.

SID: (Sits fuming, trying to stifle an insulting retort. I intervene.)

SHARPE: There are two important aspects of what happened here. One is the feelings you had, Sid, that prompted you to take over. The other is what feelings come up in you, Eva, that may lead you to encourage Sid to take over.

EVA: But I didn't want Sid to interfere.

SHARPE: Yes, that's true. But I think you may also be in conflict about this—wanting to do the dinner (or whatever) on your own, but not being totally confident that you can. So the side of you that is used to relying on Sid might show itself in some way—like in leaving him in the dark about your change in plans.

EVA: I don't know about that. I just think he should trust me more.

SID: How can I, when you don't tell me what's going on?

EVA: I didn't tell you because you spoke to me in a very dismissive fashion on the phone.

SHARPE: So, you were angry with Sid.

SID: Is that why you dumped everything on me?

EVA: I didn't dump things on you. You charged off to the supermarket without even telling me where you were going.

SHARPE: I think you're trying to change an old pattern here, and you're running into some snags, like everyone does. [I judged that Sid would be more amenable to examining his motives than Eva would be at this point. For the moment, she was staunchly entrenched in defending her position.] Sid, let's look more closely at why it's so compelling for you to take over and not let Eva work things out on her own.

SID: I don't know. It's automatic. I feel I just can't trust Eva. If I didn't take over, nothing would get done.

SHARPE: Let's suppose you had just gone about your business and let her figure it out. What if she had managed to get the dinner ready herself? How might that feel?

SID: (speaking quickly) Good. I'd feel good.

SHARPE: You don't look entirely pleased with that idea. I'm sure part of you would like to be able to rely on Eva, let her take care of things, take care of you. But there's usually another part too. [I waited, hoping he could take it from there.]

SID: I don't know. I'm not arguing the point. I can only say I feel agitated. I can't really picture what you're talking about.

SHARPE: It might feel scary. Maybe if she were competent, she wouldn't need you anymore.

SID: Uh ... deep down ... I could fear that. I'm seeing myself as not knowing what to do—being cast adrift without a purpose.

While both Eva and Sid consciously wanted a more equal partnership, each was very afraid of such a change. At the core of Sid's identity was being a caretaker. Without operating in that role, he was afraid of being of no value and having no guiding sense of self. At a deeper level, he also feared being left by Eva.

Again, we addressed his fear of directly expressing his own needs, which he frequently managed by giving orders. For the caretaking partner, recognizing needs for nurture is difficult, but even more daunting is the direct expression of those needs to the partner. In trying to articulate his longings for love and support, he felt extremely vulnerable—*Who could possibly want a needy me?* When the caretaking partner is a man, these fears are often more exaggerated because of wishes to preserve a masculine self-image. Identification with the masculine stereotype of a strong man who has no needs is usually present and requires modification.

As I pursued Eva's resistances to change, she revealed fears that greater competence might leave her without care or support. She recognized that she had patterned herself after her inadequate, helpless mother whose incompetence had at least evoked some care from her father and children. She felt helpless and panicked about the prospect of being left to cope on her own. Change in Sid was also deeply threatening. Although it is generally difficult for the child-like partner to express needs directly, instead of through emotional or physical illness, the greater difficulty is in becoming able to listen and respond to the dependency needs of the "strong" partner. While Sid had great difficulty really listening to Eva's feelings, Eva had even more difficulty listening to Sid, once he began expressing his vulnerabilities.

Exploration of Eva's trouble listening to Sid revealed a number of fears. She described being overwhelmed by Sid's needs and feeling alone and frightened, like a small child. She resented Sid's needs taking priority over her own. She felt entitled to having her needs come first to make up for being neglected in childhood. When Sid sounded weak to her, she also felt repelled. When the child-like partner is a woman, she is often identified with the feminine stereotype of a dependent women taken care of by a strong man. This identification needs to be recognized and modified. Hence, the transition into the role of an adult, giving mate is not a smooth, easy one for either partner.

Reworking of the caretaker–needful child role relationship in therapy is aimed toward enabling the partners to become collaborating adults, who can each take the parent or child role when appropriate. This basic change in their relationship requires both partners' ability to accept their fundamental needs for nurture. This entails the ability to express directly such needs with each other and to tolerate the other's expression of dependency longings. Patterns of devaluing and merging that support a parent–child collusion can often be modified by working with the couple's nurturing deficits and conflicts. However, these patterns often require specific focus and intervention, which will be discussed in subsequent chapters. Many rounds of working with the partners' fears of change, intimacy, and separateness, along with the practice of direct expression of their needs, are necessary before lasting change occurs.

Merging

"I've Got You under My Skin"
—COLE PORTER (1936)

CHAPTER 5

Closeness as Oneness

In songs, novels, movies, and real life, lovers often describe feeling as one with each other. Catherine, the heroine of *Wuthering Heights* (Bronte, 1847/1981), passionately cried out to her nurse, "Nelly, I am Heathcliff!" (p. 74), proclaiming oneness with her lifelong love. In *The Bridges of Madison County* (Waller, 1992), the most popular love story of the nineties, Francesca's beloved Robert said that "they had ceased being separate beings and, instead, had become a third being" (p. 156). In more objective, elegant prose, Freud (1930/1961) noted: "At the height of being in love the boundary between ego and object threatens to melt away. Against all the evidence of his senses, a man who is in love declares that 'I' and 'you' are one, and is prepared to behave as if it were a fact" (p. 66). Wedding vows usually define marriage as the two becoming one.

The term "merging" is used here to refer to this psychological blurring of self–partner boundaries that is subjectively experienced as a feeling of oneness. More specifically, merging is considered to encompass a kind of experience, certain patterns of relating, and the fantasies underlying both. When a number of partners with reportedly good marriages were asked to describe intimacy in their relationships, many expressed various kinds or derivatives of merging as central to feeling close:

"A feeling of oneness," said a wife of forty years. "Being psychically entwined," said a husband of twenty-three years, "so that we often know what the other is thinking or feeling. Sometimes she knows what I'm thinking before I know what I'm thinking." Another wife described intimacy with her husband as "being so close that you know what it's like to feel like the other person, to be the other person—a complete kind of empathy, that goes both ways." "Being soul mates," said a wife who was several years into a happy second marriage, "we are more alike than either of

97

us would be with anyone else." A man married for thirty-five years said: "Sharing the same beliefs, values, and attitudes and having the same kind of reactions to things—a deep sense of commonality."

These statements are ordered in a certain sequence to illustrate a developmental progression from merging as oneness, in which the partner is not perceived as separate, to merging as mutuality, in which the partners accept each other as individuals. All of these forms of merging can coexist in a well-seasoned relationship.

In child development, merging is most often associated with the earliest mode of attachment between infants and their mothers. From the infant's viewpoint, being nurtured and merging are likely the first forms of connection. Margaret Mahler and her colleagues (1975) describe this form of attachment as symbiosis and distinguish the first three to four months of life as the symbiotic phase. According to Mahler, infants begin to differentiate themselves from their mothers at about four months of age.

At what point and to what degree the infant merges with mother is a question still under debate. Some infant researchers (notably, Daniel Stern, 1985) have suggested that even the youngest infants have some ability to distinguish themselves as separate from their mothers in certain sensory aspects. However, the idea that life begins with a profound *emotional* merging between mother and baby remains widely accepted. Adults' descriptions of feeling at one with their lovers support the idea of earlier experiences of oneness.

Our first experiences with our mothers of being enfolded, soothed, rocked, and fed, with sounds of cooing, sucking, and singing (if we were lucky) would seem to combine being nurtured with bodily sensations of merging. These early experiences are likely retained as somatic sensations that later become embodied in fantasies of oneness. In adulthood, physical affection (including being held and holding) and sex are most often associated with heightened experiences of romantic love and merging.

In childhood and adulthood, wishes to blend ourselves with another are usually inspired by someone who is needed, loved, or viewed in elevated terms (like mother, father, teacher, or a lover). God and cult leaders also inspire wishes to become one with a more exalted being. The perception of the other as elevated in some way—as ideal or more powerful than the self—is necessary to achieve the desired sense of self-expansion and wholeness.

In object relations theory, the early form of merging is thought to be briefly revived when adults fall in love, but then is left behind as the partners begin to separate. Merging that continues beyond infancy or the early phase of a love relationship is generally viewed as pathological—as infantile, regressed, undifferentiated, dysfunctional. Pathological forms of merging have been variously called "fusion," "enmeshment," "symbiosis," "part–object relating," "transitional object relating," and "selfobject relating".

However, if we pay attention to our own fantasies and desires, it appears that merging with our partners in some form is essential for feeling deeply connected. In childhood and adulthood, merging fantasies and relatedness serve the same important purposes of (1) achieving a close, secure attachment with another, (2) expanding one's sense of self in some way as being more complete, perfect, and powerful than one's imperfect self alone, and (3) defending against one's fears of abandonment, separateness, and the loss an intact sense of self.

Merging as a lifelong need and positive mode of relating has only been considered by a very few researchers and theorists. In the series of subliminal oneness studies, Silverman, Lachmann, and Milich (1982, 1984) have shown this mode to be necessary for healthy development in childhood and throughout life. Heinz Kohut (1971, 1977) and many of his followers consider the selfobject relationship to be a lifelong need. In their conceptualization of attachment and separateness throughout the life cycle, Rachael Blass and Sidney Blatt (1992) also consider merging to be a normal, recurrent phenomenon.

These formulations consider merging as one kind of early relatedness that stays with us throughout life. In the conception advanced here, this mode is viewed as a set of fantasies and relationship patterns that develop and change in the normal course of a love relationship, while also being retained in their earlier forms. Earlier forms of oneness become selectively expressed, usually in a couple's sexual relationship, although many partners can feel totally joined in pursuing a common cause or interest. In the next chapter, the normal development of merging in love relationships is described, along with the common difficulties that arise as couples contend with the often conflictual tasks of deepening their union, while also evolving as separate individuals.

CHAPTER 6

The Development of Merging
Common Treatment Problems

In relationships that begin with romantic love, partners create powerful bonds of connection through merging, nurturing, and idealizing. With the evolution of each of these relationship patterns, different aspects of a couple's attachment are strengthened. Mutual nurturing by partners promotes the bonds of feeling cared for and secure. A couple's passionate attachment is created and kept alive through idealizing. Merging fosters the development of closeness and union in a relationship.

Couples in love initially experience merging in a global way, because they do not *emotionally* accept each other as separate individuals (even though their actual separateness may be intellectually recognized). When partners become aware of certain differences between them that challenge the belief in their oneness, a period of deflation follows (usually in conjunction with the disappointments of romantic nurturing and idealizing). The loss of intense feelings of closeness leaves most partners feeling temporarily deserted and alone. To avoid these painful feelings, partners often blind themselves to perceiving the differences that threaten their oneness and ideal twinship.

In an optimal developmental process, partners become able to accept each other as separate, while also sustaining a close attachment. Differences that were initially perceived as threatening often become appreciated. As the couple progresses, partners create a repertoire of ways to feel closely connected by encouraging their similarities, as well as supporting each other's individuality. Ideally, their patterns of closeness can range from the intensity of total merging during sex (and at other moments) to the comfortable companionship of taking a walk together, during which each feels deeply connected but may be occupied with different thoughts and observations. In the ideally mature relationship, the partners can move in and out of varying degrees of closeness and separateness, unhindered by crippling fears of being engulfed, abandoned, or rejected. By actively fostering their similarities and working with their differences to achieve compromises, couples gradually attain a strong sense of commonality, or mutuality, in their relationship.

This developmental progression moves from merging that is experienced as global oneness through the partners' acceptance of varying degrees of closeness and separateness, to their eventual creation of a mutual relationship. In its mature form, merging embraces both a fantasized oneness of varying degrees and kinds and the complementary recognition of varying degrees and kinds of separateness—"We are one, but we are also separate individuals."

The developmental steps from global merging to the attainment of mutuality are as follows:

- Global merging: oneness
- Deflation: recognition of differences
- Acceptance of needs to be close and separate (in self and partner)
- Regulation of being together and apart
- Attainment of mutuality

As with the other patterns of relating, this evolution occurs in the form of a spiral rather than in a one-time linear progression. The steps overlap a great deal and many repetitions of the original processes occur in the lifetime of a relationship. In the intimacy dance, partners move toward each other and may reexperience the intensity of oneness temporarily, but then one or both partners will need more distance to reestablish independence. Desires for joining will then resurface and a deeper level of connection will likely be experienced. Recapitulation of the aforementioned sequence may be formalized when couples take second or third honeymoons, in order to recapture the intensity of romantic merging, nurturing, and idealizing. However, the first round of this evolution tends to be of fundamental importance to subsequent development of a love relationship.

Life-cycle events influence the ebb and flow of partners' closeness and distance. The birth of the first child commonly disrupts a couple's intimacy. Many wives shift intense feelings of closeness from their husbands to their babies. Couples often need to work consciously to regain and develop their intimate connection. In contrast, the empty nest and retirement create an environment of togetherness that may foster or disrupt a couple's intimacy. Without the stressful demands of raising children and working, partners have the opportunity to focus more intensely on each other. However, the specter of endless time together may stimulate a partner's fears of a stifling enmeshment and the loss of his or her independent identity. In these cases, partners may generate conflict to create the distance necessary for each to maintain a sense of independence. This kind of distancing conflict is so common that the bickering retired couple has become a stereotype.[1]

COMMON PROBLEMS: POINTS OF REGRESSION AND DERAILMENT

Most couples have difficulties with each of these developmental steps and their related tasks. Many partners become derailed before or during the first step in this process by their inability to experience oneness with their lover to any significant degree. Partners who are not in love, or who renounce this profound experience of connection because of intimacy fears, may always feel lonely and unfulfilled in their relationships. At the opposite extreme are those partners who may feel so fulfilled and secure in the womb of oneness that they cannot move to the next step of accepting the partner as different and separate. They cling to the gratifications of global merging and deny their perception of differences.

For those who continue development, recognition of the partner as separate may occur to some extent, but the loneliness of deflation quickly sends one or both back to the comfort of oneness. In other instances, partners may react to awareness of their differences with anger, in the effort to ward off the depressed feelings that accompany deflation of oneness. One partner may become angrily punitive whenever the other fails to act as his or her extension, or each may try to coerce the other into compliance. Many couples become stalled in these kinds of repetitive but unsuccessful attempts to contend with the distressing reality of differences. They remain unhappily betwixt and between merger and separateness.

Once awareness of each other as separate is accepted and sustained (to some degree), the partners may run into difficulty managing their own needs for both closeness and separateness. Universally, people have conflicted feelings about varying degrees of both states. Closeness is most commonly feared because merging may result in feeling engulfed and losing one's sense of an independent self. Separateness is feared because feelings of isolation and abandonment can be aroused. Either state can incite fears of loss and rejection. Many people feel anxious with any intensity

---

[1]The bickering of retired couples may also result from other dynamics, such as using the relationship to express anger that derives from partners' feeling useless and depressed about aging and being abandoned by children, colleagues, or friends.

of closeness and any degree of separateness. One wife commented that she had a narrow comfort zone between feeling too close and too distant with her husband. She could easily feel smothered when he hung around her for very long, but then she would feel painfully anxious and lonely as soon as they were apart.

In order to be comfortable with varying degrees of closeness, partners need to feel secure in their abilities to retain or recapture a sense of separateness when experiences of merging and boundary blurring occur or might occur. This ability means that partners have developed *flexibility* in their boundary between self and other, a boundary that can become permeable when intense closeness is wanted but then easily becomes impermeable when separateness is desired. People who always need to keep their distance and maintain separateness have rigidly impermeable boundaries. Those who merge easily but have difficulty reestablishing a separate sense of themselves have inflexibly permeable boundaries. Sensitivity to feeling smothered or controlled when in close proximity to one's partner usually indicates that one's sense of self is insecurely established. Fear of losing identity or autonomy (either temporarily or permanently) may lead the insecure partner to become more distant in order to protect personal boundaries that blur too easily or for too long.

Sensitivity to feeling anxious and alone when one's partner is out of contact (either emotionally or physically) usually suggests that one's representation of a close, loving relationship has not been *reliably* internalized. Actual contact with the partner is needed to restore the sense of a close connection. When couples have reliably internalized their relationship as intimate, they are able to draw on memories (or representations) of their closeness together to sustain a feeling of comforting connectedness, even when the partner is absent (physically or emotionally). One of Gottman's (1999) findings supports the importance of this internalization. Those couples he studied who were able to remember with positive feeling their original passion and closeness had a much better chance of working out their problems and staying together than those who could not access these memories.

Partners who have not been able reliably to internalize a close, loving relationship and a strong sense of self surrounded by a flexible boundary often act out their intimacy–distance wishes and fears in the relationship. These partners often develop collusions to protect themselves from experiencing the anxiety caused by feeling too close or too separate in their relationship.

Couples who share intense needs for merged forms of togetherness and greatly fear abandonment may form a *pseudomutual collusion*[2] in which

---

[2]"Pseudomutual" is a term borrowed from Wynne, Ryckoff, Day, and Hirsch (1958).

both deny their separateness. At the other extreme, partners who share great needs to protect their autonomy because fears of engulfment and identity loss are predominant may form a *parallel partner collusion* in which each functions very separately, as though living on parallel tracks. They often describe themselves as "ships passing in the night." If not too distant, these partners often engage in oppositional argument and control struggles in order to maintain distance and their separate identities (see Sharpe, 1990).

In another common defensive dynamic, the intimacy–distance conflict is divided between the partners in a *pursuer–pursued collusion,* wherein one seeks more closeness and the other continually moves away, proclaiming needs for more space or independence. Sid and Eva (the caretaker and the needful child) engaged in this dynamic. In this collusion, the partners try to solve their shared anxieties through projection of one side of the conflict onto the partner who receives and acts out the projection. The conflict is thus divided so that one partner carries the couple's shared needs for closeness and fears of separateness, while the other expresses their joint wishes for separateness and fears of closeness. In this way, the couple maintains the exact degree of closeness and distance they unconsciously require for safety, termed "the fixed diameter of Eros" by Michael Vincent Miller (1995).

If partners become able to acknowledge and work through their needs and fears in these areas, the tasks of creating and regulating satisfying patterns of being together and separate come into the foreground. Many couples founder over the issues—"How and when will we be close, and how will we be separate?"

People vary greatly in the kind and intensity of closeness they desire. Some partners are comfortable feeling a deep, merger-like connection in only one sphere, such as the sexual or the intellectual, and that is sufficient for them to feel intimate. Others aspire to fulfilling the romantic ideal of closeness, which requires that feelings of oneness be operative in most, if not all, of the domains of connection—the sexual, the emotional, the intellectual, the moral, the recreational. In their typologies of good marriages, Judith Wallerstein and Sandra Blakeslee (1995) distinguish these intensely close relationships as romantic marriages. The success of these marriages seems to depend on the *similarity* of the partners' needs for closeness in both degree of intensity and domains of relating.

When partners need different kinds and intensities of closeness to feel connected, they have a more difficult time in finding ways to accommodate each other. A common example of gender difference is the man whose needs for closeness are met through having sex and doing active things with his partner, like playing tennis or hiking, while the woman only feels close when cuddled up and talking intimately. Women more often seem to want long, intense merging experiences through talking, holding, and touching, while many men become impatient or anxious with prolonged contact of this kind.

In the course of a relationship, partners' needs for closeness and separateness also change. For example, Eva wanted constant togetherness early in their marriage, while Sid experienced her as too clingy. He wanted to work on projects or watch sports on the weekends. However, when Eva became interested in developing her artistic talent and wanted to throw pots on the weekends, Sid began pressuring her to spend more time with him. Their original roles of pursuer and pursued had completely reversed. These roles can also flip-flop over short periods of time and in the course of a day. Just as soon as one partner stops pursuing, the other begins the pursuit. Developing a satisfying choreography of how and when to be close and apart takes a lot of practice for most couples. Many partners cannot or will not bend to meet their partner's needs. Derailment over these issues is common, often leading to divorce.

In describing their ideal of an intimate relationship, many people express the wish to feel consistently connected with their partners in a variety of ways, while at the same time supported in pursuing their individual talents and interests. This ideal is only achieved when partners continuously nurture and develop areas of commonality, attempt to mesh their differing wishes through compromise, and allow some areas in which a meeting of the minds is not possible.

The developmental steps, related tasks, and common pitfalls (outlined in Figure 3) provide a guiding framework for therapists in helping couples work with their needs to be close and separate. The first task for therapists is to understand at what point in this developmental process a couple has become derailed. Identifying the most troublesome relationship task(s) and helping the partners express their fears and wishes about closeness and separateness may free the couple enough to resume development in this area. With other couples, deeper therapeutic work may be necessary, as in the cases of two of the couples who are presented (Eva and Sid, and Lola and Max). Working with the origins of these couples' entrenched fears of abandonment and engulfment, and their enactment in relationship with the therapist is discussed in later chapters.

GLOBAL MERGING: ONENESS

Global merging and idealizing are the major psychological processes that create the intense, pleasurable sensations we call falling in love. Throughout the life of a relationship, merging and idealizing continue to be necessary for emotional and physical closeness, at least as we conceive of intimacy in our society. As noted previously, global merging echoes the

Steps in Development of Merging	Tasks for Couple/Guide for Therapy	Common Problems (Points of Regression and Derailment)
Global Merging: Oneness	Experiencing oneness with partner Establishing bond of romantic closeness	Lack of love or intimacy fears prevent merging Closeness not romantically intense Clinging to oneness
Deflation: Recognition of Separateness	Perceiving differences and separateness Overcoming hurt and anger Experiencing loss, sadness, loneliness Mourning loss of oneness and ideal twin	Denial of differences, regression to global oneness Stalled in anger: coercing compliance Stalled in depression and withdrawal Avoidance of mourning, regression to anger
Acceptance of Needs to Be Close and Separate (in self and partner)	Acknowledging needs to be close and separate within self Understanding partner's needs and fears Working through fears of closeness and separateness Internalizing a close, loving relationship	Needs and fears projected onto partner: *pursuer–pursued collusion* Partners accept closeness, deny separateness: *pseudomutual collusion* Partners accept separateness, deny closeness: *parallel partner collusion* Unreliable internalization of close relationship
Expansion and Regulation of Being Together and Apart	Finding multiple ways to be close/separate Balancing being close and separate Moving together and apart without great fears of engulfment or abandonment Developing *flexibility* in the boundary between self and partner	Failure to develop varieties of closeness/separateness Too much together or too much apart Anxiety hinders coming together and moving apart Boundary between self and partner remains too permeable or impermeable
Attainment of Mutuality	Creating and nurturing commonalities Understanding and meshing differences Compromising to create common goals Respecting differences that cannot be altered Oneness experienced selectively and temporarily	Commonalities undeveloped Partners too focused on their separate development Inability to compromise in many areas Regression to pseudomutual, parallel, or pursuer–pursued collusions

FIGURE 3. The development of merging.

106

infant's early connection with mother and promotes the couple's close attachment.

When people fall in love, feelings of oneness occur whether the initial attraction was based on a conscious perception of similarities (interests, attitudes, values) or on complementary differences, such as he being shy and she being outgoing. The ways in which couples feel alike are variable. One couple may share the experience of feeling deprived in childhood, while another couple may profoundly connect over a shared rebellious attitude toward authority. Whatever the ingredients, the feeling of alikeness or similarity tends to be experienced emotionally and globally as "We are exactly alike," even though, simultaneously, differences may be intellectually perceived and appreciated.

Both partners also tend to idealize each other in global ways if their courtship leads to falling in love. He or she is perceived as totally perfect or, at least, a perfect fit for oneself. Romantic, global merging is commonly expressed between the partners in forms of rapturous clinging, accompanied by the flush, gush, and glue of mutual sexual arousal. No one is as important as the partners are to each other. They act as one another's admiring mirror that continuously reflects back: "You are the greatest of them all." They also act as twins who think alike and feel alike; some may even dress alike. They are obsessively preoccupied with thoughts of each other and will take any opportunity to share these thoughts with whoever will listen.

There are, of course, couples who marry without falling in love (or one partner "falls" and the other does not), and these partners do not experience blissful feelings of oneness. As noted previously, one or both partners may be unable to fall in love because of profound fears of merging, stemming from fears of engulfment, rejection, or abandonment.

Commonly observed patterns of relating that express fantasies of oneness are mind reading, mirroring, twinning, and obsessive preoccupation with the partner. During the romantic phase, these patterns are predominant. While merged patterns will often be obvious and pervade the interactions of a couple in love, they do not usually appear dominant later on in a couple's relationship. However, when global fantasies of merging are not modified, these patterns continue to flourish in dysfunctional ways, usually in the context of a marked dominant–submissive role relationship.

Encapsulated in Oneness: Max and Lola

When global merging remains dominant beyond the romantic phase, the partners' experience of a blissful oneness can be transformed into feelings of suffocating dependency. Prolonged denial of a separate sense of self stunts the couple's growth and creates an environment where underground anger and anxiety flourish. Cole Porter's song "I've Got You under My Skin," which is supposed to be about falling in love, also captures the flavor of the downside of merger. Consider, for example, what it might really be like to have someone under your skin or be under someone else's skin. In the following excerpt from a midphase therapy session, Max uses his own version of the skin metaphor to describe his forty-year-long marriage with Lola:

MAX: We live inside each other's skins. That gets to be real confining sometimes. When one of us needs to stretch or scratch, you feel bound too tight to move . . . and then if you do, it hurts the other one. . . . You know what I mean?

SHARPE: Well no, I'm not sure I do.

LOLA: (*Smiles sweetly and nods. She seems to know what he means.*)

MAX: If I'm inside her skin wriggling around scratching, it's not gonna feel too good to her, right? And it's gonna bother me too, because I can't get a good scratch or stretch. Then you got to think about how it is when we're in the same skin and I want to go in a different direction than she does. Our skin doesn't stretch far enough for that. (*He chuckled and glances nervously at Lola, whose smile now looks strained.*) It gets tiresome, all of this trying to move around in the same skin, bumping each other and getting chafed. It's irritating. We get irritated with each other sometimes, don't we? (*He says this with an anxious jocularity, patting Lola on the knee.*)

LOLA: (*Her eyes glaze over and her smile fades as she takes in his wish to be more separate from her.*)

This interaction occurred well into treatment and indicated the couple's beginning to "hatch" out of their womb of oneness. More accurately, Max was the one expressing discontent with the degree of their closeness. In the beginning of therapy, this couple hardly ever acknowledged having different opinions, needs, or interests. To ensure their attachment and avoid fears of abandonment, they held each other too close for comfort and growth.

Regression to Oneness: Henry and June

While Lola and Max had remained encapsulated in oneness for forty years, Henry and June's problems illustrate a regression to global merging patterns that had not yet become seriously entrenched. In their early thirties and married for eight years, Henry and June came to therapy because of increasing distance between them. Henry was particularly disturbed by the waning of their sex life and physical expressions of affection. When June fell asleep before they could make love on the night of their anniversary, Henry became seriously alarmed and called for a consultation. Prior to the birth of their two children, the couple had been able to accept some degree of separateness in their relationship and permitted development of individual interests. June was pursuing course work toward a degree in library science when she became pregnant.

However, following the birth of their first child, June gave up her personal development and devoted herself to the care of Henry and their little boy. Henry felt that June became even less interested in sex after the birth of their second son. Before having children, the partners had tolerated differences between them to a minimal extent. But at the time of entering therapy, they hardly ever openly disagreed. Anger was only rarely expressed by Henry, who would occasionally explode over something "trivial." Such painful ruptures were quickly sealed over and forgotten by both partners. Henry and June went to great lengths to prove to themselves and the world that they were a perfect couple, always in total agreement—the hallmarks of a pseudomutual collusion.

Patterns of global merging—mind reading, mirroring, and preoccupation with the partner—were prevalent. Henry's dominance and June's submissiveness had become more marked as the years went by. This dynamic seemed reflected in Henry's high color and robustness compared with June's shadow-like presence and pale, translucent skin. It looked like June was transfusing her life energy and blood to Henry.

Each described the other in predominantly idealized terms, though in individual evaluation sessions, both were freer to express some negatives about each other and the relationship. June was afraid of Henry's temper, and she felt she had lost track of who she was. She had become consumed in her role as wife and mother, and had given up all of her previous interests and ambitions. She could not even find the time to go for a run on the beach or read, which had been her favorite activities. Henry felt deeply wounded by June's sexual withdrawal but was unable to discuss these feelings. Along with wishing to deny any problems, he was ashamed of being jealous of his sons and believed that anger at his wife was unacceptable.

In the following excerpt from an early treatment session, working with mind reading, mirroring, a dominant–submissive role relationship, and each partner's fears of being separate are illustrated. Henry opened the session, as he usually did, speaking enthusiastically:

HENRY: It's really exciting; we're going trekking in Tibet this fall. We've always wanted to hike in the Himalayas. My parents have gone before, but they've offered to take us this time—all expenses paid. Isn't that terrific? We could never afford to do this on our own. We're really excited, aren't we? (*glancing at June for confirmation*)

JUNE: (*with forced enthusiasm*) It's a great opportunity.

I had noticed that June was sitting tensely through Henry's sharing of this news, looking into space with a vague smile. The fingers of one of her long, white hands were squeezing and picking on the fingers of the other. She appeared ill at ease about this proposed trip. I commented on the discrepancy.

SHARPE: June, you're not looking as enthusiastic about this as Henry.

JUNE: (*glancing at me with frightened, doe-like eyes, speaking hesitantly*) Well . . . uh . . .

HENRY: (*jumping in*) She's just worried about a couple of minor things, aren't you babe? She's worried about accepting such a big gift from my parents. But, they can afford it. No problem at all. (*He produces a gleaming smile, wide enough for both of them, as though to say, "That's the end of that problem."*)

SHARPE: (*quickly, before Henry shifts to another subject*) June, is that your concern? (*She had gone back to staring blankly.*)

JUNE: Well, to some extent. Um, but . . . also there's leaving the kids for all that time and . . . I'm . . .

HENRY: Oh, *that*. We already talked about that, remember? We're going after school starts, when your mother can come to take care of the kids. So it's not a problem.

JUNE: (*stammering*) Well, it's not just the kids . . .

HENRY: It's such a terrific opportunity. We can't pass it up. You've got to stop worrying about minor things. Think positive. . . . Think about seeing those incredible peaks all around you. We'll have gourmet meals in the evenings under the stars . . . no responsibility, no kids . . . the Himalayan moon shining down on us. It'll be awesome. (*He flashes another wide grin, reminding me of a predator that's just wolfed down a smaller animal's dinner.*)

Throughout Henry's pep talk, June had been bobbing her head in little nods, trying gamely to look positive. The atmosphere in the room had become increasingly tense. Even though Henry sounded confident, I sensed his growing anxiety. I observed him frequently massaging and stretching a stiffening neck.

In this interchange, Henry spoke for June *as though* he knew her mind better than she did. With smiling nods of agreement and little or no objection, June tried to mirror Henry in the attempt to fulfill his wish for total compliance.

While both appeared to be striving to fulfill the ideal image of a union unmarred by disagreement, the content of their oneness fantasies differed in a significant way. In a dominant–submissive role relationship, the merging fantasy experienced by the dominant partner is "You are an extension of me," while the submissive partner experiences and enacts "I am an extension of you." Oneness fantasies of the partners in more equally balanced role relationships involve the blending together of two essentially separate people who move in and out of varying degrees of closeness and merging with only temporary loss of their separate identities.

Henry's need for June to act consistently as his echo was apparent. He ignored any signs of disagreement. With bullying behavior and condescending instruction, he coerced June to comply in order to keep alive the needed fantasy—"We are of the same mind, which is my mind."

Mirroring, a term extensively used by Kohut (1971), originally refers to the young child's need for admiring, confirming responses from his or her mother. Mirroring is "the gleam in the mother's eye, which mirrors the child's exhibitionistic display . . . and is so important in confirming the child's self-esteem" (p. 116). Kohut recognized that many of his patients who did not have a stable sense of themselves lacked mirroring from their mothers. This unfulfilled need was then enacted in the therapeutic relationship in what he called "the mirror transference." In this transference, the therapist is expected to act as a mirror to the patient by responding to "the patient's demands that he reflect, echo, approve, and admire his exhibitionism and greatness" (p. 270).

As applied to couple relationships, each partner mirrors the other partner by echoing, approving, and admiring responses. Partners who are in love spontaneously mirror one another, frequently admiring each other's greatness. In a good relationship, this kind of support continues but in modified ways that incorporate more realistic, less grand perceptions of the partner. When spouses continue to unrealistically mirror each other in a pervasive way, this behavior has likely become defensive, indicating a developmental lag or derailment. Mirroring also becomes dysfunctional and defensive when it supports a dominant–submissive role relationship, wherein only the dominant partner receives mirroring. In either event, the partners have likely formed a pseudomutual collusion in order to sustain their oneness fantasies and avoid their fears of becoming separate. Unfortunately, the high price of this collusion is stalled development of the relationship.

In previous sessions, June had mirrored Henry with the total agreement and enthusiasm he wanted. In this session, her tentative efforts to clarify her own differing point of view were something new and reflected substantial progress on her part. Previously, June had trouble distinguishing her own views and feelings from Henry's. She had now advanced to some awareness of her own mind but was extremely fearful of expressing difference.

With the hope of promoting awareness and discussion of their fears, I noted the mounting tension in the atmosphere. June timidly agreed that she felt a little tense. With some gentle probing, she admitted to feeling worried about appearing to be a spoilsport about the trip. She would love to go on such a vacation with Henry but felt uncomfortable about being with his parents and leaving the kids for so long. She was afraid to discuss these concerns with Henry for fear that he would be disappointed and hurt. Eventually we got to her fear that, if she disappointed Henry, he would get angry and abandon her. She worried that Henry was angry with her right now. She already felt anxious and alone.

Henry listened to June with growing dismay. He admitted to feeling disappointed and hurt, and struggled to suppress his anger. He'd already gotten the message that she was not thrilled about this trip. His overbearing behavior was his way of trying to deny her negativity and disagreement. He felt threatened. He wanted her to be as enthusiastic as he was. Otherwise, he felt rejected and deserted.

The initial therapeutic aim in working with global merging patterns is to create the safety necessary for the partners to expose their underlying fears. Openly expressed disagreement and anger cause couples like Henry and June to feel fearfully isolated and abandoned. Awareness of this difficulty can aid the therapist in focusing on the partner's anxiety and its likely meanings. Empathic acceptance of underlying fears, followed by exploration of their origins, gradually enable partners to modify global oneness fantasies and their expression in collusive patterns of relating.

The underlying wishes and fears that sustain defensive patterns of merging will go unrecognized if the therapist initially responds in a directive, communication-focused, or problem-solving way to this kind of material. With merged couples who use mind reading not only as an expression of wishes for oneness but as a *necessary* defense against awareness of separateness, pressure by the therapist for the partners to communicate directly—make "I" statements, direct requests, expose and explain their feelings—is experienced as traumatic, producing high anxiety, though the partners may try to comply. If a couple does comply under instructive pressure, a therapist can mistakenly think progress has been made, for the partners may temporarily look like they are interacting as two separate adults. However, this is really a step backward, because the partners' needs to sustain pervasive oneness fantasies have just been buried deeper.

Later in treatment, when partners have some understanding of their mind-reading wishes, patterns, and fears, exploration can become more refined and include communication training. Focus can turn to why certain kinds of messages, but not others, are sent in the "read my mind" mode, or why being of "one mind" is such a necessity. It is often the case that whenever one or both partners' security is threatened, there will be a regression to increased mind-reading expectations and other collusive patterns.

Treatment interventions are thus guided by the therapist's understanding that the couple's merged relationship patterns reflect attempts of each partner to secure a close attachment and the sense of a whole, acceptable self. The therapist's interventions are informed by understanding that a couple may have substantial difficulties giving up oneness fantasies and interactional patterns, because of the losses and fears involved. The treatment of global merging that has become defensive requires the delicate operation of retaining and encouraging the positive ties that bind, while slowly loosening and then removing those ties that strangle, so that growth of the partners and the relationship can resume.

DEFLATION: RECOGNITION OF DIFFERENCES: EVA AND SID

As most of us are well aware, global merging as a central mode of connecting does not usually last. Fissures begin to appear in this magical state of oneness, commonly within the first year of marriage. Blows to romantic oneness fantasies occur when partners discover they are not only flawed but substantially different from each other and, therefore, must be separate. Each partner's experience of losing the sense of an all-encompassing oneness with the other is uniquely disturbing.

Many people cannot accept the reality that the partner is not quite the soulmate imagined. Unlike those who try to keep fantasies of oneness and twinness intact, these partners recognize that they are separate. Instead of integrating this reality and moving on, they stay in a state of chronic hurt and anger, repetitively punishing the partner for failing to behave as an extension or twin of themselves.

The couple derailed in deflation continues to sustain certain aspects of global merging, particularly expectations of mind reading and a warped version of preoccupation with the partner. This kind of preoccupation has an anxious, defensive quality. Couples like Eva and Sid, who become entrenched in this mode, are constantly preoccupied with each other in an angry, devaluing way. Thus, the joyous preoccupation with each other so characteristic of people in love can become a negative, defensive means of maintaining a partially merged connection.

In the following excerpt from an early-phase therapy session with Eva and Sid, I attempted to foster understanding of their wishes to sustain mind reading in order to avoid recognizing their differences and the loneliness of being separate. In the midst of exploring why they had a particularly vicious fight, I pointed out that both had expected their minds to be read by the other and were consequently disappointed that the other hand not behaved as wished. Sid responded in an aggressive tone:

SID: Expecting anyone to read your mind is stupid, and trying to read someone else's mind is a waste of time. Eva is always doing that.

EVA: She was speaking to both of us. That includes you.

SID: Well, if I do it, it's still stupid.

SHARPE: Mind reading is a very popular mode of communicating from where I sit. It has its uses. Granted, it doesn't work very well to get anyone's needs *actually* understood and met, but it keeps a number of illusions alive and well.

SID: Yeah, like what?

SHARPE: Well, like "Love is never having to say you're sorry" . . . or ask for anything.

SID: (*Gags, recognizing the reference to* Love Story.)

EVA: (*eyes shining with wistful sadness*) Yes, if you truly love each other, you should know what the other needs and feels. And it's so disappointing when that doesn't happen.

SHARPE: Yes, it is.

SID: What a lot of rot.

SHARPE: (*hoping Sid will continue doing my work*) Why is that?

SID: I don't see what mind reading has to do with loving someone. (*turning to Eva*) If you don't say what you want, I don't know what I'm supposed to do. At least if you asked, there's a good chance you'd get whatever it is.

EVA: I don't believe that, and neither do you. You don't ask for anything, and you're mad all of the time.

SID: (*Rolls his eyes, then looks to me expectantly.*)

SHARPE: (*seizing the opportunity*) There are a lot of good reasons for wanting to keep mind reading going. For one, the need to ask out loud for something makes you realize that you're not really of the same mind. You're two different people. That recognition can feel very deflating and lonely.

Eva nodded in agreement and said she felt lonely a lot of the time. Sid looked annoyed and said, So we're different people. So what's the big deal? Their opposite responses underscored the point.

In this intervention, I took the side of mind reading in the hope of normalizing oneness wishes and fears of being separate. My empathic interpretation of their feelings of deflation only appeared to reach Eva. Since Sid rarely acknowledged feeling comforted or understood, it was difficult to tell what got through to him. However, when he strongly argued a point, he would often later appear to have integrated the insight. The technique of joining the defense can be a useful approach for engaging partners who are on the surface compliant (like Eva) or oppositional (like Sid) in recognizing and examining their defense.

Twinship and Accepting Differences: Lola and Max

Partners recognition of distressing differences between them strikes a blow not only to the oneness fantasy but also to the fantasy of the partner as an ideal twin. The twinship fantasy might be seen as a version or derivative of global oneness, since ideal twins are exactly alike but also separate entities. Wishes for the partner to be a twin of oneself are expressed in each partner's attempt to be like the other. Who initiates twinning and who follows can shift from one partner to the other. Wearing matching shirts or other items of apparel is a common twinning behavior. Extensive twinning and mirroring between partners create what might appear to be a highly mutual relationship but is really a *pseudomutual collusion* in which differences have never been processed or integrated.

For many years, Lola and Max had sustained the romantic fantasy of being just alike, of being ideal twins. Sometimes they even dressed alike. Differences between them had been suppressed by one or the other partner in the major areas of living in which cooperation is desirable, including parenting, finances, sexuality, social and recreational life, short- and long-term planning, life goals, and decisions. Open disagreement had surfaced over reactions to their youngest daughter, who had moved away. This difference rocked the foundation of their relationship, leading them to seek consultation.

In order to maintain their veneer of togetherness, or pseudo-mutuality, one or both partners needed to cede his or her identity and individuality to the other in certain major respects. Max had allowed

Lola to run most aspects of their relationship. Lola had submerged her identity to Max in the sexual arena. Submerging aspects of one's identity to the partner fulfills mirroring and twinning needs and protects each partner from feeling too different. Expressions of difference are experienced as the partner's betrayal of the twinship contract—a withdrawal of love and support. The affected partner feels suddenly alone and inadequate without the continuous supportive twinning or mirroring of the partner.

The therapist aims to help the partners accept their differences and essential separateness, work through their deflated feelings, and restructure a stronger connection that permits differences. These aims are illustrated in the following interaction with Lola and Max. In this turning-point session, I had just confronted the couple with our lack of progress. Max became angry and openly disagreed with me for the first time. I noted that the cozy, picnic atmosphere we had created was not helping us work on the difficulties in their relationship. The story of how we got to this impasse (which reflected a countertransference enactment) is described in a later chapter. While putting his lunch leftovers in a bag, Max began:

MAX: Can we still bring lunch?

SHARPE: (*about to say "Sure," but then thinking better of it*) Uh . . . Let's think about that.

LOLA: I don't think we should bring lunch. I got indigestion today. We can eat at Mrs. Gooches after our appointment.

MAX: (*looking at me for support, since I know he dislikes eating in restaurants*) Uh . . . I don't like Mrs. Gooches [a local restaurant].

LOLA: What do you mean, you don't like Gooches? We've been eating there for years!

MAX: (*getting another dose of courage from making eye contact with me*) I like eating at home a lot better.

LOLA: (*coldly*) All right, if that's what you want. We'll eat at home before we come. [She is clearly miffed and stares straight ahead, her lips pinched tightly together. Max begins shifting around in his chair. I sense he is about to retract his self-assertion and intervene before this could happen.]

SHARPE: Lola, you don't look thrilled about his idea of eating at home. What's bothering you?

LOLA: I'm not sure. (*pausing*) I guess it's that I've always hated making sandwiches, since I had to do so much of it when I was growing up for my brother and me, and then for all the kids and Max. Going out to lunch is a treat for me.

MAX: I didn't know that. (*He is quiet for a moment*) I could make the sandwiches?

LOLA: Fine. That would be fine. (*She looks like a puppet, nodding her agreement. When she stops being the leader, she seems to lose all backbone.*)

SHARPE: Lola, Max is negotiating with you. You can negotiate back. You don't have to just agree with what he suggests.

LOLA: I don't know how to negotiate.

SHARPE: Try just saying what you want, and what you think would be a fair compromise.

LOLA: (*hesitating, looking tense and miserable*) I feel so confused my head hurts.

SHARPE: Maybe you don't like this idea of negotiation and compromise. It's against the familiar way and probably feels unloving.

LOLA: It certainly feels unfamiliar. (*pausing, trying to figure out her reaction*) I think I'm upset with Max for pretending he was with me going to lunch when he really wasn't. I feel, I feel . . . I don't know, betrayed or something. (*Her eyes well up with tears.*) [I suddenly understood that Lola's blank, puppet-like behavior and odd states of confusion were a result of anxiety and her attempts to stifle hurt and anger.]

MAX: I'm sorry. I just meant to please you by going along. But what's the betrayal? Betrayal's like having an affair or something.

LOLA: I don't know. It just feels that way. Dishonest . . . I guess.

SHARPE: It's not easy to explain, because the lunch thing is symbolic of something bigger. Lola thought you felt like she did about eating out. Imagine thinking for a long time that your partner is with you and on the same wave length, and then you find out they're not. It's like the rug's been pulled out, and you feel deserted and alone.

LOLA: (*sounding both relieved and triumphant*) That's it. That's exactly how I feel.

MAX: Well I sure never intended that. I was just trying to keep my crabby feelings to myself. I think I should have just gone on doing that. (*Now he looks miserable.*)

LOLA: No, no. You need to speak up. We both need to speak up. I just want you to be truthful sooner.

MAX: Or keep my big mouth shut. We should go out to lunch. I don't mind that much, now that I've made my fuss.

LOLA: No, I think we should compromise. That's what grown-ups are supposed to do. (*She looks to Max for direction.*)

MAX: How about we eat at home part of the time, and we eat out part of the time . . . and when we're at home, I'll make lunch . . . mostly.

LOLA: (*nodding slowly, and smiling*) Sounds like a plan.

Needs for twinning are not only defensive but also express wishes to be supported and admired by someone just like oneself. This is a normal childhood need that continues to be prominent in adulthood, when a child has not been sufficiently admired and supported by parents or peers. Twinning as a developmental and defensive need is also often connected with a partner's reenactment of a childhood sibling relationship that provided crucial safety and support. At a later point in treatment, we came to understand that Lola's need to twin with Max was an attempt to re-create her early relationship with her brother, which had been crucial to her emotional survival in childhood.

ACCEPTING NEEDS TO BE CLOSE AND SEPARATE

When couples succeed in accepting their differences and essential separateness to some degree, their work in this area is far from over. Many couples are hampered by the paucity of ways they have to be connected and separate, and have overdeveloped one of these aspects to the detriment of the other. These relationships appear lopsided to varying degrees. At one extreme are those couples who do almost everything together, and at the other are those couples who do most things separately. In the course of a relationship, couples often swing between these extremes. Each partner needs to find his or her own comfort level and balance between time together and time apart. Optimally, couples are motivated to develop variety and balance. When a couple does not create deeper, more extensive ways to be connected or the partners have a paucity of separate friendships or interests, fears of intimacy and/or separateness are usually involved and will often need to be understood before partners can make active changes.

In therapy, one partner will usually bring up dissatisfaction in this area when he or she is ready to work toward a change. Some acceptance of differences and separateness needs to occur before a submissive partner can actively engage in self-development. Max now felt secure enough to discuss his wish to have more interests of his own. He began taking yoga lessons and classes in woodworking, an interest he'd had as a boy. Lola, feeling more secure in their relationship, was now able to support Max's wishes to engage in separate activities.

Like Max, June felt she had allowed Henry to determine almost everything they did. Although this couple did most things together and were socially active, they were rarely alone with each other. As June became a stronger individual, she expressed wishes to develop her own interests and a desire for more meaningful intimacy with Henry. She began taking classes in anthropology, a subject that had always fascinated her. Initially Henry felt left out and rejected. Recognition and understanding of his fears of abandonment enabled him to accept June's separate interests. Her expression of wishes for more time alone with Henry brought their sexual problems into focus. This area of their intimacy had been left to wither and almost die since the birth of their children. Both partners' performance anxieties and fears of engulfment were found to be significant impediments to an active and intimate sex life.

REGULATION OF BEING TOGETHER AND APART: EVA AND SID

Eva and Sid had a very few satisfying ways to feel connected. They participated in social obligations and sometimes went to church but had no shared interests beyond raising their daughter and maintaining a household, areas that were regular sources of conflict. Their sex life, the little I knew about it, took place in a parallel sort of way, with each partner blocking out the other's presence through fantasy and a total focus on personal pleasure. Sid openly expressed wishes for more closeness, but Eva was now focused on expanding her artistic abilities and preserving her newly developed separate identity. They had switched roles in their pursuer–pursued dynamic, but now, each partner rapidly shifted from one position to the other, as is illustrated in the following interchange:

SID: I feel like we live in one of those comedies where people are always at cross purposes and missing each other. It would be funny if I weren't in it. (*He looks at me as though expecting a response.*)

SHARPE: You'd better say more. I'm not following.

SID: You mean you can't read my mind? (*teasing good-humoredly*) Eva won't give me the time of day. We hardly spend any time alone together.

EVA: Don't blame me. When I suggested that we talk about our vacation last night, you just grunted and stayed plugged into the computer for the rest of the evening.

SID: I had to get that project done. You knew that.

EVA: When I came over to hug you this morning, you didn't even hug me back. (*rolling her eyes*) You just stood there . . . enduring.

SID: (*sarcastically*) So it's me, is it? I'm the one who's not available. Come on, I've tried almost every night this week to get together to talk or for sex and you're either too busy or too tired.

EVA: I have work to do, too, you know. I have a pottery show coming up.

SID: We're both very busy, okay? But I get the feeling you'd really rather not be alone with me.

EVA: I have the same feelings about you. Whenever I want to be close, you have something better to do.

I was impressed with their progress in directly expressing their feelings. Inability to recognize and express their needs had been a serious problem for both of them.

SHARPE: What comes through in your descriptions is both of you wanting more closeness—which is a good thing. That's what we've been working on. But it sounds like you only want to be close on your own terms. (*to Sid*) Eva should drop everything whenever you want to be together. (*to Eva*) And Sid should do the same when you want to be with him.

SID: I feel like saying, she does it more than I do it.

EVA: (*snapping*) Well, don't.

SHARPE: (*to Sid*) You seem to feel judged by what I said.

SID: Well . . . it makes me sound self-centered. I don't like to admit to that.

SHARPE: I thought we all wanted our partners to be at our beck and call some of the time.

EVA: (*smiling*) I'd sure like some of that. I guess I want to be close to Sid when I have warm feelings, but not when I don't, or when I'm doing something else. I want him to leave me alone when I'm working or studying. I want him to respect my needs for privacy and to do my work.

SID: Well, I want the same consideration.

SHARPE: You might have another thing going on, a kind of control struggle that comes from feeling rejected by each other. (*Sid looks ready to pooh-pooh this idea, so I quickly soft-pedal.*) This would probably be going on mostly out of your awareness. Unconsciously, you might feel if Eva's not going to respond to you when you want to be with her, you're not going to respond to her when she wants you. (*to Eva*) You could be turning Sid down for those reasons, too. This can go round and round. It gets to be a game, like you said, Sid, almost comical from the outside, but not from the inside.

SID: I can see some of that. So what do we do?

SHARPE: I'm going to throw that one that back to you.

EVA: If we planned ahead to do something together, we wouldn't run into these issues.

SID: I've given up trying to plan ahead.

SHARPE: Sid, you're discouraging her move toward you. Are you sure you want to do that?

For Eva and Sid to develop satisfying ways to be connected and to comfortably regulate being close and separate took a great deal more work in therapy. Eva's fears of merging and being engulfed, of losing her hard-won identity if she were to allow much closeness with Sid, had to be repetitively addressed. When Eva could initiate more closeness with Sid, his fears of engulfment surfaced. Additionally, Sid's need to dominate in order to allay deep fears of abandonment and rejection also required repeated exploration.

Once partners manage to understand their fears that hinder expanding and regulating closeness and separateness, they are continuously challenged to modify patterns they establish by the impact of external circumstances, life-cycle changes, and their own evolving needs. Obviously, a couple's ability to recognize and discuss changing needs is crucial for deepening a close connection.

Attainment of Mutuality

Partners with a truly mutual relationship actively nurture their existing commonalties and develop new ways of being connected. They solicit and respect each other's thoughts and feelings, attempt to resolve their differences through compromise, and work in partnership to achieve common goals. Thus, a small decision or their life plan is not the result of one partner going along with the other to please or placate, or the result of one partner's submerging his or her identity in the other. This behavior is indicative of pseudomutuality, a rampant condition in coupledom, often mistaken for a good relationship. Additionally, the partners come to accept that some of their differences cannot be resolved. In these ways, partners stay closely attuned and joined together. These are the positive ties that bind.

In the course of an optimally developing relationship, the global oneness fantasy appears to evolve along two distinct but interrelated paths. Along one path, a couple fosters those areas that are truly shared and works toward having enough commonalties, so that the partners feel strongly connected. "We are one," first becomes modified into "We are one, but we are also separate." Next, the twinship fantasy ("We are exactly alike") is modified into "We are alike in certain important ways and different in other ways." Mutual acceptance of areas of likeness and difference clears the way for expansion of both.

Along the other path, the global aspect of the merger fantasy, the feeling of oneness, remains in the unconscious background, keeping a couple deeply connected. Experiences of oneness ideally become consciously expressed in the arena of a couple's sex life. However, if sexuality is inhibited, a couple's needs for this intense closeness may be channeled into another arena, like the passionate sharing of a certain interest, a cause, or an intellectual, spiritual, or altruistic pursuit. (For most partners, such substitutes do not entirely make up for the lack of an intimate sex life, but they can help.)

Attaining a high degree of true mutuality in a relationship is not a frequent achievement, even for couples in long-term marriages. A reworking of all of the previous developmental steps is continuously required. The three couples discussed in this chapter are in various stages of achieving mutuality. Each has the shared experience and concern of raising children together by virtue of living together. Eva and Sid, the most openly conflictual, have developed common goals that carry both their imprints. Henry and June have not developed shared goals, because June has not yet individuated enough to know her wishes clearly, let along fight for them in a discussion. Their couple and life goals are still Henry's, though this is in the process of change.

After a long period of therapy, Lola and Max gradually moved out of pseudomutuality toward real mutuality. While Max used to feel dragged along by Lola, who had wide-ranging interests and altruistic pursuits, he became able to determine which of these activities he would share with her. His input was more frequently given and accepted even though, as he said, "I've never been much of an idea man except in the bedroom."

Idealizing

"You're My Everything"
—MORT DIXON, JOE YOUNG,
AND HARRY WARREN (1931)

CHAPTER 7

The Bedrock of Passion

When I first met Lily and Garth, they looked like the ideal couple. They were holding hands and smiling when I greeted them in the waiting room. Both were unusually attractive and looked to be in their mid-thirties. Lily had masses of auburn hair curling around a beautiful, heart-shaped face. Her green eyes glowed in a flawless, creamy complexion. Garth was "black-Irish" handsome, with black hair and blue eyes set in a dark, chiseled face. They emanated robust good health and were dressed in coordinated autumn hues. They looked like Irish models on their way to a photo shoot.

Lily and Garth had known each other for six months, were recently engaged, and still in love. They were about to move in together. When asked about their attraction to each other, they replied:

GARTH: I was attracted to Lily because of her stunning looks. When we first met, I was so dazzled I could hardly speak. She was like my child-hood dream of the beautiful princess. But when she spoke to me so sweetly, I felt instantly at ease. (*He beams at Lily, clasping her outstretched hand.*)

LILY: I sound kind of chaste and boring. What about sexy?

GARTH: Oh, God, you're very sexy . . . very exciting. We have the best sex I've ever had.

LILY: (*grinning*) That's better. . . . Sexy is the first thing I thought of about you. Sexy and confident. I love Garth's virility and vitality. He can do anything. When I'm with him, I feel so safe and happy for the first time in my life.

I watched them gaze into each other's eyes and wondered what this blissful couple was doing in my office. It is unusual for a couple to initiate therapy during the romantic idealizing phase of a love relationship. Kate and Jana, lesbian partners in their early forties, were another such unique couple. They described their initial attraction to each other in similar idealizing terms.

KATE: When I first saw Jana, she was speaking at a feminist retreat. I was so impressed. She was striking looking, with her wild black hair, dark skin, and big brown eyes. She seemed so vital and alive, yet somehow vulnerable. She has this deep, musical voice, and she could articulate *exactly* everything I believe in. I fell in love with her on the spot.

JANA: I just didn't know what love was until I met Kate. She makes me feel like I'm lucky to be who I am. She's the wisest, most insightful, accepting person I've ever known. Sometimes I think she's a female Buddha or Mother Earth. She has the power to make me feel totally at peace and connected.

These two couples, so different in many respects, were alike in initiating therapy when they were still in love and hoping to prevent destructive problems. This unusual foresight came from experiencing failure in their previous love relationships and the self-awareness gained in individual therapy. They wanted couple therapy in place *before* damage to the their relationships occurred. I thought I was dreaming when I heard this. Most couples who come for therapy in the early phase of a love relationship arrive in the painful throes of major disappointment with each other.

These interactions illustrate normal romantic idealizing in the early phase of a love relationship. Idealizing, briefly defined, is a psychological process by which one subjectively views another person or his or her attributes in ideal rather than realistic or objective terms. Romantic idealizing includes the perception of the person as the perfect lover, often as an erotic ideal as well (in contrast to idealizing someone in another kind of role, such as the wisest leader, parent, or teacher). The romantically idealized partner is described as wonderful, fantastic, and totally irresistible. He or she is not just an ordinary human, but special, heroic, enchanting. For example, in the balcony scene from *Romeo and Juliet* (Act II, Scene II) an enraptured Romeo describes his love:

> But, soft! what light through yonder window breaks?
> It is the east, and Juliet is the sun!—
> Arise, fair sun, and kill the envious moon,
> Who is already sick and pale with grief,
> That thou her maid art far more fair than she:

In a more lighthearted vein, popular songwriter Cole Porter (who special-ized in the nuances of falling and being in love) expresses idealizing in "You're the Top," his well-known "ditty that's not so pretty."

Negatives or flaws appearing in the idealized beloved may be intellec-tually recognized, but they are disregarded or rationalized as endearingly special. Garth said that he thought Lily might be a bit too shy, too bookish for his gregarious nature. But then he immediately dismissed this worry as silly, transforming it into a special attribute: "Her ability to be intro-spective will help me stay more in touch with myself."

Idealizing behavior patterns express partners' idealized perceptions. They gaze adoringly into each other's eyes, engage in much physical touching, speak in excited tones about and with each other, are interested almost solely in the other, yearn to be together all of the time, celebrate likenesses, and suppress differences, anger, and conflict. In general, the climate generated is that of an exciting, exotic paradise of "You, me, and our relationship," while the rest of the world fades into background shades of gray.

Idealized perceptions and patterns in couples can be normal and pro-mote development, as explicated in this chapter, or collusively defensive and inhibiting of development as discussed in Chapter 9.

CHAPTER 8

The Development of Idealizing

Common Treatment Problems

The importance of idealizing in the *ongoing* development and quality of adult love relationships has not been duly recognized in the literature. Most discussions begin and end with the acknowledgment that idealizing is an important aspect of falling in love (Person, 1988; Kernberg, 1995; Dicks, 1967). Henry Dicks has discussed this process most extensively and has recognized the impact of a couple's early idealizations on the subsequent development of a relationship. However, Dicks's important observations are primarily focused on the defensive role of idealizing.

From the perspective of normal development, couples' patterns of idealizing have their own life and developmental progression that not only create emotional ups and downs in the relationship but also gradually move the couple toward greater acceptance of each other and a deepening of the passionate aspects of their attachment. Idealizing and its opposite, deidealizing, operate throughout the life of a love relationship, starting when the partners fall in love, and continuing through their falling out of love (deidealizing). Hard work is then necessary for a couple to find their way into a more mature love. The whole process may recycle again and again, each time strengthening the bonds of passionate attachment. Understanding this developmental evolution in the course of a love relationship is of great value in treating couples.

The developmental progression is summarized as follows:

- Romantic idealizing
- Deidealizing
- Acceptance of the real partner

128

- Modulated idealizing
- Intermittent romantic idealizing

For a love relationship to develop, the global aspects of romantic idealizing need to become modified. Initial idealizations usually reflect our hopes and dreams that cannot be fulfilled by any real person. At some point, each partner begins to perceive flaws in the idealized other, and this intrusion of reality initiates deidealizing of the partner and the relationship. During this painful process, the partner and the relationship may be perceived in an extremely negative, devalued way—"Marrying him was the biggest mistake I ever made."

In a maturing relationship, partners become able to modulate and integrate idealized and devalued perceptions of each other, leading to acceptance of the partner as a real person, who can then be admired and appreciated for his or her unique attributes. Modulated idealizing also includes the partners' capacities to develop their own relationship ideals as distinct from those imposed by culture and families of origin. Since the partners and the relationship are continually developing and changing, the idealizing–deidealizing processes are ongoing. However, the first round of deidealizing is the most significant, since the relationship cannot move forward without it.

While partners' early romantic idealization needs to become modified, some aspect needs to be retained. Romantic idealizing in the "right" dosage, intermittently experienced, appears to be crucial to the survival of passionate love. The right dosage, however, is difficult to determine. Global idealizing maintained for too long between partners often results in a stagnant relationship, drained of vitality and passion. Likewise, little or no romantic idealizing can also result in a devitalized, passionless relationship. Helping couples find the right amount of the idealizing love potion remains an ongoing challenge. Unfortunately, no recipe will be provided here, only some understanding of the processes.

In optimal development, our first image of an ideal partner, originally formed from childhood fantasies of perfection, gradually becomes modified through our acceptance and appreciation of the real qualities of our partner. Ultimately, the admired image of our real partner becomes internalized as the ideal. In Figure 4, these developmental steps, related tasks, and common problems are outlined.

ROMANTIC IDEALIZING AND FALLING IN LOVE

Romantic idealizing is an essential component of falling and staying in love. The special alchemy that brings about falling in love can be partially

Steps in Development of Idealizing	Tasks for Couple/Guide for Therapy	Common Problems (Points of Regression and Derailment)
Romantic Idealizing	Finding a partner who matches internal ideal	Inability to romantically idealize and fall in love
	Falling in love	
	Creating bond of passionate attachment	Minimal or no passionate bond
Deidealizing	Perceiving flaws in partner	Denial of flaws, regression to global idealizing
	Devaluing partner, relationship, and self	Stalled in devaluing
	Oscillating between idealizing and devaluing	Stalled in splitting idealized and devalued images
Acceptance of the Real Partner, Relationship, and Self	Modulating and integrating ideal and devalued images	Inability to modulate and integrate polarized images
		Enactment of idealizing and devaluing collusions
	Accepting whole partner (ideal, devalued, real)	Inability to accept whole partner
	Modifying the internal ideals	Internal ideals remain too perfectionistic or too accommodating
Modulated Idealizing	Admiring and appreciating the real partner	Partner too devalued to be admired
	Creating shared relationship ideals	Can only admire unreal, idealized partner
	Integrating tender love with erotic love	Conflicted relationship ideals
		Relationship ideals determined by culture or families
		Tender love disconnected from erotic love
Intermittent Romantic Idealizing	Romantic idealizing remains accessible	Romantic idealizing inaccessible
	Admiration ignites passion	Passionless relationship
	Admired real partner becomes internal ideal	Admiration insufficient to ignite passion

FIGURE 4. The development of idealizing.

130

explained by describing the major psychological processes involved—admiration, sexual and emotional attraction, idealization and merging. Admiration and attraction, both sexual and emotional, are often the first steps that evoke falling in love. Admiration of certain traits—how a person looks, his or her intelligence, aura of self-confidence or power, sense of humor, kindness—leads to feelings of sexual and emotional attraction. This initial attraction then may quickly or slowly proceed to a more inflated kind of admiring, which we call idealization. He's not just good looking, he's the most desirable man in the world. With this shift in perception, one is on the brink of falling in love, or already well into the fall.

Idealizing is the key process that distinguishes falling and being "in love" from loving. Even if the beloved is described as "just an ordinary person," what is really meant is that he or she is the most wonderful "ordinary person" in the world. However, loving in the mature sense involves the capacity to care deeply for the real, ordinary person, *without* idealization.

The process of falling in love also includes the experience of merging with the idealized person, the intrapsychic blending of boundaries between self and partner. Speaking more poetically, there is an opening up of oneself to join ecstatically with the beloved. When merging occurs, exhilarating feelings of oneness and self-enhancement are experienced—"She completes me; she's my other half." In more theoretical terms, each person connects with the other at an unconscious level, recognizing a longed for ideal that is both fundamentally familiar (like coming home) but that also holds the potential for liberation from past wounds. Merging is the aspect of being in love that most directly causes intense longings to be with our beloved, and those characteristic feelings of a wrenching loss—like losing part of ourselves—when we are apart.

Mate Selection without Romantic Idealization

As noted previously, many people in our society select someone to marry without romantically idealizing that person and falling in love. One or both partners may admire, even idealize, the other to some extent, and there may (or may not) be some sexual attraction. However, the idealization experienced is not romantic idealization. In these cases, a partner's idealization of a prospective mate remains limited to the person's abilities to be a parental caretaker, a good provider, or a social asset (like the trophy wife).

One or both partners may be too fearful of romantically idealizing and merging to fall in love.[1] While marriages that begin without romantic

---

[1]For discussion of other fears that may inhibit falling in love, see p. 46. See also Kirshner (1998) and Kernberg (1995).

idealization do not follow the developmental progression of idealizing in exactly the way described here, many of these partners experience a similar sequence of psychological events in modified forms. There is likely an initial idealizing of the relationship and the partner in terms of their potential to fulfill specific conscious and unconscious wishes. Inevitably, these hopes and wishes are likely to be disappointed in some respects. For example, one or both partners may find it quite difficult to live with just a nice person in the absence of feeling a special attraction or the intensity of romantic love, especially in this society. Or a partner may discover that money or prestige without romantic passion does not bring the satisfactions expected. Hence, a period of deidealization of the partner and the relationship will ensue, requiring a revision of expectations if the relationship is to continue in any satisfying fashion.

Creating the Ideals, Matching to the Ideals, and Mate Selection

Understanding *how* we fall in love does not answer the big question of *why* a specific person becomes selected for romantic idealization. This fascinating question has occupied theorists, writers, and poets for centuries. It is the central question occupying theories of mate selection, a complex subject that cannot be given full justice in this book. However, object relations theory provides a framework for understanding the more complex psychological determinants of mate selection—of whom we idealize and why.

In accord with this theory,[2] we seek out an external match for certain representations of an ideal partner and ideal love relationship that we have already created in our minds. These ideals are highly interrelated psychological structures that I differentiate as *the ideal partner, the ideal self,* and *the ideal relationship.* From early childhood onward, we create and modify these ideals both consciously and unconsciously. How we experienced being loved by and loving the important people in our lives becomes encoded in representations, often unconscious, of a loved other in relationship with ourselves. Idealized versions of these internalized relationships are also formed to fulfill childhood wishes and to cope with significant deficits, both real and imagined. Children often think their mothers are the greatest, even though they may be actually quite inadequate.

Representations of oneself in relationship with an important person include characteristics of both people and their main way of connecting—

---

[2]The conceptions of Sandler and Rosenblatt (1962), Dicks (1967), and Kernberg (1995) are the object relations theories referred to in this discussion.

of how love was experienced.[3] Major modes of connecting often take the form of those described in this book. For example, to love and be loved may mean dependent merging with a nurturing mother, a need to idealize and be idealized in return, or involve needs to devalue or be devalued, to control or be controlled, to competitively win or lose. In adulthood, idealized representations of important relationships coexist with more reality-based representations.

We are drawn to a person who appears to have certain features that match most closely with the ideal representations structured in our minds. For example Lily was drawn to Garth's good looks and adventurous, outgoing personality, largely because her internal romantic ideal of a partner had these traits. I designate the *appraisal* of whether and how well a person fits the internal ideal image of a partner (interwoven with images of an ideal relationship) as the process of *matching to the ideals.*

When the match seems to fit, the process of idealizing begins. We *project* on to the chosen lover many or all of the other features of our ideal image, whether or not he or she actually has these qualities. For example, since Garth fit the basic outline of Lily's ideal partner, she assumed he had many other desired characteristics, as well, such as emotional strength and maturity. An ideal relationship that will enhance and fulfill oneself is an integral aspect of idealizing the potential partner. The idealized partner is thus most always considered in terms of what he or she does or can do for me.

Lily imagined Garth would not only take care of her like a good parent but also make her feel like a desirable woman and liberate her sexually. Jana thought that Kate would make her feel totally accepted and keep her safe from fear and self-loathing. Kate thought that Jana would free her from inhibition and guilt. Hence, the idealized loved one becomes a blend of both real qualities that approximate the internal ideal and imagined qualities projected onto him or her.

If there is considerable discrepancy between the real person and the ideal, we may deny the discrepancy and continue idealizing the person, or we may feel disappointed and begin to dismiss or devalue the person. For example, when Garth learned that a woman he previously thought he loved had an explosive temper and depressive episodes, he began to lose interest in her. Suddenly, she did not fit the image of his ideal in certain important respects—the ideal of a warm, accepting woman who would not repeat his childhood experience with a depressed, critical mother and an angry father. He quickly fell out of love.

---

[3]This concept is an elaboration of the conception of internalized role relationships described by Sandler and Rosenblatt (1962) and Sandler (1976).

Every time something new is learned about one's lover, another round of matching to the ideal occurs, which then may be followed by increased attraction and idealization or, alternatively, may initiate devaluation and dismissal of the person as a prospective mate.

Modifying the Ideals

To further complicate these events, another important process also occurs, which I term *modifying the ideals*. When newly discovered information about the person does not fit the ideal, we may modify our internal ideal to incorporate qualities we see in the real person (instead of either denying the discrepancy or dismissing the prospective mate). In modifying our internal ideal to come closer to the real person, a new tint is added to the idealizing lens through which the real person is viewed. Internal ideals thus evolve and become more realistic with experience, a process that needs to be fostered in therapy to promote the partners' fuller acceptance of each other.

For example, when Kate moved in with Jana, she discovered that Jana was quite moody. Without apparent reason, Jana would suddenly fall into a depressed, withdrawn mood. Previously, Kate had seen Jana as a dynamic woman with a great sense of humor. Moodiness did not fit her ideal image of a mate and briefly threatened her idealization of Jana. She reworked and modified her ideal image to accommodate this unwelcome piece of news, as follows:

> "At first Jana's moodiness scared me. I didn't know what to do. I would try to cheer her up. Sometimes that worked and sometimes it didn't. We talked about it, and now that I understand why she's that way, I feel much better. I know to leave her alone at certain times. Now that I know her better, it's okay that she's not the perfect model of mental health. Actually, it makes me feel better about my own inadequacies. I think I was hoping that her optimism would keep my own demons at bay."

Through greater understanding of Jana's "flaw" and gaining a perspective on her own needs (so that she could separate herself in this respect from Jana), Kate was able to modify her ideal in accord with reality. However, this modification was just one step in the long process of knowing and accepting Jana as a real person.

The complex steps involved in falling in or out of love are diagrammed in Figure 5 and summarized as follows: admiring, matching to the ideals, a preliminary fit, sexual/emotional attraction, idealizing/merging; new information, matching to the ideals, a deeper fit, intensi-

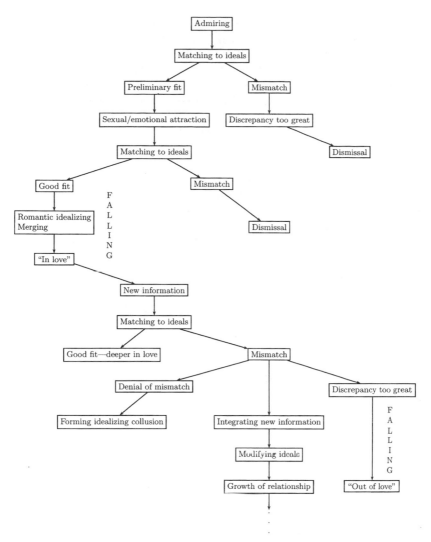

FIGURE 5. Falling in and out of love.

fied idealizing/merging; new information, matching to the ideals, a mismatch, disappointment leading to the end of the relationship or to modifying of the ideals and greater acceptance of the "real" person. In the maturing love relationship, perception of the loved person continues to evolve as a blend of real and idealized attributes. These are derived from a mix of preexisting ideals, the ongoing revelation of the real person, and continuing modification of our internal ideals.

Since these processes continue on in various forms for the life of the relationship, how partners manage these cycles in the opening phase is often predictive of what follows. Relationships end and problems develop when partners' internal ideals are too rigidly formed and are not easily modified to incorporate the less perfect aspects of their lovers and mates. This internal rigidity may result in unfortunate outcomes. Partners who deny the existence of each other's faults will often form an idealizing collusion that keeps them stuck in the first phase of romantic idealization. Those who recognize flaws in each other but do not have the capacity to accept and integrate this information often remain stuck midway in the devaluing phase of deidealization. Overly rigid and perfectionistic internal ideals may also result in a person's prematurely devaluing or eliminating a potentially good mate and good relationship.

On the other hand, if a partner's internal ideals are too insubstantial and accommodating, anyone with any number of grave faults can easily be made acceptable. This is one reason why an apparently decent person can end up with (and put up with) an abuser, a psychopath, or a grossly self-centered boor. Helping such a partner to structure more defined ideals with higher standards is the therapeutic task, rather than modulating rigidly maintained, impossible ideals.

THE IDEAL PARTNER

One's internal ideal of a partner is created from a variety of influences throughout development. Three of the major ones are discussed here. The most visible source is from our culture's stereotypical ideals of men and women, particularly the romantic ideals of a man and a woman in a love relationship. Our perception of these cultural ideals is substantially affected by our family-of-origin and life experience. Somehow we combine and synthesize cultural ideals with more personal ideals, stemming from experience with our parents, siblings, and other important people in our lives. Additionally, the particular shape of our internal ideal partner is influenced by the developmental stage of life and the state of our needs and wishes at a given time. Probably the less adequate we feel, the more inflated the internal ideal partner becomes.

The knight on the white charger is not only a romantic ideal of the young girl, but also can take shape in the mind of a disappointed women in middle age. In a recent psychotherapy session, a forty-seven-year-old woman in the throes of a bitter divorce reported to me that she felt "in love" with her wonderful attorney, who was going to rescue her like a "white knight" from her life of misery and despair.

Cultural Ideals: The Handsome Prince and the Beautiful Princess

From the time we are young children, the ideal love story is about the handsome prince and the beautiful princess. The handsome prince appears in many guises: as a white knight like Sir Lancelot, a god, a warrior; or in disguise as a ordinary man, a poor man, a frog, or a beast. The princess might be a goddess, a queen, or in disguise as a beautiful maiden (Sleeping Beauty, Snow White), a poor servant (Cinderella), or an ugly duckling who becomes a swan. Whatever the shape, the prince and princess characters have certain traits that we idealize in childhood, idealizations that persist into adulthood, influencing mate selection. Garth, age thirty-eight, saw in Lily his childhood ideal of the beautiful princess.

The prince character, who is the romantic ideal man inhabiting young girls' and women's dreams, is strong, brave, handsome, supremely confident, and competent. He is also honorable, steadfast, and kind. The princess, one type of ideal woman in a young man's dreams, is beautiful, innocent, sensitive, and helplessly in need of a strong man to adore. Until recently, the ideal of a desirable woman has been split, because sexuality was not allowed to sully the child-like innocence of the beautiful princess. Hence, a separate, opposite kind of ideal was created though not often featured in childhood stories.

The beautiful siren, like Delilah and Cleopatra, is the sexualized version of an ideal woman, seen as desirable by men and admired by women.[4] The siren has her own ambitions, seduces men, and is not very nice. Delilah seduced the powerful Samson and Cleopatra conquered Julius Caesar. In addition to being erotic, sexy sirens appear to have more fun, smarts, and power than the beautiful princess, who sleeps most of the time or is stuck cleaning house all day like Cinderella.

The ideal of a man is also split into those who are noble and those who are sexual. There is a dark prince that seems to attract women in much the same way as sexy sirens are irresistible to men. The dark prince is powerful, arrogant, and sexy. Don Giovanni exemplifies the essence of this irresistible ideal. He is selfish, unreliable, and unattainable. His major pastime is seducing and abandoning women who continue to flock to him for the experience of sexual ecstasy. Modern and more modified versions portray these unadmirable traits as protective defenses that conceal an injured, vulnerable man who can be healed through love. The woman's love eventually breaks through these defenses, transforming the heartless

---

[4]Such an ideal represents a fantasied object and does not necessarily correspond with one's reasoned or moral evaluations.

scoundrel into an ideal prince. Many stories have this theme, including the fairy tale "Beauty and the Beast."

One interpretation for the existence of these pure and impure male and female ideals is that they reflect the difficulty that both men and women have in bringing together tender love and erotic love. The handsome prince and the beautiful princess are asexual and only kiss tenderly. The sexy siren and the dark prince liberate erotic desire and passion, sweeping away the confining restraints of morality and guilt. When a sexy siren, such as Delilah, or a dark prince, such as the Beast, is transformed through love, we experience fulfillment of the wish for the fusion of tender and erotic love.

These ideals of the desirable man and woman (one pure and one sexual) are sustained and bolstered beyond childhood through their continued representation in stories, movies, television shows, advertisements, and songs that are created for adolescents and adults.

The theme of the strong man rescuing and protecting the helpless woman who will then adore him forever is perhaps the role relationship most often portrayed as the ideal of romantic love. The handsome prince and the beautiful princess are translated for adults into romantic Hollywood heroes and heroines, such as Humphrey Bogart rescuing and protecting beautiful Lauren Bacall in those articulate and winsome romances of the 1940s (*The Big Sleep* [1946], *To Have and Have Not* [1944], and *Key Largo* [1948]). More recently Mel Gibson finds, loses, and avenges the murder of his lost love in *Braveheart* (1995), and Ralph Fiennes endures torture to save his dying love in *The English Patient* (1996).

In modern times, or when we grow up, the good man should be masculine, powerful, protective, successful, or potentially successful. Handsome, brave, and noble are not so important. The feminine ideal of innocence is also not required, since the sexy siren has become integrated to some extent into the ideal of femininity. The good woman is still one who gives in a self-sacrificing way. Like Garth, men so often speak first about the physical attractiveness of their loves. Qualities of character, such as sensitivity and nurturing, seem to come second.

For those who think that romantic heroes are getting more tarnished, less heroic, and more realistic, and heroines less chaste, less helpless, and more sexy, the purist "fairy tale" tradition has been resurrected in *Titanic* (1997), the most successful movie of all time. The story has a handsome, brave hero and a romantic heroine who is desperately in need of rescuing. While the hero dies saving his beloved when the ship sinks, the couple's love is transcendent. This tragic loss of a perfect love with the perfect partner has also been idealized in stories throughout the centuries. Cultural ideals of love relationships are discussed in more depth in a subsequent section.

Romantic Ideals from the Family of Origin

More influential than the romantic ideals of our culture are those generated by idealization of our first love objects from our family of origin, since we are dependent upon them for survival from birth. However, the cultural influence is there from the start, since our parents' behavior and attitudes have been partially shaped by the larger culture. We combine these influences in personalized ways to form our internal representation of an ideal partner. While idealization of our parents is usually the most profound influence in shaping the internal ideal partner, siblings and other loved people outside of the family of origin can also importantly shape this ideal. Lily's image of an ideal partner was centrally derived from an idealized image of her father. She described him in excited, glowing terms as a handsome, energetic, adventurous man who built his own sailboat and sailed around the world. He was also outgoing, had many friends, and loved to socialize. These were precisely the traits that attracted her to Garth and made her feel excited yet safe.

Her idealization of Garth included not only his personal qualities that were like those of her father (handsome, adventurous, gregarious) but also a fantasized ideal relationship that derived from a deficit in her actual relationship with her father, who paid little attention to her as she was growing up. She imagined that Garth would act like a good father. He would support and encourage her to attain greater self-confidence, improved social skills, and a successful career as an artist.

Ideal representations of a desired mate may also be created in contrast to real disappointing parental figures. Thus, Garth, who perceived his mother as dowdy, intrusive, and socially embarrassing, was attracted to Lily, who appeared to be the opposite of his mother in every respect. She was beautiful, a social asset, and sensitive. Such ideals created in opposition to bad experience with an inadequate parent can be a constructive attempt to protect against the repetition of another disappointing love relationship.

However, this strategy does not always work. Those consciously rejected images of bad parents and bad relationships still exist unconsciously and can powerfully motivate one to seek out partners who embody the old, familiar people and the old, familiar kind of love. These images might be seen as more deeply unconscious components—the dark underbelly—of the ideals.

"You Were Meant for Me"

The popular song "You Were Meant for Me"[5] expresses the common view that the ideal partner is tailor-made for oneself. The belief that we were

---

[5]Song written by Nacio Herb Brown (1929).

meant for each other reflects (1) the wish for a mate very like oneself, a twin in certain respects, who will bolster one's sense of self and forever stave off feelings of loneliness, and (2) the wish for a mate who complements oneself, who will fill in and correct for experienced deficits in one's own personality.

In the experience of twinship, partners share certain important likenesses, such as fundamental attitudes, values, coping mechanisms, and family experience. The perfect complement implies the dovetailing of psychological needs and personality traits. Partners are consciously aware of certain of these aspects of twinship and complementarity, but certain crucial aspects remain unconscious.

For example, Garth and Lily had certain important emotional experiences and resultant coping mechanisms in common. Both felt that, while growing up, their emotional needs were ignored, and both were required to take care of an inadequate mother. Both had also learned to cope with such emotional deprivation by developing pleasing, caretaking behavior. In these ways they experienced feeling alike, deeply understood by each other, and strongly connected. They were alike in other respects as well. They came from the same social class, valued the arts and intellectual pursuits, and they loved the outdoors and travel.

Their perfect complementarity was formed by their opposite personality traits accompanied by certain dovetailing needs. Garth appeared to be self-confident and gregarious, while Lily was shy and more introverted. Both were attracted to qualities in the other that they desired for themselves. On the most obvious and conscious level, both felt Garth could help Lily be more self-confident, and Lily could help Garth be more in tune with his feelings and more at ease with himself, less frantically driven. Thus, each could help correct for the other's perceived deficits in personal development. In the early idealizing phase, they could appropriate the other's desired attributes through merging with each other.

On a deeper, more unconscious level, each sensed the other to be a potential "ideal" partner who could fulfill certain unmet needs from childhood. Garth had a great need to provide nurture and guidance to an insecure, unformed woman with potential—to be a Henry Higgins to an Eliza Doolittle. The insecure woman represented his own unrecognized insecurity and need for mothering. His unconscious hope was thus to solve his inadequacy problems by helping Lily become more secure and accomplished. In addition, the role of guiding parent was familiar to him (and was a way of being wanted and loved), having tended to his inadequate mother in many ways throughout his childhood. Lily, having had so little support from her own parents, had a great need for precisely this kind of guidance, particularly in developing her intellectual competence and artistic abilities. Garth's greatest need was to be idealized and admired, while Lily's most prominent need was to idealize a father figure.[6] It seemed like a perfect match.

More pathological attractions are based on devalued views of oneself in relationship with someone initially idealized as powerful but also denigrating in a significant way. These kinds of initial idealizations can rapidly turn to demonizations and often replicate images of parents who were viewed as powerful but also hateful in some way.

For example, Jana, as a young woman, felt weak and incapable of running her own life. She was attracted to her first husband by his apparent self-confidence and protectiveness. He was also domineering and verbally abusive, both features of Jana's father. Her husband was thus chosen on the model of her father with whom she could reenact feeling needy, taken care of, and abusively dominated by someone more powerful. In such choices, domination and abuse are misread as love and caring, since this was the only kind of caring connection a person may have experienced.

THE IDEAL SELF

Our sense of self is enhanced when we romantically idealize someone. Initially, we are uplifted by euphoric feelings. Lovers describe feeling on top of the world, more alive than ever before, "high," buoyed up with optimism. Indeed they can appear hypomanic. Allied with this euphoria is a feeling of enchantment. A magical spell has been cast over us, and we are "love sick."

Although a substantial boost in self-esteem occurs when anyone we admire admires us in return, when a loved, idealized person, idealizes and loves us in return, the boost to self-esteem is even higher. This happy exchange often results in our feeling, "If this incredible person loves and wants me, then I must be someone special." However, if self-esteem is too low, then a person may not feel enhanced by another's love, but instead devalue the lover's worth—"If he admires and loves me, he must be a nobody." Groucho Marx expressed this sentiment in the famous line: "I wouldn't join any club that would have me as a member."

Through mutual idealizing, both partners perceive the other and oneself as special. Therefore, each can feel more effective and powerful than either could be alone—"With her by my side, we can make all of our dreams come true." In addition, a greater sense of personal power comes

---

[6]In Freud's (1914/1963) concept of love object choice, Garth's choice of Lily was based on narcissistic needs, and Lily's choice of Garth was based on the need to fulfill early dependent (anaclitic) longings.

from the feeling of being supported by an idealized person—"If she thinks I'm more than I am, then I can *become* more than I am." Our sense of self is additionally enhanced through merging with our idealized partner and appropriating his or her desired attributes. Lily described this kind of self-enhancement when she spoke of Garth's self-confidence as giving her more confidence.

However, this incorporation of the partner's desired attributes lasts only as long as a state of idealized, merged relatedness exists. As soon as a deidealizing process sets in and a few degrees of separateness develop, the partner's appropriated qualities are lost as parts of the self and can become a source of competitive envy and lowered self-esteem. As Jana said of Kate during a difficult time in their relationship: "I loved her way with people, her ability to win friends. I thought I would have a lot more friends and a nice social life when we got together. Now, I hate her popularity. It just makes me feel inferior. All of these people in our lives just take her away from me. I wish they would all drop dead!"

Another source of increased self-esteem derives from the sense that the rest of the world admires and envies us for having won such a special prize. In less optimal beginnings, the partner may be idealized and selected primarily *because* she or he is thought to be a prize by others—a man with much power and wealth or a beautiful woman (i.e., the trophy wife). When the idealizing is thus more based on opinions of others, a quick and dramatic deflation of infatuation usually follows a marriage.

When we consider all that is gained through idealizing our partner, it is easy to understand the painful loss experienced when he or she begins to look less ideal and more like an ordinary human being, for the newly enhanced self is inextricably linked to the idealized partner. Thus, all of the ways the self has become expanded are lost when deidealizing occurs. Euphoric, enchanted sensations, higher self-esteem, the conception of being special, the appropriated desired attributes—all of these gains begin to slip away at approximately the same rate that the partner descends from the pedestal.

THE IDEAL RELATIONSHIP

Our initial view of an ideal relationship is quite complex in that often the consciously recognized ideals are contradictory to the unconscious ideals. Although each person has his or her own unique picture of an ideal relationship, there are certain general ideals of a love relationship that permeate our culture. I have organized these cultural ideals under three main headings: *the romantic ideal, the patriarchal ideal,* and *the equal partnership ideal.* I use the term "ideal" here to mean a model of a role relationship that is commonly held to be either the most desirable or felt consciously or unconsciously to the most accepted. The relationship fantasied to be the most pleasurable may not be the one that is considered to be "ideal" in this sense.

First to be considered is that cluster of interconnected "shoulds" forming *the romantic ideal*, summarized as follows:

The Romantic Ideal

We should be everything to each other.
We should always be first with each other.
We should always be faithful to each other.
We should do everything together.
We should have the same goals, values, and beliefs.
We should never feel disappointed in each other.
We should never disagree and strive to be of one mind.
We should have a romantic, passionate relationship.

This ideal seems to be based on the notion that early phase merging and idealizing should be perpetuated indefinitely. In this romantic ideal, there is little or no conflict, disappointment, or anger in the relationship, since each partner should automatically know and be able to fulfill all of the other's needs. Needless to say, this ideal is impossible to fulfill and creates enormous heartache, disappointment, and profound feelings of failure in couples.

The romantic ideal has its origins in the ideal of courtly love created in medieval times to amuse the French aristocracy. Over the centuries, the ideal of romantic love has drastically changed from the highly circumscribed courtly dance between chivalrous knight and married Lady to become, in our times, an all consuming way to love and live.[7] The modern-day core of this ideal—"We should be everything to each other"—is broadcast in every form of cultural expression.

Representing this ideal in its extreme are numerous lovers in novels, plays, poems, songs, and movies, who sacrifice everything, including their lives, for their love. One example is portrayed in the popular movie *Elvira Madigan* (1967), wherein Elvira and her lover starve together and ultimately commit suicide to the lovely strains of a Mozart piano concerto rather than be separated.

In our decade, the lovers in the *The Bridges of Madison County* continue the glorification of *the romantic ideal* in sophomoric dialogue, ac-

---

[7]See Miller's (1995) excellent discussion of the origins of the romantic ideal.

companied by the copious tears and wild applause of the general public. This book (Waller, 1992) and the movie (1996) seem to have brought as many tears into my office as have losses of real love relationships. They are mostly women's tears, women who feel cheated of experiencing such a transporting, ideal romance in their own unsatisfying lives.

The potent power of *the romantic ideal* is often overlooked in therapy with couples and individuals, because therapists and patients alike are more often consciously wishing to promote the ideals of separateness and individuality intrinsic to *the equal partnership ideal*. Partners who pride themselves on being separate individuals who can give each other a lot of "space" have a difficult time recognizing their unconscious fantasy of being merged and are confused by feelings of disappointment and anger when this wish is not fulfilled in reality.

For example, Garth reported:

"I have to admit it really bothered me when Lily went away for the weekend to her friend's wedding without me. We could have spent that weekend together, even though I had to work a lot, we could've been together in the mornings and evenings. I thought she should be there with me. But this is her oldest friend, and she felt obligated to go. I should understand that. I want us both to have friends and be able to see our friends. We're not joined at the hip."

The romantic ideal of relating particularly tends to rear up and show itself when couples face retirement. This likely happens because retirement may re-create many of the conditions of a honeymoon. The couple is suddenly together all of the time, without the outside work of one or both partners to structure time away and time together. Also, couples are supposed to relax, have fun together, and enjoy life while they still can—Have a second honeymoon! For many, this is not a welcome prospect and brings to mind the wife's complaint, "I married him for better or for worse but not for lunch!"

A recent case example illustrates this point. Working in individual therapy with a long-married woman in her mid-sixties, I noticed that she seemed to resist retiring, even though she frequently claimed she wanted to stop work and spend more time with her husband. She finally recognized that she dreaded the prospect of being at home with her retired husband because so much would be expected of her. She would have to live up to *the romantic ideal* (colored by shades of *the patriarchal ideal*), an exhausting and demoralizing prospect.

She pictured having to do everything with her husband. They would be together constantly, and she would have little freedom and little control. What would she do, for example, if he wanted the heat on all day and she did not? What if she wanted to go out somewhere, and he did not? What if he expected her to make lunch! She, herself, did not attribute controlling, possessive traits to her husband, who, from all accounts was an easygoing man with many of his own interests. We found that they were coming from her view of what an ideal relationship should be. And now, without work to ensure her status as a separate individual, she would have to live up to this restrictive, suffocating ideal or face the possibility that she was a selfish person with a bad marriage. Once all of this was exposed and talked through, she realized she could dispense with this so-called ideal that was far from ideal. It seemed to help free her when I said that this romantic ideal of relating was only meant to last for as long as the honeymoon. "And for many couples," I said, "it doesn't even last as long as that."

When I get a glimpse of *the romantic ideal* influencing couples from behind the scenes, I ask the partners where they think this ideal comes from. Many say it comes from how their parents related and from our culture, especially in the way Hollywood movies, television, and popular songs present ideals of a love relationship. Certainly it is in the culture, but why, against all experience of its unreality and inevitable disappointment, does it continue to flourish in our culture?

Looking for a developmental explanation, the mother–infant relationship comes first to mind as the prototype. We continue to long for the intense degree of closeness once experienced in the blissful mother–infant relationship. The romantic ideal is a grown-up version of having a devoted mother's attention all to yourself, except that both partners play the roles of adoring mother and adored baby.

However, if we cast a cold, objective eye on the reality of the mother–infant relationship, it becomes quite apparent that even this closest of bonds does not really fulfill the ideal. For mothers do not usually just relate to their babies. From the infant's earliest years, mothers also relate to other people—like husbands, other siblings, grandparents, friends—and may often go away to work or to pursue other interests. It may be the child's fantasy, that mother is always with me, there when I need her, loves and wants only me. Hence, the more likely developmental source for this ideal of a couple relationship is a fantasy we have created about the nature of the mother-infant bond, an ideal of what we did not really get but wished we had.

The Patriarchal Ideal

The romantic ideal coexists in our society with an even older one—*the patriarchal ideal*. Even though we may rationally dismiss *the patriarchal ideal* as a model by which to live and love, it still wields considerable power. When I think I have rooted out all influential vestiges from the dark corners of my mind, one of these "shoulds" will pop into my head without warning. A likely time is after enjoying a nice meal cooked by my husband. I will hear my mother's voice intrude, dispensing guilt and superiority: "The good wife cooks dinner for her husband, no matter how tired she is."

At the heart of *the patriarchal ideal* is a rigid gender-role relationship that has its origin with the beginning of family life in prehistoric times. Originally this role relationship—the man who provides and protects the weaker woman who bears children and makes a comfortable cave—had tremendous value for the survival of our species. Power in this relationship is unequal, because the man is stronger, more aggressive, and brings the food. Over the ages, from the time of the cave man to the present, man's superiority in these circumscribed respects broadened to encompass a more generalized superiority in relation to women in Western culture. This aggrandizing of the man occurred for multiple reasons pertaining to economics, politics, biology, and psychology, and is detailed by numerous social historians and feminist scholars.

The ideal husband in this role relationship should provide, protect, and make the important decisions, while the ideal wife devotes herself to meeting the husband's needs and taking care of the home. While this relationship is founded on inequality, there is an intention of an equitable exchange of needs. The husband gets nurturing and basic care, meals prepared, a well-maintained home, and care for the couple's children. His wife gives him unflagging emotional support and admiration, and should willingly respond to his sexual demands.

In return, the woman gets her needs met for financial security, a home for raising the children, a strong man to protect, guide, and shoulder the responsibility of dealing with the world and making the difficult life decisions. Ideally, the husband makes the decisions with her best interests at heart. While the wife is expected to support and agree with her husband's decisions, she may connive to get her own way by manipulating behind his back, as long as his leadership and superiority are not openly challenged. She may be adored for being beautiful or for her role as self-sacrificing wife and mother. In order to get the rewards of security, dependency, and idealization, she should not put her own needs before husband and children, nor present her own thoughts as being of equal or superior value.

Women's liberation has exposed *the patriarchal ideal* as a vehicle for the devaluation and suppression of women. Many men also find it demeaning and unfair. The cost of self-worth and individual development has become too great a sacrifice for most women to bear in exchange for financial security and the gratifications of remaining dependent. *The patriarchal ideal* is no longer held up as an ideal to the extent it once was in our popular culture. Television shows are no longer created that portray idyllic, happy couples living according to the traditional model and patriarchal ideal—*Leave It to Beaver, Ozzie and Harriet,* or *Father Knows Best.* Today, we see shows such as *Thirtysomething* or *Mad About You* that portray married partners who both work and have conflicts about who takes care of the chores and the children. Although the *patriarchal ideal* is antithetical to modern views, it remains alive in many people's minds.

I am reminded of an intelligent young man who recently began individual therapy with me for help in improving his love relationship. He described his mother as June Cleaver and his father as an upper class Archie Bunker. He was mortified to discover that he acted like his authoritarian father and treated his girlfriend as an inferior who should only agree with him. While he said he despised his behavior and the traditional, patriarchal model of relationships, he could not keep himself from acting this way. The only difference between this young man and many of the couples I see is the unusual degree of awareness he had about his behavior and internal conflicts.

The Equal Partnership Ideal

This ideal emphasizes the concepts of two separate individuals engaged in an equal partnership in which differences are assumed to exist and will require ongoing negotiation and compromise. The partners are expected to have separate interests and spend time away from each other pursuing their own interests.

From a developmental point of view, the partnership ideal reflects a more mature mode of relating. In terms of Mahler et al.'s (1975) phases in the child's development of internalized relationships, we have moved from the symbiotic (*romantic*) relationship mode of the one- to four-month-old infant to the phase of separation–individuation of the eighteen- to twenty-four-month-old toddler. This more mature, differentiated ideal that emphasizes an equal partnership, separateness, and self-development can be summarized as follows:

> We should be equals in a partnership relationship.
> Gender should not determine the division of labor.
> Roles and tasks should be defined by interest, time, and ability.
> We should be mutually respectful and faithful.
> We should have similar goals and values.
> We should support each other's individual development.
> We should *not* be expected to fulfill *all* of each other's needs.
> We should *not* always be together.
> We should have some shared activities and other separate activities.

We should express our feelings and our differences.
We should negotiate our differences and make compromises.
We should have a mutually satisfying sex life.

It can be surprising to couples and therapists alike how often the
equal partnership ideal is found to operate strictly on the surface—at the
conscious level of awareness. What is found just below this top layer is the
other, old-fashioned *romantic ideal* that rumbles around quietly or noisily,
looking for a way to get expressed. Below *the romantic ideal, the patriarchal
ideal* can often be found to lurk. Suddenly, these irrational attitudes, experienced as unmet needs, expectations, or guilty failure will bubble up and
cause a host of confusing feelings and behaviors. Couples like Lily and
Garth, and Kate and Jana, who sustain these highly conflicting models of
the ideal relationship—partnership on the surface, romantic and patriarchal underneath—have the most difficult time making sense of their reactions.

It can be very helpful to couples to explain "irrational" reactions in
terms of their conflicting ideals. When the existence of the romantic or
patriarchal ideals are presented as universal phenomena and as conflicting with a more rational ideal model, exposure and acceptance is more
easily achieved. The "irrational" feelings generated can then be productively explored and understood. The following excerpt from a therapy session with Jana and Kate illustrates the conflict between *the partnership* and
romantic ideals. Jana appears to have successfully deidealized and discarded *the patriarchal ideal* in the process of leaving her first husband and
coming out as a lesbian. Kate had known she was gay since early adolescence.

JANA: I don't know why I felt so let down and angry when Kate decided
to go to that conference without me. I couldn't go because of work,
and I really do understand that she needs to take these opportunities
to advance in her career. But I still felt upset, and we had this huge
fight. (*Jana and Kate described the circumstances causing this fight and
their angry interactions in detail.*)

SHARPE: Your reaction, Jana, sounds like it has a lot to do with a conflict
of ideals.

JANA: Uh, you mean a conflict between my ideals and Kate's?

SHARPE: No, I mean inside yourself. A conflict between one set of ideals
and another set . . . having to do with what you expect from love relationships. (*Jana and Kate look perplexed.*) Bear with me. How would you

both describe your notions of an ideal relationship, the one you're consciously aware of?

JANA: My ideal is that we should be good friends who support each other. I was stifled in my marriage. It wasn't all my ex-husband's fault, I hate to admit. We both assumed that my needs would be subordinate to his. That's how my parents operated. My mother always did what my father wanted. She got to do what she wanted by going behind his back. I want nothing to do with that kind of cowardice and dishonesty. I want us to be equals in the relationship, and I want there to be mutual respect. We should support each other for who we are and to become all we can become.

KATE: I totally agree with that. So why did you get so mad about me going to the conference? You know I have to do those things to get anywhere.

JANA: I'm sorry about my reaction. I told you that. I'm really ashamed I threw such a childish fit.

SHARPE: It might help to understand why you got so hurt. These reactions make sense when we look at them in relation to your expectations of a relationship. A lot of us have expectations that are contradictory. You've described the ideal you want, consciously—a partnership of equals. But there's another version that's probably operating behind the scenes. That one says the opposite, irrational things like "Love means we should never leave each other; we should be everything to each other. Love means we should do everything together; we should . . . "

JANA: Say no more. I've gotten rid of all that garbage.

SHARPE: Are you sure? I think most of us have quite a lot of those notions still hanging around but hidden from sight.

JANA: I refuse to believe I'm like that.

KATE: Like what?

JANA: Clingy, dependent, possessive. Like the feminine stereotype. . . . Like the romantic heroine in trashy books. . . . Like my mother. . . . You know, like . . .

KATE: Don't worry. You're not like that. If anything, you're overboard the other way. Sometimes I think you try too hard to be the other way.

JANA: What do you mean?

KATE: Well, trying to suppress natural feelings, because you think they mean weakness.

JANA: Like what natural feelings?

KATE: I don't think wanting to be with someone you love, or missing that person, is being clingy or possessive.

JANA: Well, I don't logically think that either.

SHARPE: That's my big point. None of this is particularly logical.

JANA: I do feel being needy is being weak. I can't help it.

SHARPE: Maybe that's why you got so mad, because you felt in need of being with Kate.

JANA: (grimacing) So how do I get rid of being needy?

SHARPE: I don't think you can. But, if you could accept these feelings as human, they wouldn't run you so much from behind the scenes.

Many partners resist becoming aware of the romantic ideal and the patriarchal ideal, since both seem irrational, outdated, too suppressing of individuality, and reflect a potentially frightening degree of dependency. Therapists, too, have tendencies to overlook the influence of these ideals. Most therapists, along with many approaches to couple therapy, operate according to *the equal partnership ideal* of a relationship. This kind of relationship is currently thought to be the optimal model of maturity and good mental health. Unfortunately, if this attitude is *rigidly* held by a therapist, couples consciously committed to other ideal models can be alienated. There are many couples who are content to live in a traditional marriage, and this area of agreement and satisfaction needs to be respected by therapists. More unfortunately, a therapist's rigid devotion to *the equal partnership ideal* may inhibit adequate exploration and understanding of the conflict of ideals that is operating with most couples.

Since ideals powerfully influence how we feel and behave, it is helpful for the therapist to be on the lookout for their influence in the reactions of individuals and couples and bring them out in the open to be examined in the light of day. Each partner has expectations of how the relationship should be in general and how the mate will fulfill him or her in certain important ways. Disappointments and problems arise when one or both partners discover that the other really does not match the internal ideal in many respects, and that the relationship does not match the internal ideal of a love relationship. The greater the discrepancy between the ideals and the real person/real relationship, the greater the disappointment. In these situations, the crucial process of *modifying the ideals* has not occurred, so that greater acceptance of the partner and relationship is possible. Hence, couples find themselves increasingly disillusioned and at a loss to understand why their partners and relationships that seemed to hold such promise of fulfillment turned out to be so disappointing.

In the early phase of a love relationship, romantic idealizing is an important means of securing an attachment. Mutual idealizing assures each partner that he or she is special, is better than all other contenders, and thus cannot be replaced. Being mere ordinary mortals, other people are much less important (much less ideal) and therefore cannot threaten the relationship. In mutual idealizing, both partners feel that they come first and are the one and only mate for the other. Perhaps there are echoes from mother's idealizing of her baby as the most wonderful baby in all the world. This sense of "We were meant for each other" makes for the beginnings of a special and passionate attachment. However, before a passionate attachment is really secure for the long haul, it must weather a few storms, particularly the first deidealizing storm.

DEIDEALIZATION

GARTH: We spent the weekend in Mexico to celebrate the day we first met, and everything that could go wrong did go wrong. This charming rustic inn where we stayed was a disaster. It was hot, dirty, and filled with scorpions. There was no air-conditioning. And then I got sick from the lousy Mexican food. What we did in bed was sweat and itch on sheets that felt like burlap bags. It wasn't very romantic, and things between us . . . well, they got a little tense. We sort of had a fight.

LILY: Not much of a fight, really. You were feeling sick, and you were so disappointed in the place. You just couldn't get over that.

GARTH: I spent a lot of time looking for just the right spot. It was supposed to be the perfect place.

LILY: The inn did have a lot of charm. We had a beautiful view. I kept trying to point out the bright side.

GARTH: That was one of the troubles. I can feel my stomach start to churn all over again. I feel so alone when you start that "Let's look at the bright side" stuff when I'm feeling bad.

LILY: (*her upper lip beginning to quiver*) I thought you liked me to be cheerful. I was just trying to make the best of things.

GARTH: I know. I know. I'm sorry. I do like you to be cheerful. I don't know what I'm saying.

LILY: (*looking acutely unhappy*) We were together. I thought that was the most important thing. It seems like I'm not enough to make you happy anymore.

GARTH: (*pleading*) Don't say that. It's not true. I love you more than anything in the world. It's me. Something's wrong with me.

Their anguish was palpable. I could feel them straining to keep a lid on more hurt, anger, and disappointment than they were able to openly express. Bewilderment and anxiety permeated their facial expressions and body language. They had fallen out of love, and the nourishing flow of mutual idealizing had suddenly stopped like a wellspring gone dry. Without the rose-colored glasses of idealizing, each looked at the other and saw not just the real person, but someone far more disappointing.

Through Lily's eyes, I could see that Garth no longer looked like her handsome, swashbuckling hero, but more like a regressed, peevish little boy who stamped his foot and refused to be comforted. Through Garth's eyes, Lily was no longer his beautiful, princess, his perfect soulmate, but had somehow transformed into an irritating Pollyanna who did not understand him.

When disillusionment occurs, partners do not just stop idealizing and see the real person in a balanced way. For a while, they see a devalued version of the real person, or they may oscillate between idealizing and devaluing: "She's wonderful, and I love her/She's the world's worst bitch, and I hate her." The loss of the idealized partner and the ideal relationship brings acute disappointment, anger, and sadness. The idealized self is deflated in the process, causing many, like Garth, to feel like failures.

Garth's extreme disappointment in their hotel was a metaphor (and displacement) for his great disappointment in Lily and the relationship. Lily and Garth both had particularly strong needs to fulfill impossible ideals. No criticism, anger, or conflict was allowed in their relationship. They could not really talk through their disappointments with each other, so that understanding and acceptance could expand and modulate the rigid perfectionism of their expectations.

Disappointment in both partners is intensified by a phenomenon described by Dicks as "the return of the repressed" (1967, p. 58). The partner's perceived failure to meet ideal expectations is a major factor in stimulating dissolution of psychological barriers that keep childhood hatreds and disappointments safely repressed.

When repression fails, the "ideal" relationship is flooded with all that was hurtful and disappointing in the partners' original family relations. The hated characteristics of a parent now appear to be embodied by the partner. Painful aspects of the past that each partner thought to heal through marriage with an ideal partner have become shockingly alive in the present.

Lily began to see in Garth the other side of her ideal father—the hated father figure who left her and her mother for long periods for his own self-aggrandizement and pleasure. She had been deeply injured by his neglect and disregard of her own and her mother's needs. In her marriage, she found herself beginning to sound like her mother, trying to pretend everything was fine. She tried to get Garth's approval by being a good girl, but she also used this mode as a cover for retaliation—the kind that her mother employed by being impervious to her husband's feelings.

Garth began to see in Lily aspects of his needy but insensitive mother—the mother who made him feel overburdened and choked with suppressed anger, and whom he later viewed as having driven his father into uncontrolled rages. Lily's insecurity and frequent pleas for reassurance, behavior that Garth once found so endearing, now made him feel depleted. Furthermore, she ignored his needs for motherly care. She was preoccupied with making it in her career, and her adoring gaze was now more often fixed on one of her extravagant canvases rather than on his handsome face. He felt his vitality draining away, the vitality that fed on her idealization. He wanted to withdraw as his father had done or fly into a childish rage. He so hated his father's temper that he would do anything to avoid becoming openly angry. Instead, he brooded and stayed away from home for longer and longer periods, with the excuse of work.

Their perfect dovetailing of needs had now turned into a perfectly choreographed exacerbation of their oldest, most painful wounds. He had become the selfish, absent father of Lily's childhood, and Lily had become Garth's needy, neglectful mother. They were further demoralized by seeing themselves act like wounded little children.

Given all of this insight into the meanings of their massive disappointment and suppressed anger, what kind of therapeutic intervention would be most helpful? Since the expression of *any* negativity was very threatening to them both, my first aim was to reduce their great fear of disappointed, angry feelings.

SHARPE: It's seems like you both feel very disappointed about this important occasion. I know you wanted to re-create those wonderful early days of falling love. But the pressure you felt to achieve that state might have gotten in the way of . . .

LILY: I'm sure that was true. We both wanted everything to be so perfect. It was too much pressure.

GARTH: It was a mistake. The weekend just shoved our noses in the fact that things have changed. We're not as close as we used to be.

LILY: (*with forced brightness*) Maybe we should take a longer trip together.

The conversation suddenly stopped, and they both looked tense and unhappy. I could feel them stiffling their anger and hurt.

SHARPE: I think you both feel disappointed, but you're afraid if you talk more openly, your anger will show and be hurtful.

GARTH: I know I wouldn't want to hurt Lily, but I'm not aware of feeling angry . . . just sort of down.

LILY: Just tell me what's wrong.

GARTH: (*hesitating*) This is so difficult. (*He pauses, glancing around the room as though looking for a way to escape.*) I have these critical thoughts that I'm ashamed of.

LILY: I think I can guess what they are. You thought I'd be a better wife.

GARTH: (*protesting*) No, no . . . you're a wonderful wife in the important ways. It's just . . . I didn't think I would care about the little stuff . . . like your being there and looking happy to see me when I come home. Dinner on the table. Things being clean and orderly.

LILY: (*defensively*) I made dinner every night for quite a while. You came home later and later. Lots of times you didn't call, and the dinner would be ruined.

GARTH: I'm really sorry if I didn't show enough appreciation. I should be better about calling. I forget the time when I'm busy.

LILY: My cooking dinner can improve. I love to cook. But you know I hate to clean house, and I'm much more of a slob than you are. You're such a Mr. Clean. (*Her tone has a derisive edge.*)

GARTH: Yeah, well . . . what can I say. I'm compulsive. At least I'm not as bad as my father. He would spend hours picking lint off the furniture. It's not that I want you to be cleaning. Can't we get more help?

LILY: I'm sorry, I've just been so busy. I made a couple of calls that didn't get returned, and I let it slide.

GARTH: Disorder grates on my nerves.

LILY: I guess I don't mind disorder. I like the house to feel homey . . . lived in. My mother was so obsessively clean that our house wasn't meant for people. Sometimes, she would look at my brother and me like we were big globs of dirt that should be scrubbed away.

GARTH: (*looking sad*) I know what you mean. My dad was just as bad.

Strange, isn't it? We had opposite reactions to the same kind of compulsive craziness.

LILY: (*gravely*) I'm really afraid I'm a big disappointment to you. (*Garth denies this loudly and grabs her hand.*) You fell in love with me as an artist. We connect on the creative level. But it seems like you really want to live with a traditional wife.

GARTH: I don't think so. I had that before, and I wasn't happy. You're the one I want, however you come.

LILY: At least you know the worst about me now. I feel guilty about not being a good housewife. Really guilty.

SHARPE: Why is that?

LILY: My mother was the perfect homemaker, but she was so lonely and unappreciated and dull. I just don't want that, and I don't want to spend my time that way. And I guess, to be honest, I resent Garth's wanting me to be in that role.

GARTH: But I don't, really.

SHARPE: You can want both things. Everyone wants a good housewife these days. I'd certainly like one. There's too much to manage for a couple with demanding careers.

LILY: (*grinning*) I'd like a wife, too.

GARTH: That's a fine idea. It's not that I need you to be the homemaker. I wanted someone with a career, with her own identity. Someone *not* like my mother who could only talk about the price of meat or what Aunt Betty was doing.

LILY: My mother talked about the virtues of various cleansers and how they affected different kinds of dirt.

SHARPE: (*chuckling*) You have big things in common. Your mothers were both traditional housewives and that's the model of a good wife that sticks in both of your heads, whether you want it there or not.

GARTH: (*jokingly*) No, no, I refuse to accept that.

SHARPE: What about assuming that Lily should be the one to find a house cleaner?

GARTH: (*with good humor*) I'm being ganged up on.

SHARPE: Just a little. I could nudge Lily just as well. (*I look at Lily encouragingly.*)

LILY: (*speaking firmly and flashing a brilliant smile*) I'd feel better if we both shared the calling.

GARTH: (*relieved*) Okay. God, it's good to see you smile.

ACCEPTING THE REAL PARTNER, RELATIONSHIP, AND SELF

In this session, Garth and Lily moved from trying to escape disappointment and angry, devalued perceptions of each other to being able to acknowledge these difficult feelings. In the process of exposing and sharing their disappointments, they were able to move toward greater mutual understanding and acceptance. This interaction marked the beginning of their working through the deidealization process.

As their interaction continued, a more invisible reworking of internal structures was simultaneously occurring. In this internal reworking, both partners' ideal images of each other and their relationship were being modified to allow for the integration of "imperfections" and "reality." Also, the hated aspects of their parents, now brought into the relationship, were being examined in the more objective light of an adult relationship. In the process of awareness and discussion, the polarized perceptions of parents—the ideal and the devalued—became modified and separated from the real partner.

My awareness and exposure of both partners' disappointments in the relationship as not living up to their hidden images of an ideal relationship and an ideal partner contributed to their reworking of internal structures. Both Lily and Garth were strongly influenced by the romantic and patriarchal ideals, but each had suppressed these ideals in their joint, conscious effort to operate according to the equal partnership ideal. Helping the partners to recognize their shared conception of "the good wife" as derived from their mothers' roles in a patriarchal relationship enabled them to begin deconstructing this image and reconstructing their own conception of a good wife, a good husband, and a good relationship.

Optimal working through requires that the partners acknowledge their disappointed feelings with each other. If these feelings are not expressed, they cannot be modified in any productive way. Expression to someone other than the partner is no substitute for sharing these feelings with the partner. Many relationships with friends and therapists are used to dump feelings of angry disappointment with the spouse. While the sharp edges of disappointment and anger may be blunted in this way, there can be no working through that results in a mutual understanding and acceptance *between* the partners.

Sharing of disappointments between partners will result in greater acceptance of each other's flaws (i.e., modulation and integration of ideal and devalued perceptions) under the following conditions:

1. If the partner can hear and understand the complaints, anger abates and the perceived magnitude of his or her flaws tends to shrink.

2. If the partner exhibits some willingness to alter the disappointing behavior, then anger and devaluing are lessened and acceptance is increased. Garth's offer to share the duty of finding a cleaning woman indicated a willingness to try to alter deeply ingrained attitudes.

3. When partners are faced with each other's disappointments and forced to recognize their own failings and difficult quirks, the other's faults seem less onerous and more acceptable.

To be effective in helping couples with this major transition (and other, less crucial cycles of deidealizing), a therapist needs to understand this developmental process. Then he or she can helpfully encourage and guide expression of the partners' specific disappointments in each other and in the relationship. Emphasizing the universal nature of these feelings encourages expression and acceptance.[8] In the previous exchange, the therapist's interventions were probably not essential once Lily and Garth felt safe enough to express themselves. Each had the ability to hear and understand the other's feelings. This capability is not always present. If one or both partners cannot tolerate criticism or any suggestion of imperfection, this sharing of disappointments will abort before much airing of feelings can occur, or degenerate into a devaluing, blaming interaction that only increases disappointment and disillusionment. Techniques for the management of these outcomes are discussed in subsequent chapters.

All couples wish to bypass this phase. It is the experience of multiple losses and sadness that partners want to avoid. Loss of the idealized partner, idealized self, and ideal relationship is very painful. These ideals have been with us from childhood. When they are challenged and reworked, they are lost forever in their childish, perfectionistic form. Throughout life, these ideals have been a source of comfort and a beacon of light giving hope and guidance. With this reworking, we are brought far closer to the truth than ever before—the truth that it is only flawed humans that ex-

---

[8]A few of my colleagues who have more experience in treating gay couples have observed that many lesbian partners seem to undergo the first round of idealizing and deidealizing more intensely than do most heterosexual partners. One hypothesis for this possible difference is that the early mother–daughter relationship is likely to be revived more intensely in lesbian passion. Additionally, in those relationships wherein one partner helps the other to come out (as Kate did for Jana), idealization of the helping partner tends to be profound, because the coming-out partner often experiences considerable trauma, mixed with elation and gratitude, in the process of discovering her true sexual orientation. (I am particularly indebted to Susan Richards for these observations and hypotheses.) In accord with these ideas, Jana and Kate, but particularly Jana, resisted fiercely and often felt uncontainable anguish during the deidealizing process. This kind of "complementary" lesbian relationship is fully discussed by Beverly Burch (1993) in *On Intimate Terms*.

ist on our planet. Gods and goddesses are nowhere to be found, especially among our mates.

Idealizing and Deidealizing Recur throughout the Life of a Relationship

Optimally, following the first major round of deidealization, the partner comes to be viewed more realistically but with a generally positive patina. The stories of most relationships are filled with many ups and downs, good times, bad times, and blah times. Perceptions of the partner fluctuate accordingly. Certain circumstances, behaviors, or achievements of the partner can produce great feelings of warmth, admiration, and a period of more modulated idealizing. Likewise, other circumstances and behaviors can produce another round of disappointment in the partner and the relationship. Experience of the major life-cycle events are usually times of predictable stress that involve learning something new about the partner. This new knowledge may result in greater admiration of the partner or disappointment and devaluation.

The birth of a child or the need to integrate one partner's children from a previous marriage into the relationship are changes that cause great stress and demand emotional growth of the partners. For Lily and Garth, and for Kate and Jana, the inclusion of children was quite traumatic. Kate's difficulty accepting Jana's children caused Jana great disappointment and another round of deidealizing Kate. Likewise, Garth's difficulty accepting fatherhood was a great disappointment to Lily, leading her temporarily to deidealize Garth. However, when their partners were able to grow into their new parental roles, they inspired increased admiration from their mates.

With many cycles of idealizing and deidealizing, idealized views of the partner become modulated. He or she becomes increasingly perceived as a whole, separate person with an array of distinctive traits, some of which are admirable, enviable, or merely acceptable, while others invoke feelings of disapproval, dislike, and anger. As the partner is seen for who he or she really is, the tendency to idealize globally is transformed into real admiration and appreciation. The opposite tendency—to experience extreme disappointment when the partner fails to meet an expectation—that invokes devaluing perceptions and angry feelings also becomes modified. Thus, greater understanding and acceptance of the "imperfect" aspects of the partner are developed along with modification of expectations.

MODULATED IDEALIZING: ADMIRING THE REAL PARTNER

As the partner is seen more realistically and accepted in spite of faults, the capacity truly to appreciate and admire the partner's strengths and uniqueness develops and deepens. Before the first major deidealizing process, when the partner is viewed as bigger than life, true appreciation and admiration are not possible. To admire our fantasy constructions of beautiful princesses and superheroes is meaningless. Furthermore, while being on the receiving end of the partner's idealization can feel very exciting and inflating, there is also usually an uneasy awareness that those adoring eyes are not looking at one's real self. A background voice is probably saying, "How long can this last?"

When Lily and Garth, and Kate and Jana worked through many of their disappointments and became more accepting of their real partners, each began to see and express true appreciation and admiration. Garth said, "I really admire Lily's intelligence and social sense, and the way she listens and grasps what I tell her about my work. She gives me such good counsel and great ideas. I appreciate her help so much. I never had someone there for me like she is."

Jana said, "I don't know what I'd do without Kate's ability to tolerate my moodiness, my ups and downs, the extreme reactions I can get into. Unlike me, she's so accepting and nonjudgmental. I really admire that. She can let me be who I am, but she also helps me to get a better grip and come back down to earth."

It is useful for therapists to know that when partners complain that they do not feel appreciated or admired by their spouses, it is likely that there has not been a substantial working through of deidealization. At some point along the way, the process has been stalled or aborted, and acceptance of the real partner has not occurred. In this event, it does little good to instruct couples to give compliments and verbalize more appreciation. It is more helpful to direct exploration to why admiration and appreciation have not yet evolved, or look to why such capabilities have been lost if they had once been established. The couple is likely stuck in the first or a subsequent round of deidealizing.

INTERMITTENT ROMANTIC IDEALIZING: THE REAL PARTNER BECOMES THE IDEAL

For couples to maintain a romantic, passionate intensity, it seems that a certain amount of romantic idealizing needs to occur. Day-to-day loving, supporting, appreciating, and admiring the partner are essential for a good relationship but not quite enough for a passionate one. The spouse needs to be viewed, at times, as the most wonderful person in the world if a couple is to experience those intense sensations associated with passionate love. Idealizing, in this respect, is like a love potion. It should only be administered in small doses at certain times. Too much idealizing can stifle a relationship and strangle passion. Without any idealizing, there is no spark to ignite passion.

The right dose seems to come from another transformation in perceiving one's partner. This move is toward feeling such deep appreciation and admiration of the real person that, at times, a short burst of idealizing is once again triggered in near the original form. Thus, we come full circle but in reverse, as the real partner over time has become internalized as the ideal partner. In the beginning, idealizing the partner was substantially derived from the projection of our needs and wishes. Now, as the real partner becomes increasingly known and admired, our internal representation of an ideal partner has undergone successive revisions. Eventually, the real partner becomes almost interchangeable with the internal ideal.

The triggering of idealizing derived from deep admiration or appreciation of the partner's real qualities can happen under a variety of circumstances. A commonly experienced flash of romantic idealizing can occur when watching one's partner demonstrate an admirable expertise.

For example, Kate greatly admired Jana's ability to perform and sing. Jana was a good enough amateur actress and singer to get the lead female role in a local production of *The Pirates of Penzance*. She was a smashing success in this part. Kate said: "When I was in the audience watching Jana sing, I was so impressed I got goose bumps. When she came out for her bow, I stood up and cheered like a groupie."

Deep appreciation of partners that only comes with many years of knowing each other can also lead to surges of intense warmth, attraction, and idealizing. Garth recently described the following experience:

> "Lily arranged a surprise party for my forty-fifth birthday. Boy, was I surprised. It never occurred to me that she would go that far out of her way for me. You know how she hates going to big parties, and how she really dislikes hosting. But she went to all sorts of trouble. It was an incredibly beautiful event, and she tracked down some old friends of mine I hadn't seen in years. She was a terrific hostess too, so warm and charming to everyone. She looked spectacular. I found myself watching her move around with such poise and grace, and it suddenly struck me: 'My God, she's the most beautiful, wonderful woman in the world, and I'm the luckiest guy!' "

CHAPTER 9

The Adoring Parent and the Adorable Child

An Idealizing Collusion

PART I: ASSESSMENT

Lola and Max (introduced in Chapter 6) came for consultation about having conflict over their youngest daughter, Phoebe, 26, who had abruptly moved away from their town to live with her boyfriend. Lola was quick to emphasize that their marriage was not the problem, only the wounds caused by the heartless Phoebe. In their early sixties, Lola and Max had been married for forty years and had three children. Max had recently retired. The content and quality of their interaction suggested that idealizing was a dominant pattern of relating.

LOLA: (*speaking in a low, cultivated voice*) Max and I have a wonderful relationship. We're very close and never fight. So these . . . ah . . . unpleasant words we had about Phoebe were rather disturbing. (*sighing*) But we're past that now, I hope.

Her pretty face brightened, and she favored me with a dazzling smile. Lola was petite and pleasingly plump. She was dressed in varying shades of pink, her ample bosom encased in a flowered sweatshirt.

MAX: (*looking troubled*) Lola's still down in the dumps. She was crying the other night . . . alone in the dark bedroom.

Max had an appealing boyish face and elfin ears. The couple looked adorably matched, she like a pink and white cherub, and he like a kindly, impish elf. I felt immediately fond of them and protective.

LOLA: She really did it this time. She hurt me to the core. I can't forgive her for the awful things she said to me, and I can't bear that she's wasting her life on that no good bastard.

MAX: (*nodding*) He's bad news all right. But she thinks he walks on water, no matter how badly he treats her. We told her it was a mistake to move in with him, but she wouldn't listen to us.

LOLA: (*smiling at me*) Max has always babied Phoebe and let her have her own way. She thinks Max can do no wrong. (*Her pleasant delivery clashes with this obvious criticism of Max.*)

MAX: Now wait a minute, Hon. I told her this Derek creep was bad news. I backed you one hundred percent. (*Lola's smile fades.*) I'm just not sure it's a good idea to cut her totally off, that's all. You might be hurt more in the long run. (*He nervously scans Lola's face, as he did intermittently throughout the session, then turns to me.*) You have to understand, Doctor, Lola and Phoebe are opposites. That's a big part of the problem, if you want my opinion. Phoebe is selfish and self-centered . . . let's face it . . . a spoiled brat. And maybe I'm a little responsible for that. She and Lola have a lot of conflict. They're a lot alike . . . uh . . . (*He catches himself and glances nervously at Lola, who seems unaware of his critical slip.*) What I mean is . . . Lola is like the Mother Teresa of our community. She'd do anything for anyone in trouble. Charity is her middle name. Everyone but her youngest daughter thinks she's the most caring person in the world.

LOLA: She just crushes me, and puts down everything I believe in, all those values I so carefully taught her. . . . You should hear how she talks to me.

MAX: You tell us, Doctor, but I think Phoebe has a foul mouth, because Lola is so sweet. (*turning to Lola*) I think she's jealous of your being so popular. Phoebe's never been very popular. (*looking at me*) Everybody loves Lola. (*He beams proudly, but I hear a twist of envy in his tone.*)

LOLA: (*smiling and batting her eyes prettily at Max*) It's you everyone really adores. I don't believe Max has an enemy in the world. He's so goodhearted and trustworthy. He's the best thing that ever happened to me.

MAX: (*Now that a familiar harmony seems to be restored, Max turns to me with a mischievous gleam in his eye.*) So . . . Doctor, what do you think of my theory? I don't know much Freud, except about the Eatable Conflict (*holding up a roll of Lifesavers*). (*Lola groans and I smile graciously at his pun. He offers Lola and me a Lifesaver, which I refuse, then pops one in his mouth.*)

SHARPE: Sounds very plausible. Young women can have a lot of trouble separating from their mothers. Sometimes they have to snarl and spit and carry on doing and being just the opposite of who you are. (*I watch Lola's expression to see how this goes over. She nods in agreement, but her face tightens up like a fist, as though I had just punched her.*)

LOLA: (*in a steely tone*) I couldn't do that with my mother. My mother would've killed me. Literally, I mean that.

MAX: Her mother was a little crazy.

LOLA: (*emphatically*) She was a monster. She was . . . totally evil.

MAX: (*bantering*) But that proves my psychological point, Hon. She was a monster and you're Mother Teresa, and now you're daughter is a selfish brat. See it goes like that, Hon. Bad, good, bad. (*tapping his fingertips against his forehead*) Pretty deep, right, Doctor? I should sit in your chair.

LOLA: (*She looks confused, like she doesn't know whether to laugh or cry. Her troubled face is soon transformed by another dazzling smile.*) Oh, Max, what would I do without you? (*Tears spill out of her eyes, running her mascara, but she holds on to her smile.*)

I remarked on her smiling through her tears. She liked this characterization, saying that was her personality, always trying to make lemonade out of lemons. She said she was through shedding tears about Phoebe and her mother, who had been dead for some years. As I began to inquire further about this relationship, Max shifted the focus back to Phoebe. He wanted advice and clearly hoped I would support his wish to maintain contact with Phoebe. Lola said she felt scared by her eruptions at Max. She wondered if she needed individual help, since she also felt depressed. The last thing they seemed to want was for me to find a problem in their relationship or a need for couple therapy.

Collusive Idealizing

As described in previous chapters, idealization is advantageous in the early phase of a relationship. Romantic idealizing fosters a couple's passionate connection and secures their exclusive bond. This pattern becomes collusive when a couple cannot move beyond the romantic idealizing of the early phase—a mode that only has a short natural life span because of its all-consuming intensity. Such couples find it too painful to lose their ideal perceptions of each other and attempt to keep their relationship in the opening, romantic phase.

In the initial session with Max and Lola, the main characteristics of idealizing collusions are illustrated. First to emerge is the couple's *conception of the relationship as perfect*, usually in accord with the romantic ideal. In conjunction with this idealized conception, there are two distinctive role relationships enacted by the partners of *adoring parent–adorable child and ideal twins*. These role relationships both express a couple's idealizing needs and defend against their shared fears of anger, separateness, and abandonment. Each partner defends against these fears by maintaining the following kinds of unconscious beliefs: *If I am an ideal partner, I will never be left or rejected. If my partner is ideal, he or she will never leave me or be rejecting. If our relationship is ideal, it can never be lost or destroyed.*

A couple's need to defend so rigidly against these fears creates an anxious, restrictive emotional climate. In order for the partners to keep negativity outside of their relationship, they develop a *splitting/scapegoating system* in which a third party becomes the scapegoated repository for critical perceptions and angry feelings about each other.

These characteristics distinguish the defensive aspects of idealizing from those that enhance a relationship, as described in previous chapters. Each of these distinctive characteristics appears on a continuum of defensiveness from mild to severe. The assessment of treatment difficulty usually parallels this severity and rigidity of defensiveness.

Conception of the Relationship as Perfect

Lola and Max strained to perceive and present their relationship as perfect. They described each other in the kind of glowing terms reminiscent of romantic idealizing. While they were sincerely loving and devoted to each other, their idealizing had become more of a protective mechanism than a spontaneous expression of love.

Lola and Max appeared to share the same interests, goals, values, and beliefs. They were very active in the community, engaging in many charitable activities. They were well loved for their warm hospitality and generous giving to those in need. They did everything together, hardly ever disagreed, and never fought. They seemed affectionate and, for their age, had an active sex life. Because of their high degree of togetherness, friends and family also perceived them to have an ideal relationship.

In contrast to this ideal presentation, the emotional climate generated between Lola and Max seemed restrictive, guarded, and anxious. Their extravagant praise of each other did not come across as spontaneously inspired by an upsurge of warm, loving feelings. The superlatives were repetitive, seemed inappropriate at times, and so began to seem compulsively driven. The undercurrents of anxiety and anger between them were palpable.

They expressed positive feelings with far greater ease than negative ones and conveyed considerable devotion, sometimes relating like a brother and sister, and other times like parent and child. Although they reported a regular sex life, Lola was not really interested but dutifully obliged Max in a routinized way.

Partners in idealizing relationships do not usually acknowledge their pervasive anxiety over expressing disagreement and anger toward each other. Anger directed toward a third party is usually much more acceptable. Max revealed his pervasive apprehension about open anger by compulsively scanning Lola's face, talking too much, and needing immediately to placate and make light of everything. Lola seemed to be more frightened of anger and difference than Max. She revealed this anxiety with dramatic shifts from any negative expression toward Max to extravagant, honey-coated praise.

Anger is threatening to idealizing partners because it challenges the main structures of their defense—the "ideal" representations of self, other, and the relationship—and increases their underlying fears. Feeling and expressing anger at one's partner (or the reverse) means either the partner or oneself is imperfect, and, therefore, the relationship is imperfect. Garth said: "I can't stand for either of us to be angry. It means something's wrong. One of us has done something wrong, and I can't tolerate that. It ruins my picture of how things should be."

Moreover, anger threatens the partners' merged twinship by creating a frightening degree of separateness. Lola described this painful reaction in the following way: "When I feel angry at Max because he's hurt me, I feel so alienated and like I've lost my best friend." In addition, both partners consciously think that openly expressed anger will destroy a relationship, leaving each feeling helpless and abandoned like a small child. "I can't tolerate feeling angry at Max or Max being angry at me," said Lola. "It makes me feel very alone and desperate, like my whole world is going to fall apart. I'd do anything to prevent these feelings." These profound fears of anger usually stem from the partners' family experience. In evaluation sessions, it is particularly important to explore how anger was managed in each partner's original family.

The degree of emotional restrictiveness, intensity of anxiety, and underlying hostility varies among couples presenting with collusive idealizing patterns. Often, the longer such a relationship has gone on in this mode, the more polluted the atmosphere with festering anger and cloying counterdisplays of affection. Even though Lola and Max had been together a long time, they did not generate a stultifying climate of impacted rage. Their disturbance was mild in this respect. The degree and intensity of underlying anger seems to determine pervasiveness of anxiety and emotional restriction. I have virtually felt suffocated and unable to move in any direction with some couples, whose underlying hatred is so ancient and impacted it seems mummified.

Idealized Role Relationships

The role relationships of idealizing partners tend to take two basic shapes—adoring parent–adorable child and an ideal twinship. Both of these role relationships may operate together, though one may predominate over the other. Lola and Max appeared to alternate between Lola mothering Max, her naughty but adorable little boy, and the two of them interacting as ideal twins.

The adoring parent–adorable child role relationship is intended to make up for deficits in the partners' childhood relationships with their parents, particularly in the mother–child idealizing bond. Lola and Max both had cold, controlling mothers. In addition, Lola's mother was rageful and cruel. They could never get close to their mothers or please them, even with exceptionally compliant, good behavior. To compensate for this shared deficit, Lola and Max created the missed idealizing mother–child relationship in their marriage. Lola mothered and adored Max, who acted as her adoring, mischievous little boy.

This role relationship is dysfunctional when it requires a constant supply of adoration between the partners and the roles become fixed. Any relationship that does not allow either partner to grow or move into other roles at times will ultimately create resentment in one or both partners. Therapeutic intervention (illustrated in Part II: Treatment) is thus aimed toward changing the perfectionist aspect of the role relationship, so that flaws in both partners are acceptable, and toward creating more flexibility in the roles so that the partner in the parent role can be a child at times and vice versa. Achieving this flexibility then enables both partners to act as collaborating adults when appropriate.

As noted previously, the twinning aspect of idealizing relationships stems from great needs of partners to be mirrored, to be supported and admired by someone just like oneself.[1] In addition, idealizing partners have often had vitally important relationships with their siblings in growing up. As is so often the case in families with disengaged, neglectful, or abusive parents, sibling relationships can become crucial to emotional survival. In growing up, both Lola and Max had created idealizing bonds with a sibling that substituted for this deficit in the relationship with their mothers. The positive, idealizing aspects of Lola's relationship with her

---

[1]See Chapter 6, pp. 115–118, for discussion of twinning as a pattern of merging.

younger brother, and Max's with his older sister, had been transferred to their marriage.

Pseudomutuality and Submergence of Identity

Although Lola and Max were devoted to each other, their apparent mutuality in the relationship was not a solid achievement. Their togetherness did not come about through any real sharing, processing, and synthesizing of who they were as individuals. Differences between them had been suppressed by one or the other in the major areas of living.

In order to maintain this pseudomutual veneer of togetherness, one or both partners must submerge their identity and individuality to the other in certain major respects. It is normal to submerge aspects of oneself that may conflict with the partner in the early phase of a relationship, as long as it is temporary.

Max had generally allowed Lola to plan and run their lives. Although he liked being passive and dependent, he also deeply resented never being able to do what he wanted. At the same time he had trouble formulating what he did want to do with his time. In an individual evaluation session, he revealed feeling trapped into spending all day with Lola, tagging along with her plans

Lola had submerged her identity to Max in other crucial areas. She was totally passive in the sexual arena, feeling it was best just to oblige Max. She also submerged much of herself to Max in conversation and social interaction. Not only did he dominate by talking a great deal more, but she also allowed him to control the subject and emotional tone. In their first session, I could see Lola struggle to express herself in greater depth, but Max would interfere and direct the subject or the emotional tone somewhere else. He was clearly more comfortable away from emotions and with himself at center stage as the teasing entertainer. Since Lola was also threatened by expressing her negative feelings, I could see her mixed reaction to his interference—disappointment in his lack of empathy, yet relief at being rescued from painful emotions.

Submerging aspects of one's identity to the partner fulfills merging, mirroring, and twinning needs, but also protects each partner from feeling too separate. Idealizing in the twinship mode protects against these fears, because the partners are continuously reassured of being connected and adequate.

Splitting and Scapegoating

In order for couples like Lola and Max to sustain their mutual idealizing, negative feelings toward each other need to be redirected from the spouse onto something outside the relationship—a third person, one partner's illness (emotional or physical), or an external circumstance. To achieve this end, two psychological processes are involved: splitting and scapegoating.

In an idealizing system (as in a devaluing system), feelings and representations of people are split into unmodulated extremes of all good and all bad. In their first session, Lola and Max presented their feelings and views in this way. Lola was a saint, but her mother was a monster. Max was wonderful, but Phoebe was cruel and unacceptable. Then a repository or third party is needed to contain one partner's disowned bad feelings about the other and about him- or herself. The process of attributing or projecting bad traits, feelings, or behavior onto a third party is called scapegoating, and the unlucky object selected is the scapegoat. Unfortunately, in families, a child is often selected to be the scapegoat.

SCAPEGOATING A CHILD

Long-term maintenance of an idealizing mode may not present major problems until a child is added to the dyad and pays the dreadful price for the couple's maintenance of their idealization. Such couples usually have tremendous difficulty integrating a child into their relationship, since their idealizing adjustment depends on being an exclusive dyad, wherein each partner is the one and only to the other. This problem is usually compounded in second marriages, with the advent of partners' stepchildren. The child or children are oftentimes included in the relationship by becoming one or both partners' scapegoat(s).[2]

The child is also likely to be used as a repository for one or both partners' negative self-images, since the idealizing couple defense is also intended to preserve a perfect self-image. Lola projected her disavowed wishes to be angry, demanding, and selfish onto Phoebe, and Max created a coalition with Phoebe to express his disavowed anger toward Lola. The defense mechanism of projective identification comes into play when the scapegoat is induced to act out the projected role. Phoebe was induced to act out her parents' angry feelings and to fulfill her role assignment of being a selfish, spoiled brat.

The degree of destructiveness to the child, couple, and family as a unit depends on the intensity of the hatred, anger, or craziness projected

---

[2]A child can also be used by devaluing couples, for the opposite purpose, as the repository for their idealized perceptions. In this equally destructive defensive system, one or both spouses are denigrated and the child is idealized.

by the parents. Additionally, the child's vulnerability to the projections is also a significant factor in sustaining a scapegoating system. Lola, Max, and Phoebe presented a relatively mild degree of disturbance in this respect because of the good mental health of Phoebe, who not only fought her parents' projections tooth and nail but also made great efforts to separate and individuate. I based this evaluation not only on Max's and Lola's descriptions of a feisty, independent Phoebe, but also on reports from Phoebe's therapist (who was supporting a delayed adolescent separation process).

Severe pathology in this area can be extremely destructive to a child, usually creating serious emotional disturbance or mental illness. In their study of disturbed families, Ezra Vogel and Norman Bell (1981) provide an excellent discussion of the emotionally disturbed child as the family scapegoat. I rarely see this kind of couple, because they do not usually come for couple therapy, at least not on their own initiative. These are the couples that get treatment in conjunction with their child's emotional illness in clinics, residential treatment centers, and hospitals. Treatment of these couples and their disturbed children and adolescents has been extensively discussed in the family literature by many researchers, including Wynne et al. (1958), Bowen (1961, 1966), Boszormenyi-Nagy and Framo (1962, 1965), Haley and Hoffman (1967), Zinner and Shapiro (1975), and Scharff and Scharff (1987).

When the scapegoat is chosen outside of the nuclear family, for example, the partners' parents or siblings, a boss, or other authority figure, this defense is much less destructive for the nuclear family. One couple kept their mutual idealization pure and safe by directing all of their hatred and disillusionment onto their "corrupt, evil" religious leader. Their children appeared to fare very well. While these are not optimal adjustments, they are far better than sacrificing a child. Often, more than one scapegoat is needed. Lola and Max used Lola's crazy mother, as well as their children, as a scapegoat.

SCAPEGOATING ONE PARTNER'S ILLNESS

Next in degree of potential destructiveness is the scapegoating of an illness or condition of one of the spouses. Such conditions can be a physical illness, a substance abuse disorder, or any kind of emotional problem. Lola's depression was an aspect of this couple's presenting problems. The couple attributed this depression to Phoebe's departure. However, it was clear to me that Lola's depression also related to feeling angry at and emotionally deserted by Max (in addition to resurrection of unresolved grief in relation to her mother). Additionally, the loss of Phoebe as a repository for Lola's projections of self-hate also contributed to her becoming depressed.

Idealizing couples never relate the cause of the condition to the partner or the relationship. The condition, always considered to be caused by something else, becomes the explanation for whatever feels wrong or bad in the relationship. Partners will speak of the condition almost as though it were an alien entity. Lola and Max referred to Lola's depression as "The Depression." It was The Depression that caused Lola to get upset with Max and made them to feel more tense and distant from each other. Lola's depression had resulted in a couple of shocking (to them both) rages and verbal assaults on Max. These events were alternately blamed on Phoebe's awful behavior or Lola's depression. Thus, Max and Lola really had two scapegoats: Phoebe and The Depression.

My experience with severe forms of merged idealizing relationships has mainly been in the individual treatment of the "sick" partner. In these instances, it appears that the health of one partner has been sacrificed to maintain the couple's idealizing system. Usually, these couples will refuse to consider conjoint treatment because neither feels there is a problem in the relationship. If the "sick" partner gets better and begins to separate, the other partner is often then motivated to seek help. Alternatively, the couple may enter conjoint treatment, or the treated partner may leave the "sick" relationship.

SCAPEGOATING AN EXTERNAL CIRCUMSTANCE

Least harmful is the use of an external circumstance as a scapegoat, because this process only involves simple projection onto a distant object. No destructive psychological manipulation of that object occurs, and challenging external circumstances, as long as they are not too stressful, can act as an aid in bolstering and preserving a mutual idealizing bond. For example, couples living under an oppressive regime can use the government as a deserving scapegoat for all of their interpersonal negativity and hatred. A Chinese couple I knew who hated their oppressive government and struggled for many years to come to America only developed problems in their marriage when they were comfortably settled here, without an outside enemy.

Couples who must buck larger societal disapproval, such as gay and lesbian or mixed-race couples, can strengthen their idealizing defense by scapegoating mainstream society—the establishment ("We are together against a hostile world"). Families that disapprove of a couple's union can be used in this way. Rebellion may contribute an important ingredient in conjunction with scapegoating, as with Romeo and Juliet, whose passion was inflamed by their families' disapproval.

STABILITY OF SPLITTING AND SCAPEGOATING
IN IDEALIZING SYSTEMS

A stable system, with the therapist idealized, is much more advantageous for therapeutic work, since a therapeutic alliance can be rapidly formed and sustained with the couple. In working with severely disturbed, devaluing couples, establishing and maintaining a therapeutic alliance can become the focal point of therapy, since little can be accomplished without it.

Max's and Lola's tendency to split good and bad initially worked in my favor, giving me an extra boost into their good graces and trust. Their assignment of people to extreme categories tended to remain quite stable once they categorized them. Their idealization of each other had gone on for forty years, and Lola's hatred of her mother for much longer. It seemed a safe bet that once cast in the ideal mother role, I was likely to remain there unless I too abruptly and profoundly disappointed them.

However, a couple's stable idealizing of the therapist (an idealizing transference) also presents an array of predictable problems for treatment.[3] Such global kinds of idealizing always carry with them great expectations of the one idealized, both in life and in therapy. I was dimly aware at the time of their wishes for me to fulfill their need for an ideal mother on the one hand, and to be their ideal child, who would never challenge or leave them, as the ungrateful Phoebe had done, on the other. When such expectations are disappointed, a couple is bound to feel intensely disillusioned and angry with the therapist. With Lola and Max, I was always subliminally aware that a fall from grace was inevitable and that when it happened, it would be a hard, painful fall.

PART II: TREATMENT

Working with idealizing couples can evoke the most extreme reactions in the therapist of affection, devotion, anxiety, and pain. These couples want to be special and often succeed in this quest with the therapist. The kind of relationship that therapists find themselves entering with idealizing couples is distinctive, diagnostic, and very seductive.

In the first session, I felt affection toward Max and Lola. Not only were they likable people, but they were also very appealing in their displayed warmth and responsiveness toward me. I was the object of an in-

---

[3]I say predictable now, in retrospect. I did not clearly see the ramifications at the time, for I had not yet closely studied idealizing patterns, transferences, and countertransferences in couple therapy. Lola and Max provided the inspiration for intensive study of this subject.

stant idealization, which felt very nurturing and confirming. At the end of the session, feeling a little high and pleased with myself, I was reminded of why this mode of relating is so compelling. I could feel myself drawn into their orbit, wanting to idealize them in return. In psychological terms, this is the initial transference–countertransference paradigm characteristically induced by idealizing couples (also see Sharpe, 1997).

What I intuited but could not articulate at the time was the unconscious *mutual idealizing contract* they were offering me: *"We will idealize you, make you feel special if you will make us feel special, and ensure the survival of our relationship by hiding our disappointment and anger with each other, for these feelings would destroy our relationship and expose our insecurities and fears of abandonment."* In short, this mutual idealizing pact is quite similar to the one they unconsciously made with each other at the beginning of their relationship.

This mutual endowment of specialness, or mutual idealizing, gives the therapist certain advantages and disadvantages in working with these couples. The advantage is that the therapist is given more power and authority than is bestowed by couples presenting with other kinds of patterns. The disadvantage is that the therapist may become dependent on being adored and will find it increasingly difficult to confront appropriately a couple's dysfunctional patterns. Just as the partners wish to avoid deidealization, so does the therapist. Staying enmeshed too long, or forever, in this mutual idealization is probably the main countertransference pitfall in working with these couples and can create an extended impasse or failure in treatment. Making therapeutic use of this almost inevitable occurrence is described later.

The Evaluation

The previously described six-session evaluation format[4] (including both individual and conjoint sessions) is particularly well suited to idealizing couples, because their dynamics are more complex than those of other kinds of couples. Combining treatment modalities is more likely to engage this kind of couple in treatment, provide consistency in ongoing treatment, and result in overall success. Early on in treatment, the partners allow much greater access to their negative feelings about each other in individual sessions, because they are freer from fears of provoking each other's open expression of anger. If they are only seen conjointly, their collusion to deny hurt and anger can be impenetrable.

With certain couples (particularly those with devaluing and competi-

---

[4]See pp. 19–20.

tive patterns), individual sessions may be contraindicated because they incite too much anxiety and rivalry between the partners. A strictly conjoint modality of treatment is usually necessary throughout treatment. However, because idealizing partners tend to form a strongly positive, idealizing transference to the therapist, they are able to trust the therapist's recommendations and do not inordinately fear the formation of coalitions. Unlike other kinds of couples, idealizing partners are not looking for the therapist to point the finger at the partner. Instead, they wish for nothing to be wrong with the partner or the relationship. After they have expressed their negative feelings about each other in individual sessions, the therapist can then support each partner to express them in conjoint sessions.

Therapeutic aims during the evaluation, which are quite specific, wide-ranging, and challenging include (1) softening the idealizing defense through understanding the underlying feelings and fears that fuel it, (2) identifying the developmental transitions (or other stressful events) that have disrupted the balance of the couple's relationship, (3) identifying interactional vicious circles that have been created in response to the stressors, (4) identifying the couple's fears of difference, anger, and conflict as ongoing problems in the relationship, (5) beginning exploration of the role and meanings of the scapegoat(s).

The therapist also aims to engage the couple collaboratively in working toward these goals, so that the partners can accept the existence of problems in their relationship and thus be motivated to undertake further therapy. This task is unique to this kind of couple that comes for consultation with the problem located outside of the relationship. The cause of any difficulties is projected onto a scapegoated child (or other family member) or the illness of one of the partners. The therapeutic necessity of getting the problem back into the couple relationship, so that meaningful therapeutic work can even begin, presents a difficult and sometimes insurmountable task for the therapist.

First Conjoint Session: Softening the Idealizing Defense

Although a direct challenge to their pervasive idealizing would likely alienate the couple in the first session, interventions aimed toward softening the rigidity of this defense are helpful. The therapist achieves the softening of the idealizing defense by emphasizing the normality and expectability of anxiety, anger, and conflict as a response to stressful events, such as developmental transitions. This reassures the partners that their relationship is not necessarily on the road to destruction and gives a strong message that a good relationship includes anger and conflict. This intervention indirectly challenges their idealizing belief system and must be repeated many times to make any lasting impact. Additionally, it is helpful to support any sign of open expression by partners of the feelings they fear.

In the first session with Max and Lola, I underscored that conflict between partners is to be expected, especially during stressful times. I said, "Conflict may be particularly frightening to you, since your relationship has been so successfully managed without conflict and open anger. That's right," Lola replied. "We hardly ever fight, and we've never raised our voices before." Max looked skeptical of this statement but remained quiet. Supporting the desirability of some conflict I said, "Even though having this conflict is causing you a lot of anxiety, there will be a better resolution because of facing these differences more squarely now. Because separating is so difficult for parents and children, it's not unusual for anger to become the way everyone tries to cope. It's easier to say goodbye when you're each mad at the other."

They both seemed to find solace in my words of explanation and support. They readily agreed to participate in further evaluation (including two individual sessions for each) before making decisions about cutting off contact with Phoebe or the best modality of treatment.

Individual Evaluation Session with Max

In his first individual evaluation session, I asked Max how he felt about being retired. After expressing relief in being out of the rat race, he hemmed and hawed for a while, and finally got to the point.

> "I was a little big shot at work. I had a few guys reporting to me. I've got nobody to boss around at home. Lola runs the show. Even the animals look to her for direction. Understand, Doctor, I don't mind my position. I was raised to be a number-two kind of guy, and Lola is a number-one kind a gal. We're a perfect match."

All of this was said in his usual jocular tone, but of course, Max really did mind, and I said it would be hard not to be bothered, even resentful, about his loss of status. Although he made more jokes, I could see that this statement of his underlying feelings registered. In discussing his relationship with Lola, I mentioned his lack of complaints. He indicated that while Lola might complain about him, he had no complaints about her. When I asked to hear her complaints, he responded without hesitation.

MAX: I'm a slob. Lola doesn't like that. She's very fastidious. I procrastinate getting things done. Lola's very organized and punctual. She thinks I'm a pushover with the kids and everyone else, and she does-n't like my politics. She's not just liberal, she's a flaming radical. She sees red when I let slip with one of my right-wing zingers. (*pausing*) So, that's about it . . . I think.

SHARPE: I get the impression that it's okay with you for her to have complaints but not for you.

MAX: (*grinning*) She's got a lot more to complain about.

SHARPE: (*skeptically*) Really? As far as I know, you can't live with someone without some friction and complaints. (*waiting a few beats*) So, let's hear yours.

MAX: I don't really have any. (*He sits quietly for a moment. I wait expectantly.*) Sex could be better, I guess. And I don't much like going out to lunch all the time. It drives me nuts. But Lola's not really the problem. The real problem is that I don't have enough to do with my time, and I let her figure it out for me.

Rather than exploring his problem, I focused back on his complaints. He tolerated a brief discussion about his feelings of being controlled and Lola's lack of sexual interest. He felt she complied with his needs but just to oblige him. Her lack of interest had been long-standing but seemed worse to him since his retirement.

MAX: Or maybe I'm just more horny and not looking so good to her any-more. I've gained a few extra pounds. (*He pats a slight paunch.*)

SHARPE: Have you ever discussed any of these feelings with Lola?

MAX: (*suddenly tensing*) You won't be telling her what I've said will you?

SHARPE: Not without your permission.

MAX: Well, what she doesn't hear can't hurt her.

SHARPE: You're worried that what you've said would hurt Lola?

MAX: You got it. She's very sensitive, and it's not a good idea to cross Lola. I know how Phoebe feels sometimes. Her mother can be pretty scary. (*He hesitates and I encourage him to elaborate.*) She has big reac-tions to small things. She gets very hurt . . . and angry, I think, but it's hard to tell what's going on. She goes silent, and she looks right through you with this icy glare. Sometimes she won't even speak for a day or two.

SHARPE: That sounds difficult, like you need to walk on eggs.

MAX: (*dismissing my attempt to empathize*) It's not that bad. If you play along, things are fine.

SHARPE: Sounds like you're saying Lola runs things?

MAX: (*chuckling*) Yeah, it does sound that way, doesn't it? But I have ways of controlling things behind the scenes. . . . (*hesitating*)

SHARPE: How do you do that?

MAX: Well, I've always tried to calm the ruffled feathers between Lola and the kids. Lola . . . well, Lola is kinda of harsh with the kids, especially Phoebe. I've been talking to Phoebe. . . . Lola doesn't know this . . . but I'm trying to get her to apologize to her mother. I know Lola won't make the first move. So you see, Doctor, I pull some strings; I try to manipulate things on the sly. Sometimes I cause more trouble than good. (*He grins again, rather proudly.*)

I speculated that Max had been able to tolerate his resentment of Lola's control fairly well when he worked full time and before all of the children left home. However, the circumstances of retirement had decreased Max's self-esteem and increased his resentment of Lola's domination. Phoebe's departure left him more at the mercy of his wife's increasing needs and demands. Additionally, he felt injured and angry about Lola's lack of sexual interest. Since retirement, sexual intimacy had become more important to him as a means of bolstering his self-esteem and masculine identity. He could only feel safe in expressing his needs and anger covertly, through passive–aggressive behavior such as cluttering and procrastination.

In this session, rather than promoting recognition of his contribution to problems, I encouraged Max to complain about Lola. With many couples, an early treatment aim is to stop blaming and foster self-awareness, but idealizing partners need to be encouraged to complain about each other (instead of the scapegoat) before work on who brings what to the relationship can effectively begin.

Individual Sessions with Lola

Lola's hurt and angry feelings toward Max were less accessible than his towards her. She tended to blame Phoebe for all of her negative reactions. She resisted focusing much attention on her relationship with Max. We spent much of her first individual session on her feelings about Phoebe and her unhappy childhood with a rageful, neglecting mother.

Phoebe became Lola's problem child and scapegoat for a number of reasons. Temperamentally, Phoebe had always been more independent, aggressive, and volatile than her older more compliant sister and brother. She was defiant, demanding, and had big temper tantrums. These qualities were reminiscent of Lola's mother. Additionally, Phoebe seemed to represent Lola's suppressed wishes to be childishly selfish and openly angry. As a child, Lola had been required to be absolutely compliant and perfectly behaved like a little grown-up.

Although Lola proclaimed Phoebe's leaving to be a good thing and cried, "Good riddance!," she intermittently felt a deep sadness and longing for a better relationship with her daughter, though this awareness was repressed most of the time. I thought she was depressed by the loss of Phoebe, experiencing her daughter's departure as abandonment and rejection. But she was also weighed down with unconscious guilt about her feelings of failure as a mother and her own rejection of Phoebe. Anguish about her relationship with her own mother was also rekindled.

Lola's feelings about Phoebe's alliance with Max were highlighted in the next session. When she discovered Max's "secret," placating phone calls to Phoebe, she could not so easily excuse Max and just blame Phoebe. She tearfully reported this discovery in her second individual session.

LOLA: I overheard him on the telephone sweet-talking Phoebe and even joking around with her. I was shocked. I actually yelled at him. I hardly ever raise my voice, let alone yell. I haven't spoken to him since. I don't understand how he could do this. He's always protected and coddled the kids, no matter what they did, especially Phoebe.

SHARPE: You must feel hurt and betrayed.

LOLA: Yes, yes I do. I feel he's joining with her against me. I just can't believe it. He just has to be liked by everyone at all times. (*She stops suddenly, looking acutely miserable.*) That Phoebe, she knows just how to wrap him around her little finger. She's such a manipulator. She probably put him up to this somehow.

The shift of her anger from Max to Phoebe was striking. However, I didn't feel the timing was right for pointing out this pattern to her. I sensed she would need to be less conflicted about feeling angry at Max before this displacement could be effectively confronted. I attempted to keep her focused on Max.

SHARPE: Has this sort of thing happened before?

LOLA: His going behind my back with the kids? Oh, sure. He's like a kid, too. He just can't help himself.

SHARPE: It does sound undermining of your authority . . . and angering.

LOLA: Well, yes . . . it is . . . but I know he doesn't mean any harm. He tries to fix things, and I always forgive him. He's such a good man and a good father most of the time. I'd be lost without him.

SHARPE: Yes, I know that. There's no doubt that you love Max and think the world of him. But it seems you're very uncomfortable with complaining about him or feeling angry when he does things that hurt you.

LOLA: That's true, I'm very uncomfortable being upset with Max.

SHARPE: (*attempting to interpret Lola's difficulty with ambivalent feelings*) It seems as though you fear being angry at Max will destroy your love.

LOLA: (*quiet for a moment, taking this in*) I feel terrible being angry. I hate anger. (*Her voice trembles.*) My mother destroyed everything with her anger. Believe me, there was no love anywhere around when my mother got into a rage.

Identifying Developmental Transitions, Vicious Circles, and Anger

Idealizing couples most often come into therapy because of the stress to their relationship caused by one or more developmental transitions. Pregnancy and the birth of a child, usually the first major threats to the partners' exclusive attachment, will often provoke great distress (as discussed in a previous section). A child separating at various phases and finally leaving home will upset the relationship balance, because feelings of loss, abandonment, rejection, and anger are stimulated—feelings that are particularly threatening to idealizing partners. Additionally, if the separating child is a scapegoat, this transition disrupts a couple's splitting–scapegoating system. Retirement can be threatening, because partners' expectations and needs dramatically change. The increase in time together disrupts a couple's accustomed degree of closeness. To successfully manage this transition, the partners differing needs require discussion and working out. These couples have not developed such ways to acknowledge and discuss differing needs because of their mutual idealizing contract.

The balance in Max and Lola's relationship was upset by two of these developmental transitions: a child leaving home and Max's retirement. When a couple cannot integrate the necessary changes required by these transitions, the partners' anxiety will create a vicious circle. Identifying this dynamic and its causes is one of the most useful assessments that can be made during the evaluation.

The vicious circle created between Max and Lola emerged more clearly in their individual evaluation sessions. Phoebe's leaving home provoked considerable anxiety in both partners, but especially in Lola, who was more sensitive to abandonment. With Phoebe's "abandonment," Lola became even more insistent that Max stay very close.

Max, however, had to contend with his own anxieties about retirement. He was chafing at the constant togetherness desired and organized by Lola. For idealizing couples in general, the increased time together brought about by retirement removes employment as an acceptable reason for the partners to be separate. Thus, any self-esteem gained from this source of independence can no longer continue.

In Max and Lola's marriage, it was not acceptable to *want* to be away from each other. In idealizing relationships in general, an accepted system of being together and being separate, based on each partner's individual needs and wishes, has not developed. Consequently, the more passive partner, like Max, begins to feel trapped and resentful, with so much togetherness enforced by the more dominant spouse. When the passive partner is a man, insecurities about masculinity are also likely to be exacerbated, since there is no longer a work identity to provide an arena in which to feel manly. Like Max, many men focus on sexuality as a way of meeting needs for intimacy while at the same time enhancing feelings of masculinity.

Consequently, Max could not respond adequately to Lola's needs for greater closeness. She wanted him to do everything with her. Conversely, she was not able to respond to his needs for greater intimacy in their sexual relationship, in part as a reaction to feeling rejected by Max, and in part because of her own lifelong inhibitions in this area. Each went through the motions of doing what the other wanted but with an obvious lack of enthusiasm. Max covertly expressed his anger and wishes for independence by increasing his passive–aggressive behavior. Lola experienced his covertly expressed anger and desire for greater independence as rejection, which exacerbated her need to be reassured of his love. She tried to get this reassurance through increased demands for togetherness on her terms. However, when she felt too rejected and hurt by Max, she would abruptly withdraw from him.

Lola's erratic behavior left Max alternately feeling controlled by her demands for his presence and abandoned when she withdrew. These feelings further exacerbated his own fears, anger, and rejecting behavior. This vicious circle left each partner increasingly bruised and angry. Since Phoebe had removed herself from the triangle by leaving town, attempts to diffuse their painful feelings by scapegoating their daughter were no longer possible.

Because Lola and Max were so fearful of finding fault with each other, having different needs, or acknowledging angry feelings, they could not find their own way out of this painful dynamic. The therapist can helpfully intervene by framing their differing needs and fear of anger as problems in the relationship while at the same time giving permission for their existence and expression. In giving permission, the therapist uses his or her authority to expand the couple's conception of a love relationship to incorporate difference and conflict.

In individual evaluation sessions with Max and Lola, I could identify their fears of feeling critical and angry toward each other, encouraging more open expression of these feelings, while at the same time building a therapeutic alliance with each partner. Because of their tremendous fears of conflict and need for an idealizing connection, I doubt that I could have achieved the depth of exploration and therapeutic alliance by staying only in a conjoint modality.

Final Conjoint Evaluation Session

Once the partners wounded feelings have been made accessible in individual sessions, it is then possible to interpret in a conjoint session the interactive aspects of their vicious circle, one of the first interventions that exposes the workings of the idealizing system. This intervention does not overly threaten the system but explains to the couple why their relationship has become disrupted and hurtful. The therapist verbalizes each partner's underlying feelings of anxiety, abandonment, rejection, and anger. In the final conjoint evaluation session, after first highlighting the strengths of their relationship, I continued:

SHARPE: I think two events have affected your relationship and put quite a bit of stress on both of you. One is your retirement, Max, and the big adjustment that entails. The other is Phoebe's departure and all the difficult feelings that have been stirred up by that. (*Both nod agreeably, and I wait for their responses.*)

MAX: (*to Lola*) Well, we talked some about my reactions to retirement. The doctor thinks I don't feel as good about myself since I retired. She thinks I'm having a problem being a lap dog. (*This "joke" and his chuckle are met with a chilly silence.*)

LOLA: (*sharply*) That's not funny, Max.

SHARPE: Max, I think you're having trouble telling Lola how you feel in a direct way, possibly for fear she'll be hurt and angry.

MAX: I don't want to hurt Lola. That's the last thing I want to do.

SHARPE: Well, think for a moment of what the effect might be of your calling yourself a lapdog. It sounds like you're putting yourself down . . . but I think Lola could also feel put down as well.

LOLA: Absolutely, I felt put down. Like that's how I treat you or something.

MAX: No, no. I didn't mean that. I was just kidding around.

LOLA: Some of your jokes don't always feel so good . . . like the little trick you played on me the other night . . . the call to Phoebe.

MAX: (*looking scared*) I'm in over my head. Could you help me out here, Doctor?

SHARPE: You're starting to have a fight. I know it doesn't feel very good, since you're not practiced at it. (*They avoid looking at each other. Lola stares out the window, her soft face hardened into a mask. Max, stripped of his clowning defense, seems at a total loss.*) Max you're having trouble telling Lola that you're having some problems, like most men do, with retirement and not feeling as important as you once did.

LOLA: (*coldly polite*) I can understand that. What's going to hurt me about that?

MAX: (*to me*) Could you explain this? I don't say these things right.

I obliged by speaking about the effects of retirement on couples in general, with emphasis on the man's diminished sense of control and importance. I suggested that Max, in trying to cope with feelings of resentment, sometimes expressed himself in hurtful ways to Lola.

MAX: (*innocently*) Uh . . . like what?

LOLA: Like calling Phoebe behind my back after we agreed to wait. Like saying funny things that have a mean edge, like that lap dog thing.

MAX: (*a little belligerently*) But I didn't mean any harm.

Then Max abruptly shifted to blaming himself for all tensions between them, at which point Lola proclaimed that her depression about Phoebe was the cause of problems. I said neither was the problem, but that it was important to understand the effect on them of Max's retirement and Phoebe's leaving home. I addressed Lola.

SHARPE: I think Phoebe's leaving has been especially hard on you. As we discussed, it's brought up your feelings of being a failure as a mother and a daughter. These feelings would make you need Max more. Then, when Max can't be there for you the way you need him, I think you feel rejected and angry. But you try very hard not to feel these feelings and work to suppress them, as you learned to do growing up.

LOLA: That's a very accurate description. Thank you. [Her receptiveness encouraged me to continue.]

SHARPE: To Max, your reactions may feel like being pulled close at one moment and pushed away at another, but he doesn't understand what's going on. He gets to feeling pushed around and resentful, but he tries to suppress that reaction, since you're both always working full time not to be angry at one another.

MAX: You got that right, Doctor.

I went on to say that the main obstacle I saw in their working through these kinds of feelings was their fear of conflict. Both agreed that they made great efforts not to fight. Lola said she was terrified of conflict, and I asked her to talk about her fears.

LOLA: In my childhood, I only saw destruction come from anger and fighting. I expect the same thing. If we start fighting our relationship would be destroyed. We'd end up divorcing.

MAX: I think I feel the same way, but I didn't have Lola's experience. My parents were at war, but they hardly spoke to each other.

SHARPE: So neither of you had models of parents talking to each other about what feels hurtful and why.

LOLA: (*bitterly*) What a concept.

Max and Lola continued to discuss their parents' marriages and what poor models of caring and communication they presented. I underscored their shared experience in having suppressed negative feelings as children.

In the course of this evaluation, the partners' immediate pain was eased through explanation and acknowledgment of their underlying feelings. Their old balance was temporarily restored but with an important change: Complaints and differences were now allowed into the relationship. Both had come to intellectually accept that a problem existed in their way of relating, and that this problem could improve with more meaningful communication attainable through ongoing therapeutic work. To a certain extent, the problem had been relocated from the scapegoat back into the couple relationship. Additionally, their ideal of a couple relationship had become a little more flexible and realistic.

For those couples who only wish immediate relief from pain and a restoration of the old balance, these changes may satisfy their need for therapeutic help. Other couples, like Lola and Max, become motivated to pursue more extensive therapy, recognizing that improved communication could result in less fear and a more comfortably close and satisfying relationship.

With those couples who cannot engage in self-exploration or couple work, and who persist in a total focus on the scapegoated child, family therapy may be a necessary initial approach. But when a couple like Lola and Max can be engaged to work on their relationship, a family therapy approach is not initially indicated, because it would support a blurring of who has the problem instead of keeping the problem more clearly and consistently focused in the couple's relationship.

Early Phase: Fear of Conflict and Resistance to Change

Idealizing couples like Lola and Max, who wish to please the therapist, quickly form a trusting alliance and are quite cooperative early in treatment. The idealized therapist is vested with considerable authority and can appear to make good progress in a short time. However, as therapy continues, the power of this collusion becomes more apparent. A therapist who understands this defense can appear to achieve a number of treatment aims in the early phase. However, these achievements are not really integrated by the couple for a long time. Fundamental fears of an angry conflict resulting in abandonment are so profound that partners will inevitably retreat when these changes cause negative feelings to surface and the likelihood of conflict. They will quietly, politely, but nonetheless tenaciously, refuse to give up their need to deny problems. This resistance is most commonly expressed in couples' withdrawal from therapy after any conflict is experienced or when a conflict is likely to surface. Therapists can be easily fooled into thinking they have succeeded with a couple when they have only just begun, as the partners wave a smiling good-bye, saying, "Everything's fine now, and thank you very much."

This resistance is particularly difficult to deal with therapeutically because the couple will applaud their improvement and the therapist's help and may see no need to continue treatment or to meet as frequently (i.e., "We only need to come every other week or once a month"). Other forms of resistance include cancellation of appointments, especially when angry feelings are coming to the surface, or following a difficult therapy session. If a couple does persist with therapy on a regular basis, the partners will attempt to make the couple work superficial, though one or both partners will often be quite cooperative in working with family-of-origin material, since this does not directly threaten the couple relationship. As with Lola and Max, the partners may skillfully attempt to create a social hour rather than a therapy hour.

Seduction of the Therapist: Mutual Idealization

As we settled into ongoing conjoint treatment with the general goal of improving understanding and communication, Lola and Max did everything in their power—and they were exceptionally creative—to seduce me into their idealizing system. Therapy sessions became like visits to a beloved friend or relative. They brought candy and baked goods to the sessions, enticing me to join them in a little snack. They did their best to take care of me through careful observation or cleverly inducing me to reveal personal information. For example, when they found out I like chocolate, they would bring me chocolate. Although for the most part I resisted eating their food, the therapy sessions began to seem like festive tea parties.

While I felt very important and cared for, I also felt increasingly uncomfortable with their rather driven attempts to meet my needs and in
danger of losing sight of my job as their therapist. I was aware of my reluctance to disrupt the surface harmony, jolly atmosphere, and mutual
idealization. I was hesitant to do anything that would make them feel rejected, angry at me, or disappointed in me, such as reminding them of
the purpose of our sessions, exploring the meaning of their bringing
food, or more aggressively tackling the reality of their deeper anger and
disappointment with each other. I was finally shaken out of our cozy
idealizing collusion by the following event: One day—it happened to be
my birthday—I listened to a message on my answering machine. The
message was Max and Lola singing "Happy Birthday" to me. I was momentarily touched but then upset that they had found out the date of
my birthday. I recalled that when Lola had mentioned the date of her
birthday, I had let slip that my birth date was the same. Confronted
with this lapse, I could no longer deny my collusion with their wish to
make me one of the family.

I had identified not only with the role of the longed for "ideal"
mother but also with the "ideal" daughter, who would always lovingly
comply (and never leave them, as their real, ingrate daughter had done.) I
recognized their wish for me to fulfill the role of their good compliant
child as a reaction to the loss of their daughter and as a reversal of their
own childhood experiences with depriving, narcissistic mothers. I was
particularly vulnerable to responding to this role of child because my own
mother was dying when Lola and Max entered therapy.

With an understanding of my countertransference reactions in terms
of the couple's needs and our dovetailing losses, I was in a better position
to work out of this collusion and pursue appropriate treatment. I realized
I was in collusion to avoid their deidealization of me (and me of them),
just as they wished to avoid this process with each other and had successfully done so for forty years.

Deidealization: The Therapist Steps Down from the Pedestal

Helping this couple in a significant way meant encouraging and supporting them through deidealizing each other, so that painful feelings and
critical perceptions could be fully accepted in their relationship. Their
concept of a relationship needed to make room for each partner's individual needs, imperfections, and full array of negative emotions. The partners should be able to disagree with each other and fight, if necessary,
without fearing abandonment, rejection, and destruction of their relationship. With the partners' achievement of these capabilities in a lasting way,
idealizing becomes one of many modes of perceiving and relating that en-

rich a relationship, instead of being the central mode, operating as a growth-inhibiting mechanism of defense.

With Lola and Max, as with many other couples, the deidealization process needed to start with me. I had to be the first one willing to descend from the pedestal and face the unpleasant consequences.

At our next session, I was greeted by Max carrying a bigger bag of food than usual. I waited until they had settled into their seats.

SHARPE: I thought we should assess where we are in therapy. [As they spread out their snacks for a picnic lunch, the term "therapy" sounded absurd.] I've been wondering how you feel about our progress.

MAX: (*gaily*) I've been making progress on cleaning up the garage.

LOLA: Oh, Max, she doesn't mean that. She means about us—how we're doing together, how we're communicating.

MAX: (*munching on a pickle*) Never better, thanks to you, Doctor. In a perfect world, I wouldn't mind a little more sex, but other than that . . .

LOLA: I don't feel as down as I did. It seems we're over that rough patch. We haven't heard from Phoebe in a month. That's fine with me. No news is good news.

The flow of conversation suddenly stopped, the silence punctuated by the rustling of paper bags and sandwich wrappers. They'd gotten the drift that something new was in the air.

SHARPE: Well . . . uh . . . are you satisfied, then, with how things are between you?

MAX: We've got it pretty good I'd say. I've got this beautiful doll for a wife, and she's got . . . well . . . she's got me. (*chuckling*) Who could ask for more? [Lola gave us both one of her brilliant smiles. I felt their combined invisible arms reaching out to pull me back into the fold. I took a deep breath and forced myself to stay on track.]

SHARPE: As I recall, our main goal was for you both to feel freer to communicate difficult feelings with each other, especially hurt and anger. Being able to disagree and fight was a part of it. [I sounded like a textbook.]

LOLA: Well, we're still great at not fighting. We haven't had any fights, or even any disagreements that I know of for the last couple of months.

MAX: That's a bad report for us, Hon. Think of the headlines: "The couple is failing in therapy because they won't learn how to fight."

LOLA: We can't be failing, can we? (*looking at me, wide-eyed and concerned*) You told us we cover over things that might lead to conflict. Do you think we're doing that?

SHARPE: Well, I'm not sure. I know we've been having a great time in here, and I've sort of lost track of doing my job. I'm wondering, is that because there's no job to be doing, or are we all in it together now— you know covering up and making nice.

MAX: (*in a bantering tone*) Now that sounds intriguing. Can you see the headline? "Doctor leads patients in coverup." (*looking at me a little belligerently*) I don't see how we could fool you? Aren't you supposed be able to see through us? [I felt a hostile edge to his jocularity.]

SHARPE: Sorry, Max, I've got no x-ray vision. They didn't give us that in psychotherapy school.

MAX: Is that so? You must have gone to the wrong school.

I really felt Max's hostility then. I suddenly realized I was a little afraid of Max, afraid of his ability to needle tender places. Lola, I noticed, sat frozen clutching her sandwich, her eyes shifting back and forth between us.

SHARPE: You sound angry, Max.

MAX: Angry? I'm just needling you, Doctor.

SHARPE: Yes, and I felt it. Needling is a way of being angry.

MAX: (*shrugging*) Okay, have it your way. (*He looks down, becoming engrossed in vigorously brushing imaginary crumbs off himself.*)

SHARPE: Max, I have the feeling I hurt you in some way. You were joking about failing therapy, but maybe you felt I was saying that about you— that you're a failure . . . so then you were telling me I'm the failure.

MAX: I've always said you're a smart, Doctor . . . especially for a woman.

LOLA: (*looking horrified*) Max, that's insulting. You're sitting here with two women. One of us is going to clobber you.

MAX: (*with unmistakable sarcasm*) So, I'm a little chauvinistic. That should come out. The doctor wants us to say *how we really feel.*

SHARPE: I'm getting the message, Max, that you don't like my ideas about communication, but I'm not sure why.

MAX: (*with surprising directness*) Maybe I don't believe in it. No disrespect, Doctor. I know that saying how you feel is supposed to be good communication. But I think you can hurt people doing that. That's what

Phoebe does, and look how she's hurt Lola. That's what Lola's mother did, and look how she hurt Lola.

SHARPE: So you think you'd hurt Lola if you say more about how you feel?

MAX: It's not worth taking the chance.

I encouraged him to say more about his fears. He said he was afraid that if Lola were hurt, she might shut him out. I asked if he had ever been shut out before when he expressed disagreement or anger, either with Lola or anyone else. He said he thought that might have happened, but he couldn't come up with any examples. Lola said his parents had shut him out, and maybe that was the source of his fear. Max seemed unable to go any further. I sensed he was too fearful of Lola's response to bring up her tendency to withdraw when injured. I turned to Lola and asked if she also felt threatened by the idea of working on their communication.

LOLA: I know you think we'll be better off in the long run if we could talk more easily about how we feel—all of how we feel, not just the good stuff.

MAX: So you're on the doctor's side about this?

LOLA: Well . . . uh . . . in principle I am.

SHARPE: But maybe not so much in action.

LOLA: Well, I don't know. I have fears, too, just like Max. [I was about to encourage her to say more, but Max interjected.]

MAX: We had a good thing going here, Doctor. Now you're messing it up. These sessions used to be a lot more fun.

SHARPE: You sound irritated about that.

MAX: You bet I am.

SHARPE: I'm glad to hear you say so. It helps me to know where you stand. (*smiling warmly at Max, who looks quite pleased with himself*) I think we've made some progress today, but I understand that you're both really uncertain about wanting any more of this kind of progress.

LOLA: I'm not uncertain about coming to therapy. Just scared. [I looked to Max for his vote.]

MAX: Can we still bring lunch? [I was about to say sure, but then thought better of it.]
(The rest of this session is reported in Chapter 6, pp. 116–118)

This session was a breakthrough on several fronts. Max and Lola had felt criticized and angry about my busting up our cozy social hour and mutual idealizing by focusing back on the goals of treatment. Max was able to openly acknowledge these feelings. In asking them to do the threatening work of therapy, I instigated their deidealization of me. This is specifically illustrated in Max's anger at me for not having x-ray vision and the powers to know all and provide a painless, magical cure. The surfacing of his anger enabled him to openly disagree with me about the treatment plan. To an extent, Lola also disagreed with the goals of conjoint treatment, though she was more conflicted. It is useful to keep in mind that, in general, idealizing couples will enthusiastically embrace the therapist's recommendations and suppress their negative or conflicting feelings, which then appear in the kind of social hour resistance just described.

Max's open expression of disagreement with me about our treatment plan strengthened him enough to challenge Lola's control over lunch. In the remainder of this session, Max and Lola openly disagreed about where to have lunch on therapy days and were then helped to negotiate a new plan for lunch that took both of their needs into account. This small exchange marked a shift in their usual parent–child mode of relating to a collaborative adult interaction.

Middle and End Phases

Although this breakthrough was followed by a retreat, repeated interpretation of their needs and fears kept Max and Lola moving forward (then back, and then a little farther forward). It was not long before they moved into a full-blown deidealization process with each other, accompanied by a stormy period of self-assertion and battles for control. Big fights broke out over all kinds of things, especially their differences in politics.

These conflicts were necessary in terms of their individualizing more definitely within the relationship. The intensity of their conflicts resulted from both partners' lifelong subjugation of hurt, anger, and self-assertive strivings. For quite a while, they felt overwhelmed and frightened by these intense exchanges. Feelings of rejection, abandonment, and anger about being controlled and unsupported were repeatedly revived and explored in relation to their current expectations and past experience.

Scapegoating Revisited

Given the couple's expanded abilities to manage the full range of emotions between them, theoretically, their need for scapegoats should no longer be necessary. Unfortunately, this defensive need is not always so logically or easily relinquished. When the illness/condition of a partner or the scapegoating of a child has meanings other than enabling a couple's relationship to function in an idealizing (or other) mode, each partner's particular relationship with the scapegoat needs direct therapeutic work.[5]

Since Lola's presenting depression involved repressed anger toward Max, this depression mostly cleared up with acknowledgment and expression of these feelings. However, her low self-esteem, which also resulted in bouts of depression throughout her life, was connected to her relationship with her mother (now reenacted in reverse with Phoebe). These aspects of the larger depression problem required individual treatment.

Likewise, parents' connection with a scapegoated child usually has other meanings than to secure an idealizing relationship. As noted previously, in addition to providing a dumping ground for the negativity in the parents' relationship, a child may also be scapegoated because of resemblance to a hated parent or sibling (of one or both partners) or may represent aspects of either partner that are unacceptable and disavowed. Phoebe was Lola's scapegoat for all of these reasons. Max used Phoebe to express his anger toward Lola, but she also expressed aspects of himself that he disavowed, such as selfishness, entitlement, rage, and self-assertion.

Lola and Max's relationship with Phoebe improved with attention to all of these meanings in individual and couple therapy. Family sessions were again reconsidered, but Lola and Phoebe both resisted this idea. However, Phoebe, in her individual treatment, came to understand her role in perpetuating herself as scapegoat and her position in the triangle with her parents. Her withdrawal from responding as a scapegoat and her attempts to make positive connections with her mother contributed significantly to improved relations with her parents.

Conclusion

In presenting the treatment of Lola and Max, I emphasized the opening phase of therapy, because this phase is the most difficult for therapists to manage successfully. The critical, multifaceted task in the opening phase is to enable the couple to accept a problem in their relationship and then be able to sustain that reality.

---

[5]For example, a partner's illness may have an array of meanings other than its role in sustaining a couple's mutual idealization, such as providing an acceptable way to satisfy basic nurturing needs; the management of low self-esteem, including anxiety about functioning more responsibly and independently in the world; or as a means of feeling securely connected and defending against abandonment fears (i.e., "I will never be left if I'm sick"; "I can never leave a sick spouse who needs me"). One or more of these meanings may also need to be addressed in individual and couple treatment for the illness or condition to be relinquished.

Exploring the bases of these difficulties in each partner's family of origin was not highlighted because this aspect of treatment is not relevant until couples recognize they have relationship problems, work for a time with their current fears and conflicts, and then are enabled to begin a deidealization process. The therapist's willingness to initiate his or her own deidealization is often critical in fostering partners' willingness to face this painful process with each other. At the point when deidealization is under way partners' connections with the past have greater meaning in terms of personal understanding (since they reexperience loss of the ideal parents of early childhood).

In the successful treatment of idealizing couples, the therapist combines understanding each partner's idealizing needs and allied fears, as they are expressed in certain dysfunctional interactions, with active communication training. Understanding partners' fears usually brings about reduction of these fears. Exposing and understanding underlying wishes to repair and repeat past relationship experience, particularly in connection with idealizing needs, wishes, and failures, transform the childish aspects of these needs into more mature forms.

Concomitant with interpreting a couple's dysfunctional interactions, the therapist teaches and encourages new and more functional methods of communicating. Understanding and interpretation are not enough to promote change. It is necessary that the therapist provide a substitute mode of relating through teaching and modeling new ways to interact. Particularly fostered is the direct, open expression of differences, hurt, and anger between partners, and abilities to negotiate differences once they are permitted expression. Optimally, partners' understanding of their needs and fears, *in conjunction* with the improved interaction attained by direct communication, will encourage them gradually to give up or substantially modify their idealizing collusion.

In this therapy process, the therapist revisits the same terrain, again and again, inching a little closer to the couple, a little deeper with each repetition. Gradually, partners are enabled to hang onto changes and stay more open and real with each other for longer and longer periods before once again running back to false fronts and the safe haven of a an ideal fantasy world.

Eventually, Lola and Max worked through the stormy phase of battles for control and self-assertion in order to become stronger, separate individuals in their relationship. With the confidence that each accepted and respected the other's individuality, they were able collaboratively to forge a truly mutual relationship. Since they could tolerate unflattering perceptions of each other, anger, difference, and conflict, idealized views were no longer defensively evoked. Idealizing had evolved into more realistic admiration of one another's special qualities, and idealizing expressions emerged spontaneously, much less often, and without the honey coating. Their sex life improved greatly.

Toward the end of treatment, Lola's progress in these respects was reflected in the following remarks: "We've got a pretty special relationship. Max is a good-hearted man, and we care deeply for each other. But we have to struggle at times, like every other couple I know."

PART II

Patterns of Separateness

Devaluing

"You're No Good"
—LINDA RONSTADT (1963)

CHAPTER 10

"You're No Good!"

Sybil and Klaus were the first couple who made me want to run and hide about halfway through the consultation meeting. It was twenty-nine years ago, but I remember them with crystal clarity. Of the many couples I have seen since that time, they would still take the prize for mutual torture.

They were a striking pair. She had jet-black hair and ghostly white skin, and her gaunt body was sheathed in a black cat suit. She wore an elegant pair of over-the-knee, black suede boots. I remember those boots very well, because I kept wanting to look at them instead of at her mask-like face. Her lips and nails were painted dark red, completing the Vampira effect. Klaus was immaculately dressed in an expensive business suit. He was tall and very blond, with a handsome face devoid of emotion. His eyes were pale blue—like ice chips. Just the look of this couple scared me. They seemed like brittle mannequins on the verge of shattering.

In a doll-like voice, Sybil began by saying they had "a perfect marriage" except for the occasional fights that seemed to be getting more frequent and violent. Everything was fine now, but he had hit her so hard in the jaw last week that she had to have extensive dental repair. She was smiling while telling me this. Klaus interjected, without a trace of remorse, that he only hit her in self-defense. She had attacked him first, scratching his face with those long, vicious nails. He spoke in a careful monotone, presenting himself as "the rational one." Sybil, he said, had become incensed because he wanted to go to sleep before she did. This "irrational" reaction on her part had been the preamble to other fights as well.

From this point on, I struggled to control the escalation of their arguing about who was to blame for causing the violent fights and inflicting the most physical damage. Being a novice at couple therapy at the time, I

197

tried to rescue the session by ending on a positive note. I asked Sybil and Klaus what they liked about each other.

SYBIL: (*grimacing*) You go first. I want to hear this.

KLAUS: (*pondering the question, sounding bored*) Sybil can be an interesting conversationalist.

SYBIL: Well, that's just great. So I'm an interesting conversationalist once in a while. Anything else?

KLAUS: (*thinking for a long time*) Well . . . let me think . . .

SYBIL: Come on, now. . . . We're all going to be asleep before you come up with something else. Isn't there anything . . . like I'm smart or sexy?

KLAUS: Well . . . ah . . . being a good conversationalist implies intelligence.

SYBIL: Can't you just say it straight out? Why don't you look at me? You sound like you're talking about someone you met casually a long time ago.

KLAUS: I can't just reel things off the top of my head like you do. I don't wish to sound foolish. It's necessary for me to consider how to phrase what I want to say . . .

SYBIL: You don't have any problem reeling things off when it comes to what's wrong in China, or Africa, or the government. You bore everyone for hours . . . but when it comes to me, nothing comes into your big mechanical brain . . .

KLAUS: Listen to yourself, Sybil. You attack whatever I say. I'm getting a headache from your grating voice, petty insults, and hysterical neediness. Pull yourself together.

SHARPE: (*I intervene to stop the certain escalation, but Sybil talks over me, her shrill voice rising.*)

SYBIL: You don't feel anything, do you? You're like a bump on a log, a piece of dead wood . . . a robot.

KLAUS: (*contemptuously*) You're becoming loud and irrational. I think we should end this conversation right now, before you get out of control. (*He looks to me for validation.*)

SHARPE: (*I say something–I can't remember what–to try and ward off the impending explosion. Sybil's shrieking drowns me out.*)

SYBIL: You want a divorce, don't you?

KLAUS: I never said that. I don't wish to discuss . . .

SYBIL: (*yelling, her nostrils flaring, her pale skin breaking out in red blotches*)
You bastard! You're a fucking automaton!

KLAUS: (*looking at me, his thin lips pulled back in a slight smile of triumph*)
You see? This is what happens. This is how she goes out of control . . .

SYBIL: Fuck that! He's a goddamn sadist . . .

Even in my blind youth, I had no problem seeing how he drove her crazy, and how she got herself slugged. Sybil and Klaus created their particular hell with an arsenal of devaluing techniques applied with sadistic precision.

The term "devaluing" has a very unpleasant connotation. Devaluing behavior appears repellent and can cause great pain, especially when used in global, intensely hostile forms, as by Sybil and Klaus. Devaluing is used here to refer to those feelings and behaviors that reflect a hostile, negative view of the other person. The 1963 song "You're No Good" (made popular by singer Linda Ronstadt) reflects a universal response to being disappointed in love. As discussed in the previous chapters, when flaws become apparent in the romantically idealized person, the disappointment is often managed by an exaggerated or global form of devaluing.

Couples use a broad range of terms to describe the experience of feeling devalued, including insulted, ridiculed, belittled, put down, blamed, mocked, scorned, humiliated, demeaned, denigrated, and degraded. Devaluing the partner can be conveyed through the content of what is said, tone of voice, and facial and bodily expressions. One partner can devalue the other with nonverbal behavior, ranging from abusive violence to constant coldness and indifference. Covert forms of devaluing are just as hurtful, if not more so, as those that are openly displayed. Covert expressions can be harder to identify and treat, because the intent to devalue the partner is not as obvious as it is in verbal abuse. Additionally, a devaluing intent is often unconscious or vigorously denied. One of the most hurtful is to conduct an extramarital affair obviously, especially one whose discovery is arranged in some humiliating way.

In the previous interchange, Sybil and Klaus overtly devalue each other in very destructive ways. Name-calling and character assassination are used, accompanied by body language and tone of voice to amplify the verbal insults—sarcasm, scorn, condescension, scoffing, and mocking. Sybil frequently sneered and grimaced, while Klaus conveyed haughty disdain in his posture and facial expressions.

While other couples are not usually as talented at mutual denigration, many who come for couple therapy often express themselves in this mode. Treatment management of this problem is often difficult and sometimes a Herculean task. I have found that understanding the developmental and defensive meanings of a couple's devaluing is the most helpful way to approach this interaction.

DEFENSIVE DEVALUING

Devaluing is used on occasion by everyone to defend against those painful feelings that are likely to lower self-esteem—rejection, envy, shame, guilt, humiliation, inadequacy, and failure. In general, devaluing another person temporarily raises one's own self-esteem and restores a sense of personal power by putting down the other. In effect, the attempt is to expel feelings of inadequacy and put them into another person ("I'm not a failure, you are"). The processes of projection and projective identification are aspects of devaluation. Those who use devaluing as a major defense tend to have extremely vulnerable self-esteem and great difficulty containing critical feelings about themselves and others. Such individuals are described by Kernberg (1975) and Kohut (1971) as narcissistic personality disorders.

Devaluing used as a collusive defense in a couple relationship is also motivated by additional factors. Sybil and Klaus used devaluing to retaliate for feeling attacked. In addition, they had become each other's receptacle for any and all negative feelings, repeating abusive childhood role relationships. Finally, intensified devaluing became their distancing device to pave the way for separation and divorce.

Blaming is one of the most common patterns of devaluation. Blaming between Sybil and Klaus was mostly confined to the subject of proving the other one at fault for their physical violence. However, in other devaluing couples, blaming is the dominant pattern that infiltrates almost every interaction. Blaming is a form of criticism that implies the hostile accusation of fault and typically reflects some degree of projection. Because blaming is so distinctive and such a common, difficult treatment problem, a chapter is devoted to understanding and treating this pattern.

Chapter 11 describes the normal development of devaluing in a love relationship and presents the treatment of a couple, Alex and Marla, with devaluing problems in the mild to moderate range of difficulty. Such couples with primarily "normal" developmental difficulties respond favorably to mainly an interpretive approach. Couples who become collusively entrenched in a devaluing/blaming mode of relating require a more varied and longer-term treatment approach that involves multiple levels of exploration and interpretation, integrated with certain cognitive-behavioral techniques. In Chapter 12, the treatment of a blaming collusion is presented, with Eva and Sid returning as the case example.

CHAPTER 11

The Development of Devaluing
Common Treatment Problems

All partners have to contend with the problem of how to manage negative feelings about themselves and each other. The more extreme one's angry and hateful feelings, the more difficult they are to contain, and the more likely that they will be expressed in hurtful ways. Additionally, when boundaries become blurred, it is often difficult to determine whether angry, critical feelings are about oneself or the partner, or both. One young woman expressed this confusion in the following anguished terms: "I have so many bad feelings I don't know what to do with them. I go back and forth between feeling either I'm no good or he's no good. The pressure inside makes me say something critical. Then I feel like a bitch, like it's me, I'm the bad one. Either way I feel awful."

She went on to express the common wish of wanting to get rid of her bad feelings "by throwing them out in the trash." Unfortunately, this solution is not feasible. Marriage may provide us with the next-best solution by giving us someone, our beloved partner, who can absorb the negative feelings we have about ourselves and others, who can act as our own personal garbage can. Used in this way, devaluing preserves our own self-esteem but at the high cost of a good relationship. However, this is only one of the roles devaluing plays in intimate relationships—the role that is most often highlighted in the literature.

Devaluing also plays a more positive role in couple relationships. When development progresses in an optimal way, our tendency to view ourselves and our partners in exaggerated ideal or devalued terms undergoes transformation. As described in the idealizing chapters, devalued images gradually become modulated and integrated with ideal images. We then become able to see and accept the negative aspects of ourselves and our partners in more objective ways. This achievement paves the way for partners to be able to express angry or critical feelings to each other in modulated, respectful ways. The well-being and progressive development of a relationship depends upon partners' abilities to perceive and respectfully communicate negative as well as positive feelings. However, a considerable developmental process is required for partners to modulate their negative views and express them respectfully. Therapists often try to circumvent the necessary developmental process by teaching couples the principles of good communication. This approach alone frequently does not work, because partners need to develop first the capacity to *perceive* each other realistically, in order to sustain *expressing* themselves in balanced, thoughtful ways.

In the course of a love relationship, partners' devaluing each other evolves from exaggerated forms to realistic and appropriate perceptions that result in the ability to give and receive criticism constructively. This developmental progression is summarized as follows:

- Global devaluing
- Devaluing to create separateness
- Acceptance of flaws (in partner and self)
- Devaluing as a distress signal
- Respectful criticism

This evolution occurs in close relationship to the development of idealizing. Modulation of one tendency is usually accompanied by modulation of the other. A couple needs to experience all of these aspects of devaluing many times in order to be able to *sustain* the desired outcome. Thus, in optimal development, this rough sequence of events is recapitulated throughout a couple's relationship, each time occurring at a higher level of organization.

Exaggerated, global forms of devaluing (of both self and partner) are periodically reexperienced, but usually with less and less destructive impact and for shorter periods of time. One of the more gratifying outcomes in working with this problem is to observe the developmental process and see couples revert to an angry, devaluing interaction but very quickly recover perspective on their own and continue the fight in a respectful fashion. Of course, no matter how "healthy" partners become, they will get angry and fight. Angry fights, however, can be appropriately confined to what has been hurtful rather than resorting to devaluing putdowns.

This developmental process is highly subject to regression and derailment. It is also substantially influenced by life-cycle events, individual development, and each partner's experiences of success and failure. When devaluing becomes and remains the most prominent mode of relating (often in conjunction with controlling or competing), this pattern represents a couple's collusive defense against a spectrum of mutual anxieties (detailed in Chapter 12). Phases in the development of devaluing, with their allied tasks and common pitfalls, are outlined in Figure 6.

GLOBAL DEVALUING

Some couples come for consultation and treatment early in the life of their relationship because of waning romantic love. They may appear in the therapist's office in the last throes of an idealizing mode of relating, desperately clinging to their ideal perceptions. More commonly, they appear in a devaluing mode, wherein disappointment is acutely and painfully recognized. They are not yet entrenched in this pattern as a long-term adjustment and may only require minimal help to work through this developmental transition.

The discovery that one's partner is not as wonderful as one had imagined, but just another flawed, needy person (though, likely, with some good points) causes varying degrees of disappointment and anger in most people. The more exaggerated the original idealization, the greater the disappointment and resultant negative perceptions. The partner who was ideal may look "all bad" for a time and possibly forever, as repeatedly expressed in the song "You're No Good."

Once disillusionment occurs and the deidealizing process takes over, partners often manage this transitional phase by angrily devaluing each other for a time. One partner may engage in this behavior more than the other. If this devaluing mode remains dominant beyond six months or a year after the deidealizing process begins, it is likely an indication of a more entrenched kind of problem, as in the case of Sybil and Klaus. They had engaged in abusive interactions for most of the two years of their marriage.

A circumscribed developmental problem can usually be easily distinguished from the more difficult and pervasive problem of collusive devaluing. Though all couples who devalue may initially display a superficially similar kind of interaction, the therapist does not react to couples in transition with anything like the disturbing countertransference reactions evoked by couples in collusion.

Disillusionment in the partner, expressed by global forms of devaluing, is often triggered by conflict over including third parties in the relationship—friends, activities, work, in-laws, having a child. Separating from parents to allow partners to see their connection as the primary relation-

Steps in Development of Devaluing	Tasks for Couple/Guide for Therapy	Common Problems (Points of Regression and Derailment)
Global Devaluing	Engaging in deidealization process Viewing partner and relationship in exaggerated negative terms	Denial of "all bad" images and angry feelings Stalled in global devaluing
Devaluing to Create Separateness	Recognizing need to devalue in order to be more separate Accepting needs to be separate in self and partner	Stalled in devaluing in order to create and maintain separateness Projection of needs for separateness onto partner
Acceptance of Flaws (in partner and self)	Recognizing devaluation of partner as a defense against inadequacy Relocating negative images from partner (or self) to original sources Modulating and integrating devalued and ideal images	Self-esteem too vulnerable to accept flaws in self Persistence of need to view partner as "all bad" to sustain self and others as ideal Enactment of devaluing/blaming collusions
Devaluing as a Distress Signal	Understanding episodic devaluing as signifying one's own or partner's distress Developing perspective (observing ego)	Inability to attain an objective view of episodic devaluing Overreacting to partner's anger or criticism by attacking or withdrawing
Respectful Criticism	Identifying partner's behavior as hurtful or undesirable Confronting partner's undesirable behavior in a respectful way Appropriately expressing anger Acknowledging and apologizing for one's own hurtful behavior	Denial of partner's hurtful/undesirable behavior Too fearful of anger or rejection to confront partner's undesirable behavior Too fragile to accept criticism or apologize

FIGURE 6. The development of devaluing.

204

ship is an integral part of this process and often constitutes the presenting problem. One or both of the partners are still too tied to their parents, who loom as more important than the spouse. Wallerstein and Blakeslee (1995) consider separating from the family of origin to be the couple's first developmental task. The impingement of a third party and the emergence of a love triangle challenges the couple's romantic closeness and frequently becomes the focus of resentment and devaluing.

Partners who devalue as a reaction to the initial deidealization of each other usually respond to developmental explanations and interpretations of their reactions with great relief, a renewed sense of closeness, and a surge forward in emotional growth. The following is an illustration.

Alex and Marla

This attractive, professionally successful couple; both in their early thirties, came for therapy because of increasingly frequent fighting. Marla had become depressed, and Alex was having temper tantrums. Both feared that divorce might be the only solution. They had been married for two years and reported feeling happy together for the first year, in spite of the many differences between them. We were able to trace the beginning of hurt feelings to the six-week visit of Alex's parents, who had subsequently moved to their town. A constant theme of their current fights was the daily "dropping by" of Alex's parents.

In the third conjoint session, Marla complained vehemently that Alex's parents were coming by too often and without calling first. She complained that her house no longer felt like it belonged to her, and she was particularly upset about a day on which they hung around for three hours when she was sick. She thought Alex should do something about this intolerable situation and speak to his parents about calling first. Alex responded that he resented the problem being dumped on him. At this point, their interchange escalated.

Alex scolded Marla, saying she was an adult and should act like one by telling his parents to leave if she wanted them to leave. She should "just get off her lazy ass, stop vegetating in the corner, and do something about something for a change." Marla quickly retaliated by stating that it was Alex's place to deal with his parents, not hers. She accused him of being afraid of his parents, insinuating that he was a coward. "He caters to their every whim," she said bitterly, "but when it comes to me, he acts like an angry tyrant or a spoiled brat." Alex countered by saying that he was sick and tired of her moping around and doing nothing. If anyone was spoiled, it was Marla.

I intervened at this point. Although there were many possible routes to take with this interaction, I thought the initial approach should address their shared pain in experiencing the normal, developmental aspect of their conflict. The relative newness of the marriage, the conflictual issue of establishing boundaries in relation to parents, and the nature of their devaluing interaction all suggested that the couple was in the throes of a painful deidealizing process.

SHARPE: You both sound so let down and disappointed in each other, like you've lost all the good, all the closeness in your relationship. (*A brief silence follows. Marla looks thoughtful, and Alex shifts around in his chair.*)

MARLA: Well, it does seem we're more often angry than close. We're not like the team we used to be.

ALEX: *You're* not the same as you used to be. You used to be so lively and fun. We had such a good time. Now you're always depressed and want to be left alone to read.

MARLA: How do you even know what I'm doing? You're never home.

ALEX: (*He is about to defend himself or counterattack. I quickly intervene.*)

SHARPE: It sounds like there's been a major change in your relationship. You used to see each other in more positive—even ideal—ways, and now the less attractive sides of yourselves are showing.

ALEX: Yeah, that's for sure.

SHARPE: People often feel angry, tricked, or even cheated when they begin seeing the not so appealing sides of their partners.

ALEX: (*angrily*) The package I bought is not what I got! I want the person I married back again.

MARLA: I'm still me! I didn't deliberately fool you. I told you I had problems with depression. I've had problems with depression all my life.

ALEX: (*sadly*) Yeah, but . . . I guess I thought I'd fixed that. . . . I used to make you happy. Just our being together used to make you happy. (*His tone shifts from anger to anguish as he allows his feelings of loss to surface.*)

MARLA: I know . . . I know . . . and it did. (*looking wistful*) But it's not because of you I got depressed. I just get to feeling worthless and isolated at times. I don't know why.

SHARPE: Something may have happened in the relationship to set off those feelings. As I recall, you started feeling depressed when Alex's parents visited for that six-week period of time.

MARLA: (*nodding thoughtfully*) I started to feel alone and angry . . . like a left out little kid. (*pausing*) I guess it felt like I was losing Alex. He wasn't, isn't the same around his parents as when it's just the two of us.

(*turning to Alex*) It's like you do everything to please them, but then you're irritable and snappish with me.

SHARPE: Maybe you feel, in those instances, that his connection with his parents is stronger than his tie with you . . . that his relationship with them comes before his relationship with you.

MARLA: I hate to say it, but that's how it seems. When his parents came to town, he just stopped paying attention to me.

ALEX: That's not true! You're the most important person in my life. (*pausing, searching for a way to express himself, then in obvious emotional turmoil*) They just make me feel so uptight, especially my mother . . . uh . . . I don't really know why. I'm sorry, if I've taken it out on you. I wish they'd never moved here!

In the course of this interaction, I observed Alex move out of the role of child with his parents and back into the couple relationship.

Because the end of the session was near, I confined myself to a few summary statements highlighting the normal developmental aspects of their conflict. I underscored the universality of couples' feeling disappointed early in a marriage and fearing this meant their relationship was doomed. I said I thought that the six-week visit of Alex's parents occurred before they were really solid in their relationship as a couple and suggested they had not been ready to give up the one-to-one kind of closeness and include others so extensively. I noted the difficulty, common to all couples, of including and excluding others, especially parents who were insensitive to the couple's needs for privacy (usually because of their own conflicts over separating from a child).

If the partners can take in these explanations and react with relief and acceptance (as did Alex and Marla), they are likely to reunite as a couple with greater understanding and less need to idealize or devalue each other. Achievement of this kind of modulation and subsequent integration of exaggerated "all bad" and "all good" perceptions takes varying lengths of time for different couples. Even when these processes occur rapidly, it takes many years of living together and jointly surmounting a multitude of challenges to stabilize these capacities.

DEVALUING TO CREATE SEPARATENESS

Partners also commonly use devaluing as a means of becoming more separate. In the evolution of a love relationship, one or both partners will feel the need to move out of the initial and subsequent periods of romantic closeness to reestablish independence. This developmental process occurs in adult love relationships much as it does with children and their parents. However, because wishes to be more separate are usually conflicted and fraught with a certain amount of anxiety and guilt, partners often need the impetus of anger and devaluing each other.

Alex and Marla responded to their conflictual needs for greater separateness by devaluing and distancing behavior. Like many couples, they had considerable anxiety about maintaining autonomy in an intimate relationship, yet also longed for closeness. Devaluing, in this sense, may be viewed as a transitional state between oneness and separateness.[1] Fears of being more independent from one's partner and feelings of guilt about abandoning one's partner are also expressed in devaluing behavior. These reactions are illustrated and interpreted in the following excerpt from an early therapy session with Alex and Marla:

MARLA: Because you have to exercise and have a great body, I was left with all the work to do for the dinner party.

ALEX: I apologized for being late. And I helped a lot with the clean-up. But I don't think that my lateness should have been an excuse for you to act like a pouting child. You looked like an angry prune face most of the evening. You insulted our guests.

MARLA: They weren't *our* guests, they were *your* guests. They're your friends, not mine. Frankly, I thought they were bores, and you got into that whole boring number you always do with Frank, talking about the good old days in high school.

SHARPE: Sounds like you felt left out.

MARLA: Yeah, I was. The three of them went to high school together. I could hardly share in that experience.

ALEX: I'm sorry I was insensitive about that.

MARLA: I never wanted to do that dinner party in the first place.

ALEX: You never want to do anything.

MARLA: That's not true. I suggested we go to the beach together on Sunday, but you were too hung over. I'd like to do more things with just the two of us.

ALEX: You know, I really don't get that impression. When I try to be with you in the evenings, you get on the phone with some friend or your sister. (*turning to me*) Last night she spent an hour on the phone talking with her sister. She sees her sister almost every day.

---

[1]This aspect of devaluing is discussed in Chapters 5 and 6.

MARLA: It was only a half hour. She was having problems. I'm surprised you noticed. You're usually glued to the tube or plugged into the internet.

ALEX: (*sounding reproachful*) We used to cuddle and watch TV together.

MARLA: I just don't like some of those stupid sitcoms you watch. [I could see their interaction had gotten into a repetitive pattern of blame–defend–counterblame.]

SHARPE: I'm listening to this blaming going back and forth and wonder what you're feeling hurt and angry about. Have you noticed how similar your complaints sound?

ALEX: We're always doing this picking and sticking each other. It's a real drag.

SHARPE: I get the impression that you both feel abandoned. Marla, you feel pushed to the side because of Alex's friends, or his work out program, or the TV, and Alex you sound like you feel deserted in the evenings in favor of Marla's friends or sister.

MARLA: I do feel deserted these days. We don't seem to be getting together much. We're like ships passing in the night.

ALEX: That's not all my fault. I feel you're not very available either.

SHARPE: Maybe you also need to keep up this friction, this bickering and blaming, to create distance from each other, in order to feel okay about doing some things separately.

ALEX: What do you mean?

SHARPE: It seems like you both want to be together, but you also want to do some other things on your own and with other people. The problem is that you haven't worked this out so being together and being apart is acceptable and comfortable. You don't think it's okay to want to be more separate at times, so you each blame the other for having this need.

MARLA: That's really strange. I know I do what you're saying. I feel I have to get pissed off at Alex in order to call my sister. It's weird. Why can't I just call my sister?

SHARPE: If you didn't get pissed off—see him as that neglectful boob watching TV—you might feel guilty for deserting him.

ALEX: I still don't get what you're talking about.

MARLA: That's because watching sitcoms has made you stupid.

Even though Alex never quite admitted to getting the point, the couple's bickering and blaming decreased markedly after this session. Their energy became productively rechanneled into more directly communicating their wishes to be together and to do things separately. Both feared being merged and losing autonomy, but they tended to project their wishes for more separateness onto each other. The partner was then viewed as the rejecting one who wanted distance, permitting each to devalue and separate without guilt. Paradoxically, they were impelled to arrange for more time spent together, now that they felt freed of the obligation to be always together. After working toward improving their communication for a few more weeks, Alex and Marla terminated, feeling relatively pleased with their progress and relationship.

Devaluing as a Way to End a Relationship

Devaluing is also used for the more extreme purpose of creating the distance and anger necessary for many partners to end a relationship. Many relationships end with the first experience of disappointment between partners. Devaluation then often becomes a *mode of separation and divorce.* Anger and devaluation fuel countless partners through the separation–divorce process and serve to keep terrible feelings of loss and sadness at bay for a long time after the event (see Wallerstein, 1997). I will comment only briefly on the assessment of this pattern, since the subject of treating separating or divorcing couples is a huge and complex topic, beyond the scope of this book.

An example of devaluing to bring about the end of a relationship is illustrated in Nora Ephron's *Heartburn* (1983). In this story, the husband covertly devalues his wife by conducting an extramarital affair about which everyone but his wife knows. After she finally finds out, he continues the affair but in a flagrant way that finally wounds and enrages her enough to end the marriage. In couple therapy, Sybil and Klaus's devaluing, which at first appeared to be an entrenched collusion, then intensified to become a mode of separation and divorce.

This shift may be hard for the therapist and the partners to recognize at first, since therapists and the majority of couples who initiate therapy are consciously oriented toward improving the marriage. The therapist's countertransference can often reflect the as-yet-unconscious wishes of one or both partners. My image of Sybil and Klaus as "brittle mannequins on the verge of shattering" foretold of a relationship in its death throes, though I did not heed this indicator at the time, being caught up in a novice's grandiose fantasy of saving impossible marriages.

Another clue to this shift is persistent lack of motivation in one or both partners to improve the relationship, or active resistance to any possible improvement. In this situation, the therapist becomes aware of working much harder than the couple to save the relationship. However, it is sometimes very difficult to tell whether such couple behavior indicates a serious wish to separate or reflects deep ambivalence (of one or both partners) embedded in a chronically devaluing relationship. Progress is thwarted in both situations.

A more tangible indicator of a wish to end the relationship is a pattern of poor attendance at sessions by one or both partners, either repeated cancellations or extreme lateness, despite the deterioration of the relationship. However, once again, these behaviors can also reflect one or both partners' resistance to exposure and change. Yet when all of these indicators appear and do not yield to a range of therapeutic interventions, it is reasonable to suspect that at least one partner is consciously or unconsciously heading out of the relationship.

When the therapist suspects that serious separation–divorce wishes underlie persistent devaluing in a deteriorating relationship, therapy can be constructively advanced or terminated by confronting and encouraging the exposure of these wishes to end the marriage. Had I been more experienced when treating Sybil and Klaus, I might have been able to read the numerous indicators, expose these wishes, and short-circuit the couple's need to act out and create a full-blown, destructive drama (using me as the scapegoat) in order to separate.

Therapeutic Pitfalls

A common therapeutic error is the failure to recognize that devaluing may be developmentally normal, reflecting a reaction to disillusionment or a wish to be more separate. The therapist may err by focusing on major difficulties in the couple's communication rather than addressing their underlying developmental trauma and resulting feelings. Partners will not really be motivated to learn better skills if they fear their love is dying.

Alternatively, the therapist may belittle or dismiss difficulties inherent in the couple's developmental process, "therapeutically" chastising the couple for having these problems. This intervention may be rationalized as confronting the couple (or one partner) with reality. For example, the therapist may point out that one or both partners are expecting too much from the other or from marriage, and they must, in effect, face reality, grow up, and give up unrealistic fairy tales of "happily ever after." This might be called the "boot-camp approach." The boot-camp attitude might be only implicitly conveyed by the therapist's minimizing a couple's anxieties and disappointments.

While the ultimate therapeutic aim is to enable the couple to integrate more realistic perceptions and expectations, an unempathic or critical approach to the couple's pain is analogous to a parent reprimanding a child for being jealous of a sibling and insisting he or she be more mature and without jealousy. Not only does such a devaluation make the partner or couple feel put down, but it also impedes the natural process of grieving and working through of anger, sadness, and loss that are normal aspects of disillusionment.

This attitude also fosters a resigned, cynical defense (actually, a disguised devaluing defense) that many of us unhappily carry through life and love. Often, the impatient dismissal of developmental process is the result of a countertransference, reflecting the therapist's own incomplete working through of the deidealization and restructuring processes in his or her own love relationships. Once a therapist can recognize his or her own judgmental or dismissive attitudes toward a couple's struggles and begin exploring why they exist, this countertransference can be brought under control.

ACCEPTANCE OF FLAWS (IN THE PARTNER AND ONESELF)

In the course of any enduring relationship, many hard times, successes, and failures must be weathered. In this weathering, the partners' strengths and weaknesses are more pointedly exposed and tested, often leading to another reworking of each partner's self-image, image of the other, and image of the relationship. A partner may become more admired and appreciated but also feel envious of the other's success or acutely disappointed in the spouse's apparent failure. A heretofore unrecognized weakness or deficiency may be exposed that cannot be easily integrated, because it challenges a previously cherished and needed image of the partner or oneself.

Alex and Marla: The Second Time Around

Two years later, Alex and Marla returned for treatment. Their relationship had gone well for most of that time, until shortly after the birth of their baby daughter, Meg. When Meg was six months old, Alex left his job as an attorney with a prestigious firm to start his own law practice. His new business did not immediately bring in much income. Marla had cut back to working only part-time, in order to care for their baby, further straining the family's finances. Alex feared he would need to borrow money from his parents or give up his own business and go back to working for a large law firm. This time, the couple came for therapy with their roles reversed. Alex was the one who was depressed, and Marla was openly furious with him. Their interaction was pervaded by devaluing and anger, both partners blaming the other for their predicament.

In this instance, the couple's devaluing was caused to a great extent by each partner's feelings of inadequacy and failure. Recall that devaluing is often used to protect one's self-esteem by projecting the fault onto the other—"I'm not inadequate, you are." Both partners were also experiencing a second round of disillusionment in each other, in the relationship, and, now more acutely, in themselves. Although financial problems superficially appeared to be the precipitating cause of their feelings of failure and consequent need to devalue, the beginning of greater distance and disappointment began shortly after Meg was born. Alex felt Marla had deserted him for the baby, and Marla was very disappointed in Alex as a father. He participated very little in Meg's care. However, feelings engendered by the baby were not immediately revealed.

Marla openly expressed her disappointment in Alex at not succeeding in his role as the family's main provider. He had made a gross error in judgment and had risked the family's financial well-being. She had been supportive when he started his own practice, based on assurances that their lifestyle would not be appreciably affected. When financial difficulties became apparent, Marla had tried very hard to remain supportive and not openly blame Alex. However, she could not sustain this resolve and increasingly perceived Alex's poor judgment and depression to mean he was weak and a failure.

Marla was having great difficulty integrating this new image of a vulnerable, depressed husband with her former image of Alex as strong, manly, invincible, and reliably optimistic. The sudden intrusion of this new, weak image threatened her security. Disappointment in her weak father was resurrected and became confused with her perception of Alex. She also felt overwhelmed because she needed to increase her hours at work, while also caring for the baby. A depressed Alex, who was unable to be supportive, seemed like an unexpected second child needing care. Financial problems frightened her, reminding her of her childhood. She had not bargained for this kind of marriage. She had wanted financial security above all.

She felt angry, anxious, unable to cope, and like a failure herself. She thought she should be better able to take these troubles in stride and support Alex when he was down. Instead, she felt like fleeing the marriage and dumping Alex. Expression of her disappointment, anger, and anxiety began to take the form of devaluing and blaming Alex (as had been her mother's pervasive mode of relating to a weak, disappointing husband).

Meanwhile, Alex was struggling with depression and a tremendous blow to his self-esteem. He had never failed at anything before, nor had he ever been really depressed. He, like Marla, viewed his depression as indicating that he was weak and inadequate. To defend against these intolerable feelings of failure, he began finding fault with Marla, criticizing her mothering abilities, poor housekeeping, and weight gain. Prior to their financial troubles, he had perceived Marla as an excellent, conscientious mother. Both partners thus felt like failures, especially in their roles as husband and wife. Their mutual blaming was a defensive effort to maintain self-esteem at a higher level, at the cost of a supportive relationship and the other's self-esteem. In a relatively short time, this formerly restored good marriage had again turned very sour.

Devaluing as a Defense against Inadequacy

Couples like Alex and Marla, who appear with this kind of blaming problem, first need help to identify the "failure" feelings that exist in conjunction with the stressful circumstances. Feelings of failure or inadequacy may be caused by a reality-based failure or may result from distorted perceptions. One or both partners may have really failed at something because of a personal deficiency or problem—a mistake in judgment, a lack of knowledge or skill, a personality problem. Feelings of failure also commonly come from perceived failure to meet one's internal standards. These are the failures that often involve perfectionistic standards. Alex was coping with a real failure in having made an unrealistic career and financial plan. Marla was coping with a failure to meet her own internal standards for being a good wife. The couple also shared the responsibility for poor financial planning, even though Alex was taking the lion's share of the blame.

Exposing each partner's feelings of failure in an empathic way is the first step toward helping them accept and integrate appropriate responsibility and modulate distorted views of each other and themselves. Projection of fault then becomes unnecessary, blaming is no longer needed, and development can hopefully get back on track.

When Alex and Marla could integrate these disappointments in themselves and each other and become mutually more accepting and supportive, other hidden feelings of inadequacy gradually emerged. Marla confessed to feeling like a failure in mothering her baby Meg. She could not forgive herself for the angry feelings she experienced toward Meg, even though she never acted on them and loved her dearly. She had internalized her mother's general perfectionism and experienced any shortcoming as a shameful defect. To the outside world, she appeared to be an excellent mother, caring and conscientious. Without Alex's support of her mothering, Marla's feelings of inadequacy in caring for Meg were more difficult for her to manage, and feelings of being a disappointment to her exacting mother were resurrected. She had been displacing her negative angry feelings toward Meg and her mother onto Alex.

Alex, we found, not only felt like a failure in building his practice but also perceived himself as having failed in his former job. Alex had, in fact, been very successful but he had detested the constant pressure to perform at a certain level. In general, he felt he had not measured up to the promise of his youth. In high school and college, he had been an academic star, the kind of kid who would be voted most likely to succeed. With both partners, these more hidden feelings of failure had fueled the escalation of blaming interactions, mutual self-preoccupation, and withdrawal. It took longer in therapy and a more secure therapeutic environment for them to reveal these vulnerabilities.

Devaluing as a means of protecting one's self-esteem is often accompanied by both partners' underlying unacknowledged feelings of emotional deprivation. These feelings are both defended against and indirectly expressed by angrily blaming and criticizing the partner. Couples like Alex and Marla, who have difficulty with the direct expression of needs in general, are more vulnerable to the adoption of a devaluing and blaming mode as a "hidden" expression of emotional need. They had not been able to deal with the impact on their lives of having a baby, particularly to acknowledge the emotional drain, anger, and disappointment about the change in their relationship. Prohibited from feeling anger or blame toward the baby, they blamed each other.

While devaluing and blaming may temporarily make one feel less of a failure (by making the partner more of a failure), it also very effectively prevents getting necessary empathic support and nurturing from one's mate. Exposing these feelings and identifying the vicious circle of blaming and emotional deprivation allowed Alex and Marla to understand themselves and each other at a deeper level.

Relocation of Negative Images and Feelings

As noted earlier, Alex's and Marla's feelings of inadequacy were initially largely projected onto each other and expressed in blaming interactions. Therefore, relocating those feelings of failure back into themselves was a necessary first step. A second step was finding the other possible sources of these feelings. The major sources of displaced negative feelings about the spouse are usually the couple's children or original families. As noted, both Alex and Marla displaced angry feelings about their baby onto each other. In addition, Marla's view of Alex as weak was magnified by seeing him as like her weak father. Inadequate views of herself stemmed from her relationship with a perfectionistic, critical mother. Alex's feelings of failure were magnified by his parents' image of him as an ideal son who could do no wrong. Anger toward his parents for these unrealistic expectations had been displaced onto himself and Marla.

Partners also commonly use each other to displace bad feelings caused by people outside the family. When an interaction with a boss, colleague, friend, or neighbor has made us feel put down and unable to respond self-assertively, we may express our anger and attempt to restore the injury to self-esteem by putting down our partner. Using the mate as a whipping boy or girl can easily become a daily occurrence if the partners do not recognize this displacement and find more constructive means of managing their stressful encounters with others. When dumping of this kind is confronted (by a therapist or a partner) and the real source of hurt or anger is found, then partners can use each other for help in managing a difficult interaction or relationship. Using the partner as a supportive friend instead of a scapegoat enhances rather than spoils the relationship.

A couple's recognition of these kinds of displacements usually siphons bad feelings away from the relationship and puts them back where they belong, where they can be understood, modulated, and integrated. Good mental health does not prevent these projections, displacements, and transferences from occurring in a love relationship, and all couples must engage in this sorting process. Since anger at our mates is often caused by their hurtful actions, this process is further complicated by the task of determining when our reactions are justified and when they may be fueled primarily by our distortions. Often, both factors are operative in that our partner has, in fact, behaved hurtfully, but our reaction is intensified by projection, transference, or other displacement.

DEVALUING AS A DISTRESS SIGNAL

Although Alex and Marla had been able to modify their intense negative reactions to each other, Marla continued periodically to devalue Alex in unprovoked outbursts even after he had restored their finances with a brilliant success in his private practice. With antidepressant medication, marital therapy, and a business success, Alex's former optimism and good mood were completely restored.

In a session toward the end of treatment, Alex recounted that Marla had called him "a stupid, clumsy ape" the previous night. He wanted this kind of attack to stop. He also wanted an understanding of why Marla attacked him in this way, without any apparent cause. He reported that they had been getting along quite well and had spent a nice weekend with friends and his parents. To me, Marla's ambush looked like a signal of some kind of distress about the relationship, herself, or Alex. Marla responded very well to sensitively expressed confrontation.

MARLA: I've been trying to think about what happened. I'm sorry for blowing up at you. You didn't deserve it, and I did apologize.

ALEX: I know, and I appreciate that. But this happens too often—you lash out at me in some demeaning way—and it's like . . . out of the blue.

MARLA: I could say I was strung out because of Meg and took it out on you, but I know that's not the whole story. (*She pauses as though weighing the pros and cons of taking a risk.*) I think I didn't feel very good with any of the people who were around this weekend. I felt bad . . . left out and unimportant.

ALEX: (*looking bewildered*) But we were with old friends and family.

MARLA: *Your* friends and *your* family.

ALEX: I don't get it. The Shanes are *our* friends. My parents and *your* in-laws, who adore you.

MARLA: No they don't. They adore *you.* You're their golden-haired boy. Your mother puts up with me because she has to. She never thought I was good enough or pretty enough for her handsome "all-American boy."

ALEX: That's not true. She thinks you're wonderful. She's told me so many times.

SHARPE: I think Marla is trying to say something else. (*turning to her*) I don't think your point is to complain about Alex's parents—uh . . . not this time. (*Marla smiles*) I think you're trying to tell Alex that you feel envious of him at times, and it's very difficult and painful for you to expose this.

MARLA: (*beginning to cry*) I hate admitting this, but I've always envied Alex his ease with people and popularity with everyone. I'm not at ease socially, and I was never popular.

SHARPE: We also know he's the favored son, and you didn't feel favored in your family.

MARLA: (*nodding in agreement, crying harder*) And I envy that, too. His parent's are all over him with love and affection. Mine hardly ever call me, let alone come to visit. It's Alex's family that's stood by us during this hard time. And Alex's friends.

ALEX: (*looking pained*) I didn't know you felt that way. I can understand. Really I can. I'd want to punch me out too, if I felt like that. I think my brother feels like you do.

MARLA: (*looking vulnerable*) I feel so petty and childish. I'm sorry.

I could feel myself beaming at Alex and Marla. He had learned so well how to respond empathically (having no apparent natural talent), and she had made impressive progress in being able to recognize and admit fault.

SHARPE: It takes courage to admit envy, especially when it's about someone you love. (*I pause, wondering if I should stop here or raise another possibility.*) I was wondering, Marla, how you feel about Alex's business success. That could add another layer on the envy cake.

MARLA: Oh no, don't say that. How could I envy him that? His success saved us. I was beating him up for being a poor provider.

SHARPE: I think you know by now that feelings aren't just all one way or logical. You could be envious, proud, and grateful all at the same time.

MARLA: (*quiet for a time, seeming to take this in*) You know what I really envy? It's not so much his success as his courage to take the risk he took, in order to do what he wanted to do—to be true to his ideals. I don't have that kind of courage.

ALEX: You practically killed me for doing that. You thought I was self-centered and reckless for leaving the firm.

MARLA: I know, but I also admired your guts.

While the content of this interaction involves Marla's use of devaluing to ward off envy and protect her self-esteem, it also illustrates the couple's achievement of additional relationship capacities. Both partners used this devaluing event as a signal that something was wrong but not understood. At this point, both partners were secure enough with each other and themselves to consider and explore what Marla's destructive behavior meant. Devaluing had become an *interpersonal signal of distress* for the couple.

An outburst of angry devaluing also commonly occurs when one or both partners have accumulated an overload of negative feelings. Many partners have difficulty with the regular discussion of hurt and angry feelings about each other. They are inclined to let one after another little injury or annoyance pass by without comment. However, these little wounds do not go away; they accumulate. When too many bad feelings have accumulated (each person's capacity varies), any small provocation may set off an angry outburst or devaluing attack. If a couple can view this behavior as possibly signaling an overload of negative feelings that need to be jointly processed and understood, then the accumulated anger can be eliminated from silently polluting the relationship. However, when couples have not yet developed this kind of *relational perspective* or *observing ego*, they are unable to see the devaluing outburst as a distress signal and may get caught up in a destructive fight or angrily withdraw from each other.

RESPECTFUL CRITICISM

When partners become able to see themselves and each other in a relatively consistent, realistic way (in spite of inevitable frustrations and disappointments), distorted views of the partner as no good or unworthy rarely occur, and when they do, they do not last very long. In their stead evolves the ability to perceive faults in our partners without losing sight of their positive qualities. In the interpersonal realm, criticisms can be made in a constructive fashion and received without undue anxiety or injury. Alex's confrontation of Marla's hurtful behavior, and her ability to receive and discuss this criticism, exemplifies the transformation of devaluing to constructively giving and receiving criticism. As therapists, this is an outcome we strive to attain with our couples. For couples, this development can profoundly improve the quality of their lives together.

Alex and Marla, like many couples, used devaluing and blaming both developmentally and defensively. Their problems are among those that I view as relatively normal and typically experienced by many couples in trying to create and sustain a good relationship. With problems in this range, the therapist can stay in the gratifying role of guide and interpreter, clearing the psychological debris that obstructs a clear developmental path.

However, the therapist has a vastly more difficult job with couples who chronically devalue and blame as a collusive, entrenched defense. As described in Chapter 12, treatment can be a long, arduous journey through a dense psychological jungle, requiring the therapist to use every known treatment skill, while sustaining the patience of a saint.

CHAPTER 12

The Judgmental Parent and the Guilty Child

A Blaming Collusion

Eva and Sid (introduced in Chapters 3 and 4) began a midphase therapy session with the following exchange, illustrating a typical blaming interaction:

SID: We have a non-existent sex life, you know . . . and I'm getting tired of it. (*glaring at Eva*).

EVA: What do you expect? We have no intimacy in our relationship. (*She speaks in a breathy, little-girl voice, taking the high road of moral superiority.*) You don't hug me. You don't even know how to hug. (*turning to me*) His idea of a hug is a sort of grab and squeeze exercise, as he runs out the door. There's no feeling in it, no sensuality. (*sighing*) And I'm a very sensual person.

SID: No you're not! You just stand there like a bedpost when I try to hug you. You could do something for a change . . . like lift your arms and hug me back. (*his tone is sarcastic*) Maybe it would last longer if you did something. . . . You know, like *par-ti-ci-pate*?

EVA: (*She emits a bored sigh, her big blue eyes focused on me, pleading for her innocent victimhood.*) There are a number of problems that interfere with my *participating*, as he calls it . . . and he knows what they are. (*She glances at Sid, then quickly averts her gaze, as if he were a disgusting bug.*)

SID: (*protesting, rolling his eyes*) I don't believe this. This really is unfair.

You said I was overweight, so I've been working out regularly the last
year, and lost fifteen pounds. You can't say my weight is the problem,
or that I'm the problem? [Although Sid had a bulky, muscular build,
he did not look overweight. He was strong-featured and reasonably attractive in a dark, Mediterranean way, but Eva appraised him with
scarcely concealed aversion.]

EVA: (*taking a deep breath*) You're always perspiring. . . . You're always, uh
. . . damp to the touch. And your perspiration has an odor . . . a very
peculiar odor. (*Her pert little nose pinching up, she turns to me.*) I've
asked him to shower more often, but he just won't do it.

SID: (*His swarthy complexion is gleaming with sweat. He lifts his arm, as though
to wipe his forehead but instead points an accusing finger at Eva.*) You get
on your high horse of judgment, as though you're some kind of
beauty queen. Maybe you used to be, but not anymore.

EVA: (*curling over to conceal her nicely rounded body*) Don't you dare say anything about my weight.

SID: (*exasperated*) It's not even about your weight. Your weight is fine. But
you slop around the house in those torn jeans, with your hair looking
like a rat's nest. And what you do with your time is a real mystery. It's
not taken up with being a wife or a mother, that's for sure.

EVA: (*clutching at her heart, wailing*) I don't know how I can go on living
with your cruel mockery and criticism. (*Her big eyes well up with tears as
she looks to me for rescue, but more importantly, to point the finger of blame
at Sid.*)

Instead, I handed her the Kleenex box and wondered what to do. I
knew it was past time for me to intervene. There were many possibilities,
and by this time, somewhere in the vast midphase of treatment, it seemed
I had tried them all. I felt defeated and worn down by listening and trying
to change their compelling need to devalue and blame. Unlike many couple's sporadic use of the devaluing arsenal to express anger, revenge, and
to ward off personal feelings of defectiveness and failure, Eva and Sid interacted in this mode most of the time. Mutual denigration and accusation were their favorite pastimes, their major defense, and their most
meaningful connection. This painful, destructive activity had become the
heart and soul of their marriage of twelve years, even though Eva and Sid
began their relationship in passionate love, then seeing each other as the
ideal soulmate.

Eva and Sid were experts at mutual devaluing, though not as extreme
as Sybil and Klaus. However, their greatest vulnerability was a shared in-
tolerance to feeling blamed, that is, condemned as responsible for an er-

ror, for a failure, and particularly for one another's unhappiness. Not surprisingly, they managed this vulnerability by projecting fault and blaming each other. Blaming (and assuming the blame) is one of the major patterns of devaluation, one that is most common, painful, and destructive to couple relationships. It can also be the most difficult to modify or eradicate when it becomes an entrenched pattern of defensive interaction.

There are three features that distinguish chronic blaming from other patterns of devaluation. First is the global, negative judgment of the partner as basically bad (often with the intent to wound) that accompanies most accusations of fault, no matter how small. Blame stresses fixing responsibility for a fault or error on another person, with the implied judgment of a deeper and irredeemable fault—something fundamentally unworthy or bad. Expert blamers find multiple ways to convey this larger message, and the one blamed, already feeling fundamentally defective, ashamed, and guilty, is exquisitely attuned to receive it.

Second, blaming incorporates and feeds on the partners' shared underlying assumption that they are responsible for each other's happiness and unhappiness. Each has not only the responsibility to make the other happy but also the power to do so. Hence, if one is not happy, it's the partner's fault.

This tie of mutual responsibility that so strongly binds (and blinds) blaming partners to each other is the disillusioned remnant of romantic idealizing and merging—the fantasy of oneness and perfection. Love, in this fantasy, means all of one's needs and wishes will be met, and all of ones defects and wounds will be healed by a perfect partner in a perfect relationship.

The third feature distinguishing chronic blaming from other devaluing patterns is that it expresses the enactment of a certain needed role relationship between the partners. I describe this relationship as *the judgmental parent and the guilty child*. This role relationship can be distinguished from that of couples who chronically devalue without blame as a central ingredient. They more often enact the role dovetail of *superior parent and inferior child*, which does not contain the core of judgment, guilt, and the accompanying ball-and-chain of total mutual responsibility.

In couples who blame reciprocally, like Eva and Sid, the roles of judgmental parent and guilty child flip-flop frequently. In the majority of their verbal exchanges, these role changes are evident. One partner accuses like a judgmental parent and the other may accuse back, but his or her internal feeling is that of a bad child who feels both wronged and guilty.

In unilateral blaming, the roles appear to be more fixed in that only one partner verbally blames and enacts the role of judgmental parent, while the other appears to accept the blame, consistently enacting the guilty child role. Otherwise, the central dynamics are similar, since both partners are usually found to experience internally both roles and associated feelings. For example, the partner who quietly appears to absorb the blame may find a silent way to judge and induce guilt by enacting the role of the injured, innocent martyr.

Couples who unilaterally blame often become reciprocal blamers when the partner who passively accepted the blame starts openly fighting/blaming back. This was the case with Eva and Sid. Their history prior to treatment indicated that Sid more often enacted the judgmental parent role and Eva that of the guilty child. Since I have found couples who reciprocally blame to be more difficult to treat because of both partners' constant reactivity and volatility (even though they may be more differentiated), I have chosen to present an in-depth treatment of this type of couple.[1]

The distinguishing aspects of blaming, (1) judgment of the partner as fundamentally bad and often intentionally wounding, (2) the assumption of total mutual responsibility, and (3) the judgmental parent–guilty child role relationship, are what make defensive blaming very often more difficult to treat than other forms of devaluing. Blaming, when it comes to dominate the couple relationship, has deep roots in each partner's fundamental sense of self, others, and relating.

Even though the discussion focuses on blaming, the motivations for this couple's defense, treatment strategies, and transference–countertransference issues are applicable in many respects to other forms of chronic devaluing.

WORKING WITH THE MEANINGS AND STRUCTURES OF BLAMING

One of the first difficulties encountered in working with couples who chronically blame is that they do not see their blaming as a real problem. As Lansky (1980) noted, couples do not usually come for treatment in order to stop blaming, even though each partner suffers greatly from the other's real or imagined accusatory attacks. Blaming, along with other forms of devaluing, has somehow become acceptable behavior or, at least, behavior that is tolerated, like a low-grade infection.

I think I have run the gamut in trying different ways to approach chronic blaming. If you try to bypass the blaming problem and work on the content of what the couple is presenting (such as parenting difficul-

---

[1]For discussions of treating unilateral blaming/devaluing collusions, the reader is referred to Lansky (1980), Solomon (1989), and Francis (1997).

ties, lack of sex and/or affection, feelings of anger and alienation), discussion and exploration become impossible because most interactions degenerate into blaming. If you try to work on communication, blaming takes over even more quickly. If you try to reach under the blaming armor and work empathically with the partners' painful feelings and their origins, a softening of defensiveness will likely occur, but only briefly, and then the blaming comes back full force, as though no understanding was gained.

Identifying Blaming as a Problem

Sooner or later, it is necessary to address the blaming behavior directly with the couple and identify it as a major problem that is both a cause of their presenting complaints and a symptom of underlying pain in their relationship. Identification of blaming as the viper in the bosom of the relationship, is an attitude that I aim to cultivate as early as possible in treatment, while also underscoring its protective function.

Of course this identification of blaming as a big problem needs to be done without making the couple feel judged and blamed for blaming. The therapist, from the start, needs to be wary of being perceived as the judgmental parent. This transference will occur at some point, no matter how nonjudgmental the therapist attempts to be, but is more workable when it develops later in treatment, after an alliance is well established.

An intervention that sets out the negative effects of blaming in the context of a typical wounding interaction is a useful initial approach (detailed in the next section). However, it is equally important to discuss with the partners the importance of understanding the *reasons* for their blaming, for as noxious as the effects of blaming are, this compelling activity protects the partners from what they intuitively fear will result in greater pain and anxiety. Blame both destroys intimacy and protects the degree of intimacy that is tolerable to the couple. My hope, for a successful outcome in couple therapy, is that blaming becomes an unnecessary defense and develops into an infrequent kind of interaction that acts as a signal of personal or relational distress.

I have found that five basic aspects of this defensive pattern need to be understood with the couple for treatment to be successful. These are arranged in a rough order, according to their degree of therapeutic accessibility, from most to least accessible (in my experience): (1) blaming as a defensive reaction to feeling injured by the partner; (2) blaming as a reaction to disappointment in the partner and the relationship; (3) blaming as a means of preserving the perfect self and expelling (but not losing) the bad self; (4) blaming as an expression of the needed role relationship of judgmental parent and guilty child; (5) blaming as a mode of connection to defend against fears of intimacy.

Unmasking and understanding these meanings of blaming, in my view, are the heart of the therapeutic work. It is useful to begin with the meaning that is usually the most obvious, pertinent, and accessible to a couple's understanding. This is the couple's defensive use of blaming as a response to feeling injured.

Blaming as a Defensive Reaction to Injury

In the context of a typical blaming interaction, such as the opening exchange between Eva and Sid, I try to point out how each partner devalues and blames the other as a response to feeling injured, most often caused by being devalued or blamed by the partner. However, this hurt is usually not acknowledged by partners to themselves (let alone to each other). *Blaming becomes a way to anesthetize the pain and a disguised means of retaliating for being wounded.* I have found it important to go into detail with the partners about these interactions and their feelings, because most of the time they are only subliminally aware of the hurts received and the hurts delivered.

For example, in the opening interaction with Eva and Sid, I would have stopped the interaction and elicited how each one felt. (I did not intervene in this way because another kind of intervention, which I clarify later, seemed more pertinent.) However, since this interaction is typical of so many that occurred in the early phase of treatment, I can imagine the responses. Sid would say he felt angry and rejected. Eva would describe feeling accused of being a failure. I would then pursue what exactly caused these feelings—the partner's words, tone, manner, with the aim of exposing their methods of devaluing and blaming. Sid would report being sensitive to Eva's expressions of physical repulsion—her disgusted tone and manner, her shudders and sighs—and her painting him as an abusive brute who is responsible for all her problems. Eva is most often hurt by Sid's accusations of incompetence and judgmental tone. She feels he blames her for the failure of the marriage.

I would home in on the shared aspects of their reactions to feeling blamed and feeling like failures—Sid's feeling of being a failure as an attractive man, and Eva's feeling a failure as a competent wife and mother. Blaming back is a way of trying to ward off the injury of being the one at fault, the one who has failed. I point out the vicious cycles that occur between the partners, with blame causing injury that provokes retaliatory blame that leads to greater and greater degrees of woundedness and withdrawal from one another. I describe how blaming results in their feeling wounded and emotional starved, thus preventing both from getting the understanding they need.

I would note that each is particularly sensitive to being blamed and wonder why that might be. If possible, I bring in what I know historically and encourage each partner to discuss experiences with feeling blamed and like failures in their families of origin and in other aspects of their lives. With this approach, I try to instill the conviction that the work of therapy is to understand feelings instead of blaming, and that direct, respectful expression and reception of each other's feelings is what needs to happen for intimacy to develop in their relationship.

This kind of basic intervention needs to be repeated over and over again for a long time to make any sustained impact. By itself, it does not effect lasting change. We may get the rest of that session to work productively, but blaming in full force is likely to be back in the next session as though no therapeutic work had occurred. This is the "Teflon" response of entrenched blamers. Nothing sticks for very long.

It is helpful to be prepared for the intractable nature of this mode of relating. Collusive blaming does not noticeably yield for a long time, no matter how empathic, accurate, or well-timed the therapist's interventions. Sometimes this defense seems to me like an alien entity, or like the mythical Hydra, whose many heads would regenerate every time one was severed. No matter what, it seems to bounce back, come back, grow back. It is easy to feel helpless, discouraged, and demoralized in working with chronically blaming couples.

However, in those cases in which blaming is not an entrenched defense, this kind of intervention, and what I next describe, can lead partners out of blaming and into constructive means of communicating.

Blaming as a Reaction to Disappointment in the Partner

As described in Chapter 11, devaluing and blaming can be considered a normal reaction to a major disappointment in the partner, the kind of disappointment that challenges a previously held view or representation. The first round of such a disappointment occurs in the early phase of a love relationship. Beyond this first deidealization, episodic blaming reactions can also occur as a response to stressful events later in the marriage. Couples who become chronic blamers have not been able to overcome the first hurdle, the first round of disappointment in the partner and the relationship. Subsequent disappointments have simply stoked the embers of disillusionment and added fuel to the ongoing blaming fires.

Eva and Sid's entry into therapy was instigated by their first outbreak of physical violence. Because physically abusive behavior was not acceptable in their jointly held value system, both suffered a severe disappointment in the other, in themselves, and in the relationship which now appeared even more devalued and hopeless. However, their shame and disappointment about this loss of control, which led to an escalation of blaming interactions, represented an acute aggravation of a chronic blaming relationship that never overcame their first experience of disillusionment with each other.

Neither Eva nor Sid could accept a "flawed" or imperfect partner. While both partners had begun the process of deidealization by being able to perceive each other's flaws, neither had moved beyond the point of seeing the other's flaws in an exaggerated extreme. These exaggerated, negative perceptions also remained totally unintegrated with their idealized perceptions of each other.

Sid, for example, could rage on about his profound disappointment in the inadequate, self-centered Eva, but then, at another time, present her as the beautiful princess who, by some lucky miracle, stooped to marrying a clumsy frog such as himself. In states of dramatic anguish, Eva could detail each and every crude, brutish insensitivity of Sid's, and at another time, in another mood, speak of him as her strong, brave knight in shining armor, who saved her from a life of chaotic degradation. (These idealized perceptions were rarely spoken aloud, but they were still maintained by each in unmodified form.) Hence, the partners had entered into but not emerged from disappointment and disillusionment with each other, the initial phases of the deidealization process.

The inability to move beyond disappointment and blame stems from the partners' powerful needs to defend against true acceptance of an imperfect partner, an imperfect relationship, and an imperfect self. In other terms, the partners share the need to sustain, in unmodified form, the romantic fantasy of oneness or merging. Criticism and blame of the partner can be seen as attempts to change and mold the partner into the longed-for perfect image. The irrational belief that drives critical blaming is expressed as follows: "If my partner loved me enough and understood the error of his or her ways, then he or she would change to meet my requirements of perfection."[2]

In treating this aspect of the blaming defense, I try to expose partners' disappointment in each other, present and past, their difficulties in accepting certain realities about each other, their feelings of personal failure, and their clinging to the belief that if the partner is punished, criticized, and blamed enough, he or she will one day transform into the desired, perfect partner. Intervention can most effectively be made in the context of the partners' reviewing the history of their relationship, or when one partner is beginning to reveal disappointed feelings. For exam-

---

[2]The wish for the mother and father of childhood to be punished for their disappointing failures, to abjectly apologize, and to become all-loving and caring is also contained within this fantasy.

ple, I found a good entry point when Sid reviewed how ideal the first couple of years of their marriage had been, when Eva always appreciated his efforts, was uncritical and supportive, and when they always seemed to be of one mind (that is, Sid's mind).

Addressing these two meanings of blame—as a reaction to injury and/or disappointment in the partner—will usually substantially modulate or eliminate blaming problems that are not collusively entrenched. However, the problem of a blaming collusion requires the therapist to move more deeply into the structure and origin of the partners' internalized interpersonal relations.

Blaming to Preserve the Perfect Self and Expel the Bad Self

Disappointment in the partner and the relationship leads to yet another disappointing recognition—facing the deflated image of a flawed self. It is difficult (but not impossible) to sustain the image of a perfect self if that self is in a flawed marriage with a flawed partner. But this is what blaming partners try to accomplish. Couples who blame have married in the hope that the partner and the relationship will repair, or at least conceal, great deficits in the self and also preserve the fantasy of a perfect self. When the partner and relationship fail to meet these expectations, blaming becomes a way to try preserve the ideal self by putting all the badness and fault onto the partner. The partner becomes the repository for all that is bad, so the self can remain good and blameless.

The kind or content of the blaming varies, however, according to the specific needs of the partners to preserve certain conscious self-images. For example, Eva not only openly acknowledged but also dramatically displayed her chronic low self-esteem, feelings of inadequacy, and failure. However, she blamed Sid for these problems. She attributed or projected the *cause* of her inadequacy onto Sid. It was Sid's fault—his criticism, abuse, impossible demands, and anger that kept her from feeling confident and being successful. In contrast, Sid presented a superior and competent self-image. His underground fears and feelings of inadequacy were directly projected onto Eva. She was the failure, the weak one, the inadequate one, the bad, irresponsible one. And as long as she played this part—remained weak, needy, and incompetent, he could shine by comparison and not have to face similar but deeply hidden inadequacies within himself.

In both cases, blaming preserved a desired self-image. In the case of Eva, it was the self-image of the martyred victim/saint who could be perfect were it not for the brutish Sid. Thus, hidden underneath her inadequate self-image, another grandiose self-image of perfection remained unmodified—"If it weren't for you, I could be or do anything!" And for Sid, his conscious self-image was also of the martyred victim/saint who main-tained perfection in spite of the draining weight of a needy, defective Eva—"You're the inadequate, anxious, needy one, not me!" Behind his grandiose, supercompetent self-image was the equally unrealistic opposite self-image of an unlovable, oddball loner who was terrified of rejection and abandonment.

Blaming also becomes a major mechanism for inducing the partner to act out the assigned "bad" role. Sid is blamed so much for being an in-sensitive, controlling, belligerent brute, that he becomes increasingly con-ditioned to act like one (it is easy for him to fall into this role, because it fits the image of his father and his father's relationship with his mother and him). Eva is so often blamed by Sid for inadequacies and dumbness that she conforms more and more to these expectations. Since Sid's criti-cal view of her also fits aspects of her own self-image and is reminiscent of her role in the original family, she can easily become a creative, dramatic screwup.

The first two kinds of intervention described lay the groundwork for deeper work—exposure of each partner's need to blame the other in order to avoid or expel internal feelings of "badness." In accord with Lansky (1980), I have not found it helpful to interpret this defensive behavior to the couple; for example, "You are attacking or blaming him or her be-cause you feel anxious and inadequate" or the more palatable "You want him or her to feel inadequate in order to experience what you feel as a way of communicating, a way to feel less isolated, a way to get revenge." Inevitably, in the conjoint format, the partner being singled out feels ganged up on, blamed, and becomes defensive. When I've tried to include both partners and interpret the couple's projective system (often called an interpretation of "collusive splitting" or projective identification), I have found that, at best, the couple accepts what I say as intellectually informa-tive, but there is no visceral punch or emotional insight.

I think such interpretations fail because the partners lack adequate internal structure. Being able to accept such interpretations requires one to have some capacity to accept imperfect behavior, feelings, and motives, and therefore be able to accept some responsibility for a fault or failure, without an intolerable drop in self-esteem. Consequently, the therapist must first help each partner develop a more individuated, flexible, accept-ing sense of self, and, in particular, a less punitive conscience.[3]

---

[3]Adjunctive individual therapy for each partner would be ideal for these problems, but many blaming couples (including Eva and Sid) will not accept this recommendation, at least not until late in treatment, because going to individual therapy means to them that it is the self, and not the partner, that is flawed.

The kinds of interventions that are more effective and developmentally appropriate are thus those geared toward helping the partners develop capacities to introspect and tolerate "unacceptable" thoughts and feelings, with their accompanying anxiety. One such method is actively to direct certain aspects of the couple's communication, both in the session, and outside the session with an assignment. The following techniques can only work if there is a collaborative alliance with the partners and at least a recognition by them that their pattern of blaming is important to understand and change.

The assignment is that the couple stop all criticism and blame of each other for the next week and that each partner pay close attention to what kinds of feelings precede the urge to criticize or blame, as well as what feelings come up as each tries to control the urge. I emphasize that the main importance of this assignment is the attempt to stop an automatic behavior, in order to see more clearly what motivates it. I allow that it probably will not be possible to stop all such expressions but underscore that it is awareness of feelings that is most important aspect of this experiment. The goal is to set a limit on the blaming acting out, so that the underlying feelings have a chance to emerge with a tolerable degree of anxiety.

In session, I instruct partners to try to discuss their feelings about the latest incident or subject raised, without blame or criticism of the other, telling them that I will stop the action each time I hear criticism or blame, and that if I do not catch it, I would hope one of them would do so. I suggest that if either feels the urge to blame or feels blamed, stop the interaction and say something. We then examine why the blaming urge or act occurred. In order for the therapist to be attuned, it is necessary to divorce oneself to an extent from the content or story line of the communications, since it is easy to miss the more subtle devaluing maneuvers and injuries.

The usual effect of these interventions, if well timed and well executed, is that the partners (or at least one of them) report feeling anxious, hurt, guilty, envious, or self-critical just before a criticism or blaming attack on the other is launched. Eva reported that she had felt the urge to attack Sid for his reckless driving but stopped herself from doing so. She found it very difficult to keep from acting on the powerful urge to blame and criticize. It helped, she said, to try and focus her attention on how she was feeling. She became aware that she felt upset and guilty that she had forgotten to bring the map for the day trip they were taking. Dwelling on her mistake, she could easily slide into feeling like a disorganized dope and a generally inadequate mess. Focusing on Sid's shortcomings (his bad driving) masked her bad feelings about her own monumental shortcomings.

Sid was not quite so cooperative. He did try to do the assignment, which he found difficult but worthwhile. He could stop himself from being critical for the most part, but this led to no revelations about himself. He just thought that being more respectful toward each other was a good aim, and that they should continue that way. (I told him that good intentions were fine, but they might not be enough to sustain respectful behavior.)

However, it was possible to reach Sid in a session, where he could not so easily run from his feelings. I stopped him in the act of attacking Eva for not helping their daughter with her homework. In exploring why he felt the need to blame Eva just at this point, it came to light that he had felt tense all morning due to an important business meeting he had following our appointment. I wondered if he could see a connection between feeling anxious about this meeting and criticizing Eva. Finally he got the point, but not happily. His self-concept was of being strong and self-confident. He hated to admit to self-doubts and personal insecurity. "That's why I'm so good to have around," said Eva, jokingly.

The Judgmental Parent–Guilty Child Role Relationship

At the center of blaming relationships is the judgmental parent–guilty child role relationship. This role relationship, containing both projection and transference elements, assigns one partner to the role of critical parent sitting in judgment of the other, who feels like a guilty yet victimized child. This role relationship can be played out in either of two forms: reciprocal or unilateral. At the time they came for treatment, Eva and Sid enacted the reciprocal type role relationship, wherein both partners play both roles.

In order to make a lasting impact on partners' collusive blaming relationship, it is usually necessary to expose and explore the childhood role relationships that are being reenacted and to find the sources of each partner's hidden sense of shame and guilt. To foster understanding in the couple, it is helpful for the therapist to recognize that the compelling need to blame the partner and the fear of blame from the partner derives from both each spouse's identification with a harshly judgmental parent or sibling, and excessive guilt and shame. This fundamental sense of badness—a hidden "all-bad" self—within each partner constantly fuels fears of judgment, rejection, and abandonment.

In treatment, a collaborative working alliance is necessary for exploration of the judgmental parent–guilty child role relationship. Without such an alliance, the exposure of vulnerable feelings and each partner's painful disclosures of family-of-origin material can and will be used as weapons in their "Who's the bad one?" warfare. When the therapist determines that a good enough alliance exists, exploration of this aspect of the couple's blaming relationship can begin. The first steps are to identify the role relationship and elicit the partners' feelings about it. The couple can then be guided toward an exploration of family-of-origin antecedents.

I had initiated this kind of work with Eva and Sid. We had gotten to the point where both partners, but particularly Eva, intellectually understood something of how their pasts influenced their relationship and self-images. Over a number of sessions, the following information was revealed: We found Eva's inadequate, victimized self-image to be derived from an identification with her chronically ailing and bitter mother, who responded to her husband's self-righteous attacks with hysterical weeping and greater inadequacy. Eva and her older sister feared their minister father's judgmental attacks and prolonged withdrawal. Eva also needed to play an inferior, compliant role with her domineering sister, who had been Eva's most consistent maternal caretaker.

Sid was not as amenable to explorations of feelings about his family of origin. With considerable anxiety, he could manage to look briefly at his relationship with his father. He was appalled to discover that he had identified, in part, with the critical, judgmental father he so deplored. He also revealed that in coparenting his four younger siblings, he tended to be bossy and critical. However, he refused to discuss his mother in anything but glowing terms.

For both Eva and Sid, enacting the judgmental parent stemmed from an identification with the blaming aggressor in Sid's father and Eva's father and sister, respectively. This identification reversed childhood roles, freeing each from the anguish of being the bad child. In this role, revenge is taken on the spouse, who alternately represents the shameful child self and the hated parent.

Both Eva and Sid were amenable to exploration of these aspects of their motivations but balked at my attempts to elicit the origins of their guilty-child feelings, though Eva acknowledged that in the impoverished climate of her original family, abusive attention was better than no attention. She also recognized that victimization as punishment relieved her guilt. What her guilt was about, however, did not become clear until later.

Exploration of family material petered out at this point but seemed to result in some improvement in the relationship. Blaming interactions were less frequent and intense; however, a series of stressful events seemed to provoke a return to intense anger and blaming that forced me back into the ungratifying mode of putting out fires and dispensing Band-Aids. Disheartened and frustrated, I felt pressured to act as the parental judge who would determine who was "the good one" and "the bad one." I felt my responsibility for their unhappiness grow into an increasingly heavy burden as I became less and less able to effect any positive change.

Therapist Identification with the Roles of Judgmental Parent and Guilty Child

As a great believer in the influence of unrecognized countertransference enactment (see Renik, 1993; Jacobs, 1986), I examined how I was affecting the relationship among the three of us. I considered that I might be encouraging their competition by unconsciously acting as the judgmental parent and siding with one partner over the other. Eva was very bright and insight-oriented, which made working with her more gratifying, but Sid seemed more highly motivated to improve the marriage. I felt more sympathetic with Sid in some sessions and with Eva in others. But I thought that, on balance, I had maintained neutrality fairly well, both internally and in action. I thought they were equally impossible (in their own unique ways), and I was fond of both and committed to them.

At this point, I failed to see certain obvious reasons for this setback. Had I not been blinded by countertransference feelings, I might have recognized that I had come too close to exposing the sources of their guilty selves and had threatened Sid's idealization of his mother. They were also probably angry with me for the exposures I had thus far effected, but they took this anger out on each other instead of me. Additionally, I knew that when any couple, particularly a blaming couple, effects an improvement that generates warmer feelings, the partners' fears of intimacy are intensified and backsliding is predictable.

Looking for a way out of this protracted stall, I seized upon the treatment plan as the problem—a handy scapegoat. (When in flight from countertransference, blame and change the treatment plan.) What was needed, I reasoned, was a stronger alliance with each partner. If they could trust me more, their need to compete for me as the judgmental parent would be reduced. I would then be in a better position to sustain the needed in-depth work. Also, I thought that this kind of merged couple, so fearful of developing a sense of separateness and responsibility, could more easily look within in the absence of the blaming partner and the competition engendered by the triangular format of conjoint therapy.

To achieve these ends, I suggested we intensify the treatment by including individual sessions for each partner. They agreed. The disastrous effects of my mistake were immediately evident. This separation of the partners into dyads with me was so anxiety-provoking that both spent their individual sessions detailing how excruciatingly awful the partner had been that week, rather than focusing on examination of themselves as I had hoped.

Prior to my seeing Eva, Sid would leave a long message on my answering machine, recounting her irresponsible behavior of the week, with the obvious expectation that if he could not be there, I should be the one to bawl her out. (He also left messages during her sessions, presumably as a way to include himself by talking on the machine.) Eva started calling me at home in the evening and on weekends in tears, with dramatic stories of how brutish Sid had been and how his attacks were driving her insane. I felt pressured to do something heroic to save her from so much abuse (such as adopt her or drive over to her house and beat up Sid).

Everything I had wanted to make better, I had made worse. The weight of guilt for all of this painful uproar lay heavily on me, finally forcing me to reexamine my feelings. I had been trying to run from their transference to me as both the judgmental parent who had all the responsibility for causing their pain and the guilt-ridden child who was powerless to do any good. I was also angry at them for making me feel this way. I recognized that Eva's and Sid's feelings in relation to each other (transferred from their families) had now been transmitted to me (by way of projective identification).

I entered the next conjoint session, armed with the insight I had not been able to access earlier. Both Eva and Sid looked exceedingly alienated and strained. Sid glowered at Eva. Eva sat rigidly, staring straight ahead as though in a trance. The atmosphere crackled with tension. Because I sensed that any moment Sid would erupt into hostile blaming, I seized the floor.

SHARPE: We're having big problems. I know you're both very upset. But rather than going into your most recent conflict right now, I think we should talk about what's been going on in a more general way with the new therapy plan.

SID: It's not working. Things are a lot worse. I think it just works better when we're all together at the same time. It's more efficient that way. And you don't have your time wasted hearing the same story twice.

SHARPE: (*smiling*) Believe me, they're not the same stories.

Sid chuckled, and Eva smiled tenuously. This momentary connection through humor drained some of the tension out of the atmosphere. I asked Eva for her view of what's been happening among the three of us.

EVA: Uh . . . I'm uncomfortable saying this, but I had a lot of bad feelings. I knew Sid was reporting on me, and I was afraid he was convincing you that I'm the problem . . . the crazy, bad one. I had to defend myself by reporting on him.

SID: (*to Eva*) We've been driving *her* crazy. (*and then to me*) All that time you had to spend on the phone . . . without being paid. Sorry about that. (*He smiles sheepishly*)

SHARPE: Well, I expect you could be mad at me for coming up with this plan that made things so much worse.

SID: I don't think it was you who made things worse.

SHARPE: Well, I came up with the plan. I made a mistake and it caused a lot of pain . . . and I'm very sorry about it.

EVA: (*eyes widening in dismay*) I don't think it was a mistake. Just because *we're* all screwed up doesn't mean that you . . . you know . . . made a mistake.

SHARPE: I get the feeling you're both trying to protect me from taking the rap here . . . spare me from taking the blame.

SID: Okay . . . your idea *was* a mistake. (*hesitating*) And, I guess it makes me a little nervous. I want you to have all the right answers, so you can guide us properly.

SHARPE: Sounds like you wish l was perfect. Maybe it feels scary to rely on a therapist who can make a mistake.

EVA: (*loudly*) This is making me really uncomfortable. I don't like this conversation . . . *at all.*

SHARPE: Why is that?

EVA: Sid's beating up on you. . . . It seems like you're in my position . . . the screw-up, the one who always makes mistakes, and it must be making you feel bad.

SHARPE: (*aware of the truth in this, avoiding a direct response*) Maybe you could feel mad or worried too, about me making mistakes . . . like that might make me a bad therapist?

Eva looked at me blankly; she didn't want to hear this. Sid came to the rescue.

SID: (*angrily to Eva*) I don't see how you could possibly construe that I was beating up on Dr. Sharpe. I just repeated what she already said . . . that she made a mistake.

EVA: (*her voice shrill and rising*) What's so bad about making a mistake? Why isn't making a mistake okay? It's human. (*She begins to cry.*)

SID: (*disgustedly*) Oh, give me a break. This is getting *way* out there . . . *way* out of proportion.

The atmosphere had charged up again with uncorked, swirling emotions. I felt my next words were very important. I was tense with the worry that I'd say the wrong thing, make a mistake, and blow the opportunity.

SHARPE: Making mistakes *is* human. [I was reassuring myself as well as them.] But I think there's a lot of fear in this room about making mistakes and then feeling judged as being bad. We all feel it. It seems like one mistake, or bad thought, or bad deed, makes you all bad and causes great injury, and you won't ever get forgiven and can't forgive yourself. (*Both listen intently. Sid stops cracking and massaging his neck. Eva's eyes glisten with tears.*)

EVA: (*sobbing*) That's how I feel. I can *never ever* feel okay. I can't forgive myself for the mess I've made.

SHARPE: What mess? What unforgivable mess have you made?

EVA: (*sighing despondently*) Oh everything. (*Gradually her sobs subside. She sits up straight and begins speaking strongly, as though confessing to an assembly.*) I'm a wicked, selfish person. I've betrayed everyone . . . my sister, my mother, my father, and myself.

As Eva revisited her childhood with her emotions now more connected to the story, it emerged that she felt a deep sense of guilt and shame about having actively competed with her sister for her parents' favor. Her hostile, competitive behavior had been left out of the earlier version of the sibling story. Her shame and guilt came into the foreground because of intensified competition with Sid for my allegiance. She was reenacting with Sid the relationship with her sister and mother in particular.

She knew her mother was disapproving of her sister's weight and admired Eva's thinness and beauty, so Eva encouraged her sister to eat fattening food. Envying her sister's academic success and diligent study habits, she particularly enjoyed leaving boxes of candy and junk food on her desk. She also provoked her sister into rages, manipulating these attacks so that her mother would punish her sister for bullying the younger, angel-faced Eva. She became aware that she repeated these tactics with Sid in relation to me and the rest of the world. She felt particularly guilty when she thought she might be succeeding in winning my favor over Sid and fooling me into accepting her angelic, innocent-victim persona.

She also felt guilty for secretly currying her father's favor, while at the same time pretending she was on her mother's side in her parents' marital war. She was the mother's confidant, her favorite. She also managed to be the father's favorite. She felt enormous guilt for displacing her mother in relation to her father when she was an adolescent. In high school, Eva often became the stand-in for her mother at church and social functions (because of her mother's many illnesses). Although her father rarely gave verbal praise, she knew he was pleased with her looks, because he liked to be seen with her by the members of his congregation, who frequently exclaimed that she looked "just like an angel," and was such a fitting companion to his saintly handsomeness. She felt honored to be in her mother's place and excited to get so much attention. On these occasions, she was glad her mother was sick and sometimes wished she would just die. Guilt and depression plagued her for these thoughts, until she found the oblivion brought by drugs, promiscuity, and bulimia.

Eva was considerably helped in terms of attaining a more integrated self-image and higher self-esteem by understanding and becoming more accepting of these competitive, "bad" aspects of herself. Her need to blame Sid and regress to states of dysfunction markedly decreased. The focus of her anger and blame shifted from Sid to her parents and sister, but especially to her father (who had been the more idealized parent). With this relocation of negative feelings to their original source, she began to function more responsibly and adequately, even showing signs of competence in running the household.

With the example and spur of Eva's revelations, Sid was more willing to speak about competition, envy, and guilt in relation to his siblings. He had done much of the caretaking of his four younger siblings and, with great difficulty, revealed shame and guilt over his periodic punitive treatment of them. In particular, he felt he had hurtfully dominated a younger brother and sister, who were preferred by his father.

He balked at examining his feelings of being favored by his mother over his father. However, he did acknowledge the strain of trying to live up to his mother's image of him as the perfect son. To maintain this image and his mother's preference, he did his best to hide his shortcomings and "bad" behavior. He was perpetually guilty over this dishonesty and for blaming his siblings to divert attention from his own mistakes. Reluctantly, he acknowledged that some of his behavior with Eva and me reflected this old pattern.

Blaming as a Defense against Fears of Intimacy

When anger and blaming begin to subside, the partners' underlying fears of intimacy come into the foreground. It is now possible to work on them more directly. While everyone can be said to fear experiencing these painful feelings, partners engaged in collusive blaming have these fears to a profound and pervasive degree. A blaming form of merged relating is necessary to keep loss and abandonment fears at bay. However, if the partners begin to experience positive forms of merging—mutual warmth and sharing, sensuality, sexuality—these feelings incite fears of engulfment, that is, fears of losing identity or autonomy. This difficult conflict is solved to a certain extent by the development of a blaming relationship in which merging is maintained but negatively toned, thus providing a degree of separateness.

Conscious awareness and expression of the intimacy fears tend to be divided in a characteristic way between partners. One partner tends to be more preoccupied with fears of abandonment, while the other seems to be ruled much more by fears of engulfment. For example, Sid's needs to control, dominate, and maintain superiority were all fueled by abandonment and rejection fears. Eva's behavior, on the other hand, seemed primarily to be ruled by fears of engulfment. A great portion of her behavior was geared toward resisting and thwarting Sid, resisting physical closeness and sex, maintaining distance by the use of her various physical and mental problems (fatigue, depression, anxiety). A significant motivating force behind these "distancing" behaviors seemed to be to preserve a very precarious sense of self.

As any experienced therapist knows, these positions can quickly reverse when one partner changes direction or tampers with the unconsciously agreed-upon set distance; that is, whenever Sid would back off, be less available, less bossy, less in pursuit of Eva, she would experience panic. Her fears of abandonment would surface, and she would immediately take action to quell this painful anxiety with tactics to bring Sid closer by becoming more needy and dysfunctional to elicit caretaking, or more defiant to elicit his judgmental anger and control—the judgmental parent role. Similarly, when Eva would take any initiative to be closer to Sid, to initiate physical affection or sex, he would freeze up, react like an automaton, or flee on some work pretext. In those instances, his fears of engulfment would emerge, and he would run (probably from images of his suffocating mother), thus restoring the old balance.

Eva and Sid's relationship finally began to improve as we were able to understand the origins and meanings of their role relationship and self-images. Gradually, our sessions changed character and were no longer permeated with anger and blaming. For a while, they were pleased with their progress and for the first time reported having fun together on a trip. However, after Sid and Eva spent one month relatively harmoniously, without fights and with minimal negative interactions, both arrived in my office looking oddly subdued and a little lost. With little enthusiasm, they reported they were getting along okay. When I noted this flatness, both expressed feeling disconnected and somewhat depressed.

SID: I remember your saying a long time ago that our fighting and blaming were our way of feeling connected. I see that now. We're only passionate with each other in our anger. Now we have no passion.

EVA: There's this feeling of flatness and emptiness between us. I feel even more lonely. [Great, I thought. Couple treatment is successful and now the marriage is dead.]

SHARPE: Giving up your fighting leaves you with a big loss. And it'll take a while to adjust. It's scary too. You're probably not sure that it's safe to feel connected in positive ways.

SID: (*sadly*) I don't think we know how to do that.

I then realized how empty it must feel to give up their only known mode of relating.

When devaluing and blaming are on the wane, the partners' feelings of loss and abandonment are usually the first to make their appearance, along with sadness and anger about experiencing these feelings. It is helpful for the therapist to acknowledge the pain of this process and give verbal shape to the partners' feelings. Loss of perceiving the therapist as perfect is usually an aspect of the couple's sadness and is important to interpret. Exploring links to feelings of loss and abandonment in relation to each partner's family or origin is also helpful if the couple is receptive.

Both Eva and Sid were lonely children who felt abandoned and neglected by their parents. Eva, however, was the only one who allowed herself access to these feelings. At one point, I interpreted: "Your feeling of loneliness and disconnection from Sid are magnified by the lonely feelings you had as a child, without parents who could nurture you." Although Sid could not acknowledge similar feelings, he seemed to benefit vicariously from Eva's expression of feeling lonely, neglected, and angry about her parents' use of her as a narcissistic extension.

The partners' recognition of feeling abandoned and disappointed by each other, the therapist, and their parents enables them to advance developmentally. Yet these changes strike a fatal blow to the romantic fantasy of merger, one of the underground mainstays of a blaming relationship. It is extremely helpful for the therapist to interpret the couple's depression over this major loss—the loss of the fantasy of oneness.

If abandonment feelings are not addressed in treatment, the couple very likely will return to blaming. The couple will return temporarily to blaming in any event, but if the therapist empathically interprets the feelings of loss that accompany progress, an important context is created for understanding the inevitable episodes of backsliding.

Fears of rejection and engulfment tend to resurface when the couple has been able to attain some positive experience of greater warmth and intimacy. These feelings of warmth activate wishes for positive merger, which are threatening because of the fear of not being able to reemerge as an intact individual from an intimate experience. This fear is particularly intense for people who do not have secure identities and flexible boundaries.

Such fears must be exposed and processed before intimacy can be sustained without constant upheaval. The person fearing engulfment is particularly fearful that positive feelings will lead to compliance and sub-mission—a surrender of the self, as occurred in the past with the partner and in the family of origin. He or she needs to be encouraged to maintain self-assertion in the presence of positive, warm feelings. Thus far, self-as-sertion has only been possible with the fuel and armor of angry, hateful feelings toward the partner.

Experiencing warm feelings for or from the partner can also provoke fears of rejection and abandonment. It is often difficult to determine which fears or feelings are in ascendance, since they can oscillate rather rapidly. The therapist not only needs to be alert to the upsurge of all intimacy fears as blaming subsides, but also to actively aid the couple in sorting out which fear or feeling is occurring in what context and for what reasons.

If greater closeness does not seem to be developing in the relation-ship, even though the peace is largely sustained, this détente usually means that the couple wants to avoid the pain of experiencing and work-ing through these intimacy fears. If this avoidance persists, the partners will most likely revert back to blaming in order to feel connected in some way. This was the case with Eva and Sid, and was the occasion for the in-terchange that I related at the beginning of this chapter. Although this opening dialogue sounds like an early-phase blaming interaction, it really marked a regression from the period of improvement that I have just de-scribed.

In that session, after I handed Eva the Kleenex box, I eventually found my wits and interpreted to the couple that this interaction was a backslide, a return to blaming, because they needed to reestablish their old familiar sense of connection to counter feelings of loss and emptiness. When I got no argument, I went on to interpret that the content of their interaction (Sid's complaint about no sex and their blaming each other for that lack) said to me that each wanted more closeness but was afraid to al-low that to happen. Their blaming each other was a way to avoid their fears of closeness. To my surprise, they accepted these interpretive com-ments without defensiveness. I suggested that we look at their fears. Eva was the first to respond.

EVA: I'm afraid to get close to Sid, because I'm afraid of being hurt and losing everything I've gained. I finally know better who I am, and I don't want to lose that.

SHARPE: Starting with hurt, how would you be hurt?

EVA: If I let down my guard and feel closer, I'm afraid he'll criticize me and the pain will be much worse.

SID: But I haven't been criticizing you. I'm criticizing you now, today, for not coming closer. You stay so distant. You're always reading, or writing in your journal, or doing your pottery. This sounds stupid, but I feel jealous of your goddamn pots.

EVA: (*nodding*) I totally understand that. I'm jealous of your business and your workout program. If I try to hug you, you push me away and say you have to go to work or go work out. It feels terrible to be pushed aside like that, like an annoying insect.

SID: I don't do that.

EVA: (*firmly*) Yes you do. You did it just yesterday, when you came home from work.

SID: Oh, yeah. I was in a hurry. I'm sorry. (*pausing*) Well, you're the one who wanted me to have a great body.

EVA: Are you paying me back for criticizing your body?

SID: (*answering quickly*) Oh, no. I've just gotten compulsive about it.

SHARPE: I'm impressed with how clear and respectful you both are in talking about what hurts you. But it does sound to me like you both feel rejected and protect yourselves by staying distant, but also maybe unconsciously pay each other back for feeling rejected.

They responded to this interpretation favorably with a useful discussion. I, then, pressed on, taking advantage of their sustained openness to introspection.

SHARPE: Eva, I don't want us to lose track of something else you said about getting closer. The part about losing your sense of who you are.

EVA: Uh huh, I feel really scared about that. (*She is quiet for a moment, thoughtful.*) If I start to feel better about Sid and warmer, I'm going to want to please him. I'm afraid I'll lose myself if I slide back into accommodating. It's so much easier to do that, just be what Sid wants, than keep struggling to figure out who I am.

SID: (*listening carefully*) I really don't think you have to worry about that. You haven't done what I've wanted in a long time.

EVA: (*smiled sadly*) I know, but you don't love me as much as you used to either.

SID: That's not true. I probably love you more. (*hesitating*) And . . . I do respect what you've accomplished.

EVA: (*looking surprised*) I can't believe I'm hearing this.

SID: (*softly*) Well, it's true.

I felt like celebrating. All of our hard work was finally beginning to pay off, and I said so. Much of our three years together had been frustrating, torturous, and messy. In order to do the necessary in-depth work, I had to build internal structures to handle it. But now, it seemed I was witnessing the birth of an intimate relationship and possibly the chance to have more fun working in-depth, without the exhausting labor of containment and structure building. I knew this improvement was not a cure, and there would be continued backsliding for a long time, but I was heartened by their apparent leap forward in development.

SID: (*apprehensively*) Are you saying we're all done, then?

SHARPE: Well, not really . . . that is, if you want an intimate relationship. The hardest part *for you* is just beginning.

Controlling

"My Way"
—JACQUES REVAUX, CLAUDE FRANÇOIS,
GILLES THIBAULT, AND PAUL ANKA (1968)

CHAPTER 13

Who's in Charge?

Often, a couple arrives for therapy still fuming over a fight that started on their way to the appointment. Being stuck together in a car seems to incite couples to engage in a certain kind of conflict, namely, a battle for control. On this occasion, arriving late and apologetic, Rina and Zack (introduced in Chapter 1) continued their freeway fight in my office.

RINA: Sorry we're late, but Zack took the wrong turn.

ZACK: I did not take the wrong turn. I deliberately exited at Birmingham to take the Coast Road. The Coast Road is better at rush hour.

RINA: No, it's not. I told you not to do that. The Coast Road is always worse than the freeway. Everyone knows that.

ZACK: That's absurd. I'm the one that goes south to work every day. I think I know more about the traffic in that direction.

RINA: Traffic was stopped dead on the Coast Road.

ZACK: No, it wasn't. It was moving. It had to have been moving, you were snapping at me to stop tailgating. I couldn't tailgate if traffic was stopped.

RINA: (*sarcastically*) Oh, very clever. (*turning to me*) Then he yelled at me and threatened to stop the car and get out.

ZACK: I shouldn't have yelled, but I was fed up with her directing and criticizing every move I made. I thought she should take over and drive, since she knows so much better how to do everything.

RINA: No, I don't. I really don't think that. I just have trouble being a passenger.

ZACK: That's an understatement!

SHARPE: So what happened?

RINA: I shut up, and he kept driving. We didn't speak a word to each other until we got here.

SHARPE: Sounds like an improvement.

For Rina and Zack, these kinds of conflict could easily escalate into wounding battles. We had been working on stopping the escalation as well as understanding the causes. The central theme, no matter what the subject, was a struggle over who had control, verbally expressed in arguments about whose way was the right way. Each partner would make certain moves to try and control the other or resist the other's control.

In this instance, Zack started out being more in control, because he was driving the car. Anxious about feeling vulnerable and out of control, Rina tried to take charge by directing Zack. Zack kept his leadership by ignoring what she advised and doing what he wanted. Increasingly anxious and angry about his disregard, Rina shifted to criticizing his driving, again trying to run things, but also punish him at the same time. Anger mounting, Zack suddenly shifted tactics from passive aggression to direct confrontation—"I'm stopping the car. You drive." Rina backed down, letting him take charge without further challenge. His forceful power play and her yielding were new moves for both of them, finally allowing one of them to be in charge at least temporarily.

This familiar kind of interaction highlights control conflicts as a central theme in couple relationships. Patterns of controlling are defined here as behavior used to influence, direct, or regulate the partner's behavior, as well as those actions used to resist or thwart the partner's perceived control. The attempt to control one's partner or resist his or her control may be motivated by (1) satisfying one's needs to effect a certain outcome or (2) needing to feel more in control or powerful. The need to feel more in control may stem from feeling personally out of control (anxious, overwhelmed, disorganized) or from needing to feel effective, powerful, or loved through getting others do what one wants. All of these motives may be operative. Controlling behavior can be seen on a continuum from extreme and unmodulated to mild and modulated.

At the extreme, unmodulated end of the continuum are those immature methods of control that involve *dominating* and *coercing* another to comply with one's wishes through intimidating threats of anger, physical force, rejection, or abandonment. The goal of such behavior is not simply to effect a desired outcome, but to feel powerful through exerting power over others. These ways of controlling can be very frightening and are often experienced as demeaning by the other person, because the one who attempts to control in this way relates to the other as an extension of him- or herself and not as a separate person.

Occupying the middle range are those overt attempts to control another by means of demanding, bossing, advising, nagging, whining, pouting, and other pressuring kinds of behavior. The more covert forms of manipulating to get one's way are also in this category, along with the various covert forms of resisting the partner's perceived control. These covert methods of controlling and resistance often involve withholding love and approval to get one's way or to feel powerful.

Adults using these methods are usually insecure in their separateness and effectiveness, tending to perceive the partner as more powerful. Feeling weak, they must resort to overly strident means of making an impact, regress to childish whining and pouting, or hide control needs behind covert methods of manipulation or resistance. Such ways of controlling revert back to those methods used by children and adolescents who try to establish themselves as separate individuals in relation to more powerful parents.

At the most mature end of the continuum, one partner directly expresses to the other a need, a wish, a complaint, or an idea in a respectful way, hoping to effect a certain outcome. The aim is to *influence* the partner to do something by asking and consulting, or to *persuade* him or her to think differently by means of reason or rational argument. Implicit in these methods is the understanding that the other's needs, wishes, and views are important and will be taken into account. There is no expectation of immediate or total compliance, or capitulation from the other, nor a primary need to feel powerful through controlling others. Negotiation and compromise are understood as integral to the management of differing needs.

Children are capable of a rudimentary understanding of other's needs by the age of three or four and gradually become able to modulate expression of their own desires and needs for control. The fact that so many adults and couples in our society primarily use the less mature methods of self-assertion and control calls for an explanation. Either these capacities are not taught or modeled by parents in childhood, or partners regress to early childhood feeling states and behavior, or a recapitulation of parent–child modes of relating occurs in love relationships in the process of developing intimacy (see Sharpe, 1984). Both of these explanations are likely operative.

Most therapists hope to enable patients to express their needs and exercise their influence with modulated methods of self-assertion and control. However, straightforward teaching of these methods through communication training is usually not effective until underlying control conflicts are somewhat resolved and the partners begin to perceive each other as separate individuals whose needs are equally important.

Control is an expression or exercise of power. To feel in control of oneself and one's life circumstances is to feel powerful. It is necessary to feel we can influence our partners to some extent not only to get our needs met but also to feel we have power in our relationships and are loved. Partners' controlling wishes and behavior take many forms and can be functional and growth promoting or dysfunctional and growth inhibiting. Usually, the modulated, overt methods of controlling, such as influencing or persuading through direct requests, rational argument, or offering a quid pro quo (giving something to get something) are functional and necessary for a relationship. However, the less mature, more extreme efforts to control the behavior of our partners usually stem from insecurity and feelings of powerlessness.

Another way to gain or express power in a relationship is to display competence and superiority. In this sense, the aim is not to influence directly or control the partner to do something one wants, but to show oneself as capable. Competence may be demonstrated in a variety of ways, such as being successful in a career, making money, or being a good mother. Feelings of superiority and the perception of another as superior may derive from a person's having particular attributes, such as exceptional attractiveness, high intelligence, or musical talent. Feeling oneself to be competent or superior may then be used to effect or to resist control. These ways of expressing power can also be used functionally or defensively.

In the interchange between Rina and Zack, a mixture of these aims appears in Rina's assumption of having superior knowledge about freeway traffic. This superiority is conveyed in her condescending tone and telling Zack what to do. Zack counters by saying he knows more than she does, using experience and reason to justify his superior position. While these power aims often go hand in hand, in this interchange, the primary goal of both partners is to gain control. Proving superiority is secondary and used as another tool in effecting or resisting control. Competing to prove superiority (or prove the other inferior) can also be the primary aim, with or without a control agenda. Since this pattern is important in its own right and reflects a different set of needs and fears, it is examined separately in Chapter 17.

Both ways of expressing power—exerting a degree of control over others and proving oneself competent and superior—are aspects of building up a stronger sense of self in relation to others. When one or both partners' desires for separateness and personal power are greater than their needs for connection, patterns of controlling or competing may dominate the foreground of a couple relationship. It is important, then, to assess whether these patterns are in the foreground as an expression of normal relationship development or have become primarily defensive. Needs to control others or prove superiority are defensive when they are driven by feelings of insecurity and inferiority.

Everyone struggles at one time or another with the conflict of wanting to be in control versus wanting someone else (the partner) to be in control. Excessive needs to control the partner are usually caused by fears of losing control of oneself and being controlled, and may also reflect anger over feeling unnurtured. Excessive needs for the partner to be in charge usually stem from fears of taking responsibility and failing, and wishes for caretaking. How partners manage the interpersonal and intrapsychic aspects of control in their relationship is crucial to their well-being.

This introduction focuses on describing patterns of controlling behavior and their legacies from childhood. The next chapter presents the couple's development of a true balance of power, highlighting the difficulties and points of derailment that couples frequently experience. Rina and Zack exemplify couples that have not been able to develop a workable balance of power. They became stalled in a phase characterized by battles for control. Since their control battles had become defensive, therapy was more difficult, requiring in-depth treatment. Interpreting the control conflicts as they played out in the relationship with the therapist is illustrated as an effective kind of intervention.

PATTERNS OF CONTROLLING AND BALANCE OF POWER

Often, couples engage in repetitive interactions about controlling and resisting control. Each partner takes a characteristic role, such as one controlling and the other resisting. Many relationships operate mostly in this one-way groove. In the previous interaction between Rina and Zack, Rina tries to control Zack and he resists. However, further knowledge of this relationship reveals that in other situations in which Rina has initially taken charge, Zack will try to usurp control and she will resist. These transactions often have the flavor of parent–child control struggles. When either Zack or Rina takes the dominant position, each sounds like a bossy, controlling parent delivering instructions to a child. Responding in the oppositional child role, Zack can revert to the behavior of a rebellious adolescent, and Rina can explode like a two-year-old having a tantrum.

When control struggles are prevalent in a relationship, the partners have not been able to work out a true balance of power. Those partners who succeed in achieving a workable balance of power have usually become able to (1) agree to clearly defined areas of control, and (2) feel safe and secure with the other partner's control and with taking charge themselves. (Each partner can lead and follow without undue anxiety). Optimally, they can shift their positions in accordance with circumstances and the needs of one or both partners. Fundamental to being comfortable with leading, following, and sharing power is (3) the capacity to cooperate.

When a couple clearly demarcates areas of control, the partners define who will be in charge of certain areas or domains. Ideally, these decisions are made according to each partner's interests, abilities, and time rather than gender stereotypes or how their parents operated. For example, one partner may handle the finances and another the food preparation and grocery shopping. If responsibility for a domain is shared—such as cooking, cleaning, or child care—then who will be in charge of what aspect is defined and agreed upon, such as an agreement that each will cook every other night and the noncooking partner will clean up. Ideally, many of these kinds of agreement can be very flexible and made on a daily or even hourly basis. However, for couples who have significant control conflicts, too much flexibility does not tend to work very well, because the need for constant decisions creates too many opportunities for conflict.

In relationships with ongoing power struggles, the partners usually do not have clearly defined domains of control. One or more important areas have been left unclarified, usually because no agreement can be reached. A frequent problem is partners' disagreement on important aspects of how the children will be parented, so that there is no agreed-upon clarification of responsibility. In this event, both partners are likely to get involved in disciplining their child in conflicting ways, making a confused mess that leaves the child essentially without clear guidance.

The partners may appear to have made such agreements, but one or both may break the agreement by crossing boundaries and getting mixed up in trying to control the other's domain. This is what happened in the instance when Rina tried to control driving the car, when Zack was the driver. Conversely, one partner does not take charge of his or her area of control or does a bad job, so that the other has to take over.

These problems—broken agreements regarding domains of control and responsibility—can be a result of an agreement that is not really agreed upon by both, but has been formulated by one partner and submitted to by the other. Additionally, broken agreements usually stem from one or both partners' inability to feel safe and secure in allowing the other partner to be in control. Alternatively, one or both partners may feel insecure being the responsible one in charge. Consequently, the partner who fears being controlled tries to take charge of everything and may continually undermine and challenge the other's authority. Sid took this role with Eva, while Rina and Zack alternated seizing control and undermining the other.

The partner who is overly anxious about being in charge will find ways to get the other partner to take over. Eva, through irresponsibility in her job as a homemaker, specialized in getting Sid to take over. The situation can get more complex, since the partner who fears taking charge may also fear being controlled, and so resent and subvert the other partner's taking responsibility for his or her turf. A common simple example of these combined fears would be the wife who says to her husband, "I'm afraid to drive, will you please drive?" But then, finding herself anxious under his control, she tries to direct every aspect of his driving (as did Rina). Partners who both have difficulties in taking charge and following direction often end up floundering and functionally paralyzed. Unable to chart a course or follow a course of action, they drift around like a rudderless ship at the mercy of any stiff breeze or strong current that may provide a temporary direction. Children, or the pressures of external circumstances, often end up running these headless families.

A major task of partners in a committed love relationship is to develop a satisfying balance of power wherein both feel they have enough say, enough control in the relationship in an ongoing way. What constitutes enough power for each partner will vary from couple to couple. Some people feel they need to control everything to feel safe. Others do not want the responsibility of taking charge of anything, preferring to be led, advised, and guided through life. (Theoretically, these two getting together—the perpetual leader with the perpetual follower—should be a perfect match!) More commonly, people want some of both—to lead in certain areas and to follow in other areas, or sometimes to lead and sometimes to follow according to interest, mood, energy, or self-confidence level. Most people will say that having enough control or power in a relationship comes down to the feeling that they have equal rights and an equal voice in determining what transpires.

However, feeling equal with one's partner in terms of control may be an unattainable ideal. While power, from an objective view, may look to be equally divided between partners, it often does not feel equally divided to one or both. As most of us have experienced and many authors have noted, the partner who has the most power is the one who is least fearful of losing the relationship. This position of greater security and power can shift back and forth between the partners many times in the life of a relationship.

Developing a True Balance of Power

Most discussions of power in relationships focus on couples' pain and dysfunction when their power balance has become disrupted or never been achieved. But the question of how a couples arrive at a comfortable management of their wishes and fears about control in the relationship has not yet been addressed.

Theoretically, there may be good relationships in which this working out of power needs is managed so smoothly that the whole process is hardly discernable. There are other relationships that may look smooth because no power struggle or jockeying appears to exist, but only because one partner has simply submitted to the other's domination. Eva submitted to Sid's domination in the early years of their relationship. Max generally submitted to Lola's control, and June to Henry. In these relationships, stability in terms of power has been achieved but not an equal balance, since one partner's role and development have been left out of the process.

From this viewpoint, the perfect match of a perpetual leader with a perpetual follower does not seem so ideal, since the follower has likely foregone developing as an autonomous person. This pattern brings to mind those unformed people in cults who blindly follow gurus to their death, such as the Branch Davidians who followed Koresh in Waco, Texas, or the 900 followers of Jim Jones, who committed mass suicide in Jonestown, Guinea.

A true balance of power in a love relationship is defined here to mean that both partners' wishes and needs have been equally taken into account in determining the management of every aspect of the relationship. Each partner having an equal say does not mean every decision is constantly discussed and negotiated. The balance element involves each partner's agreement to a certain division of power and labor, along with the understanding that each feels such a distribution is fair. Ideally, the system for power management created by a couple should be very flexible and able to shift in accord with the changing needs of each partner and the relationship.

A couple's achievement of a true balance of power is not usually an automatic, seamless, or very quiet process. Some conflict and fireworks are usually necessary in working out each partner's needs for self-assertion, dominance, submission, and associated fears. Like the other patterns of relating, a couple attains the necessary capacities to manage control wishes and fears through a developmental, interactional process occurring over time. To complicate the process, every couple also has the legacy of power struggles from childhood to rework and master in the current relationship.

The Legacy from Childhood

From the moment of birth, we attempt to control our environment and our destiny. Equipped with the ability to cry, we can demand food and attention. Looking adorably helpless, cuddly, and dependent are other means of inducing needed care. In growing up, we develop other ways of controlling—the winsome methods of cooing, smiling, and being cute, along with the less appealing techniques of kicking, biting, hitting, grabbing, or screaming. A milestone in the development of power is the two-year-old's learning to say "No!", along with other negativistic and highly effective methods of thwarting, opposing, resisting, or having a full-blown temper tantrum. At this point, a child's controlling behavior is motivated not only by getting a need met but is also by the desire to exercise control for its own sake to feel powerful.

As verbal skills advance, we attempt to control through demanding, whining, wheedling, and nagging. At a higher level, we learn to reason, argue, and bargain (although in many other cultures these behaviors are immediately squashed). Covert tactics of manipulation (such as pouting, sulking, scowling, withdrawing, withholding, resisting) are also developed, especially when parents suppress direct expression. We hope that somewhere along the way, making polite, direct requests takes precedence as one of the more palatable civilized means of influencing others and getting one's way.

Eventually, if development is optimal, we learn to express our needs and exert our influence in more modulated ways, while taking others' needs into account. By the time we commit to an adult love relationship, ideally, we have learned to share power, to feel comfortable being in control and being under another's authority when appropriate, and to deal fairly and squarely in creating a balance of power with our partners. However, our capacities in these respects depend a great deal on our experiences with controlling and being controlled in childhood.

As previously noted, all of the control methods we have used in childhood are likely to reappear in love relationships. When I first started working with couples, I was struck by the parallel with parent–child interactions. Marital power struggles in particular so often resemble a two-year-old or an adolescent struggling with a parent (see Sharpe, 1990). We also learn how to control and be controlled from our parents' relationship and their attempts to control us. The particular power struggles we have had with our parents leave an indelible stamp, especially if working out a comfortably fair and flexible power balance was never achieved.

A universal legacy of childhood that remains with us throughout life is the feeling of being small, helpless, and in need of a strong parent to take care of us and take charge. Being cared for becomes linked to being under another's control from early on, continuing in varying forms through adolescence and adulthood. Adolescents will provoke their parents to set limits so that they will still feel safe and cared for, even though they must resist those limits in order to preserve and build autonomy.

Many adults do not feel cared for if their mates are not telling them what to do or generally taking charge of them.

However, at a certain point in development, around age two, control by the parent does not just feel like needed care and protection, but rather feels like one's budding individual self is being stifled and suppressed. The toddler begins to assert his or her autonomy by saying "No!" incessantly, along with many other forms of resistance. Control battles, especially with mother, begin about this time. Thus, we carry another legacy from childhood: the link between parental control and loss of autonomy, and feeling stifled and discounted as an individual person.

A universal conflict arises between wanting and needing parental control as care and guidance and wanting to be independent and in charge of oneself. This conflict is usually described as the dependence–independence conflict, first expressed when the child works through the phases of separation–individuation with the mother (described by Mahler et al., 1975) and later in the adolescent separation process eloquently detailed by Peter Blos (1979). Even with the best of parental intentions and care, most of us are highly susceptible to regressing to childhood feeling states in love relationships—feeling too controlled and not having enough autonomy, or not being controlled enough and feeling uncared for and alone.

When parents have been particularly unable to respond sensitively to their child's varying needs for care and control, the child may develop more than the usual sensitivity to control needs and fears. The effects of experiencing undercontrol or overcontrol by parents are often reenacted in the marriage relationship in ways that can become dysfunctional or destructive.

Battles for control often appear as the presenting problem of many couples. The power struggle may be focused on one "deadlock" issue, such as having a child, or involve only one domain, such as parenting or sexuality, or may pervade many or all domains and interactions in the relationship. Whether couples' control struggles represent a normal expression of the partners' attempts to manage power needs and fears in their relationship, reflect a regression or temporary derailment in that process, or have become an entrenched, defensive pattern can be determined by understanding where and how they have run into trouble along the rocky road to developing a true balance of power.

CHAPTER 14

The Development of Controlling
Common Treatment Problems

In forming any relationship, each person's wishes to control—to influence the other person and effect outcomes—immediately come into play. The earliest prototype of controlling to forge a connection is the infants cry that brings mother close with her loving care. When people first meet, each person's sensors are activated, searching out a fit or a balance of power—who will lead and who will follow in which domains. Unlike Rina and Zack's freeway fight, this process may unfold quite smoothly.

Rina first met Zack at a party, where he took the lead by initiating a conversation with her on the patio. He was attracted by her dark good looks, beautiful smile, and vitality. They had an animated interchange, finding out they had much in common. Rina was immediately impressed with Zack's wit and intelligence, though he seemed somewhat shy. Soon, she took charge of the conversation by asking him about himself. Taking the more passive position, she then listened attentively while Zack relaxed into telling her about his love of music.

It would appear that control of this interaction shifted easily from one to the other in an agreeable exchange of leading and following, in accord with gender stereotypes. Zack appeared to take charge in a more active and overt way, while Rina influenced events in a more covert, passive way. The subtext of control continued as Rina began to wish that Zack would call her for a date but felt she could not be direct about this desire. Instead, she behaved seductively in order to intensify his interest and assure him of a positive response. In asking for her phone number, Zack again appeared to be the one taking charge, but Rina had played an equal role in covertly engineering this outcome.

In their first meeting, Rina and Zack hardly resembled the belligerent married couple fighting about driving and traffic. But in both interactions, control played a central role, though with very different motivations. In their first conversation, Rina and Zack wanted to effect another meeting—a further connection. Each one's move to encourage the relationship dovetailed with the other like a smooth dance. In contrast, their efforts to control each other on the freeway had nothing to do with building a connection, but, rather, had the opposite aims of fostering self-assertion, domination, and separateness.

In the course of a love relationship, partners' needs to control, fears of control, and wishes to be controlled are expressed in a variety of ways in their efforts to work out a balance of power. In the beginning of a relationship, partners' needs to control are often geared toward effecting a connection with each other, although a struggle about one partner's reluctance to commit can also be a central theme. When a committed relationship is established and wishes to be more separate emerge, one or both partners' need to assert themselves will usually come into the foreground. Many partners become frightened by self-assertive, dominating wishes and repress them in order to avoid conflict. When derailment occurs at this point, partners often become more distant to keep self-assertive and angry feelings from surfacing.

In an optimal developmental process, the partners' control efforts become focused on effecting their independence, and the couple may for a time engage in arguments or mild battles for control. While control battling is a normal aspect of development, a couple's struggles are often intensified and prolonged by the reenactment of control battles from partner's childhoods. The partner who asserts control is often experienced as a dominating parent by the other partner, who may react like a submissive or resentful child. When these reenactments go unrecognized, derailment occurs and the relationship stagnates in battles for control.

In order for partners to move beyond control battling, they need to recognize and accept all aspects of their wishes and fears in this domain— needs to dominate and submit, fears of controlling and being controlled, and feeling out of control. Differentiating one's own control conflicts from the partner's conflicts is an important part of this process, so that futile efforts to control oneself through trying to control the partner (or be controlled by him or her) can be relinquished. Conflicting wishes to dominate and submit, along with fears of self-assertion and engulfment, originate in the partners' family experience and in cultural stereotypes of a man–woman love relationship. In order for each partner to accept needs both to dominate and submit, some revision of his and her gender-identity and gender-role expectations is often necessary. When the partners are able to integrate all aspects of their control conflicts into their self and relationship images, each partner can be comfortable in taking control or yielding control in the best interests of the relationship. In other words, the partners become able to cooperate and create a workable balance of power.

Figure 7 outlines the steps, associated developmental tasks, and common points of derailment in a couple's development of a true balance of power.[1]

CONTROLLING TO FOSTER CONNECTION

As couples fall in love, their wishes to secure a deeper connection are usually the primary aim, and each partner wields his or her influence to effect this bonding. Typically, each bends over backwards to try and please the other and appear as appealing and accommodating as possible. It is as though there is a jointly shared denial of control as a need or a potential conflictual issue. While wishes to be separate and independent still exist, they are suppressed as much as possible, so that the couple can establish a strong connection.

There is another common pattern of courtship wherein each lover acts out one side of the control conflict. One person ardently pursues the other, who resists becoming involved in spite of being strongly attracted. This resistance usually stems from fears of being controlled and losing autonomy (often called "fear of commitment"). Competitive interaction and control struggles may be aspects of this courtship pattern.

In opening phases of this type, one person expresses desires for connection, and the other person expresses fears of losing autonomy. This dance often continues in reverse. When the one fearful of losing autonomy finally commits, the former pursuer is suddenly confronted with his or her own fears and begins running for the hills. Couples can spend their entire relationship acting out this shared internal conflict about connection, control, and autonomy.

From the beginning of a relationship, one partner frequently emerges as the more dominant and controlling, while the other is more submissive and compliant. Often, this kind of fit in terms of leading and following is desired by both partners and is an important aspect of their attraction. This dovetail may not present major problems unless these positions become rigidified and extreme, as when a couple constructs a

---

[1]As with the other patterns of relating, the developmental progression is not linear but recapitulatory. Additionally, partners' working through of these processes on their own or in therapy often overlaps and may occur simultaneously.

Steps in Development of Control	Tasks for Couple/Guide for Therapy	Common Problems (Points of Regression and Derailment)
Controlling to Foster Connection	Aiming and modulating control to win partner Experiencing partner's control as love and caretaking Suppressing differences	Fears of being controlled/losing autonomy interfere with commitment Partner's love experienced as control Control conflicts expressed in pursuer–pursued dynamic
Controlling as Parental Domination	Controlling to feel like a powerful parent Reacting angrily to partner's perceived "parental" control	Denial of differences, anger, and wishes for autonomy Submitting to win and keep love Stalled in rigid role relationship: Dominant parent–submissive child
Controlling to Foster Autonomy	Asserting individuality and wishes to dominate Engaging in argument' Reworking childhood control struggles Supporting partner's needs for autonomy and control	Too fearful to assert self, take charge, or argue Stalled in parent–child or child–child control battles: Controlling parent–oppositional child collusion Too insecure to support partner's self-assertion
Differentiation of Self-Control from Partner Control	Recognizing overcontrol of partner as attempt to manage own anxiety and needs for nurture Recognizing need to control or submit in order to feel loved and secure Developing capacity to delay gratification	Overcontrol of partner continually used to manage personal anxieties and nurturing needs Submitting to partner used to allay anxiety, avoid responsibility, and ensure connection
Modulation of Wishes to Dominate and Submit	Recognizing wishes to dominate and submit within oneself Understanding impact of masculine and feminine stereotypes Revising gender identities to include both wishes to dominate and to submit	Projection of wishes to dominate or submit onto partner Ruled by gender stereotype of dominant man–submissive woman Gender identity too insecure to revise
Controlling in Service of Cooperation	Attaining capacities to take charge and yield control to enhance the relationship Working out a true balance of power: Defining areas of primary responsibility Negotiating meaningful agreements	One or both partners too insecure either to take charge or to yield control True balance of power never achieved or stabilized

FIGURE 7. The development of controlling.

dominant–submissive role relationship in order to function as a merged unit. One partner determines what transpires in most or all areas of their lives, and the other partner automatically submits, often without really knowing what he or she wants as a separate person.

If a couple remains in a dominant–submissive relationship, development in the control domain stops at this point. The couple may have achieved a stable balance of power, but at the expense of growth. Continued development of a true balance of power requires the relinquishment of rigid defenses erected to manage needs for control, care, and autonomy. Eventually, in these relationships, the lopsided control relationship usually becomes less satisfying and begins to erode. The dominating partner can become overwhelmed and resentful about having too much responsibility (as did Sid), often instigated by the arrival of children. Sooner or later, the submissive partner is likely to become very resentful over feeling powerless and discounted as an individual person (as did Eva). Women's liberation prompted many women to break out of this kind of submissiveness to a dominating husband.

CONTROLLING AS PARENTAL DOMINATION

In the beginning of a relationship, one partner's ardent pursuit is generally experienced by the other in a positive way. When a besotted lover insists that he must see his beloved and that she put off other obligations so they can be together, she is likely to respond with intense pleasure over being so wanted and desired. She willingly cancels her other plans to be with him. However, later on in the relationship, such demands—that she drop everything to be with him—begin to feel like suffocating, self-centered control that make her feel resentful and resistant.

When Zack surprised Rina with a trip to Mexico to celebrate their engagement, she was delighted. His taking charge made her feeling cared for and loved. When he surprised her in the same way to celebrate their first anniversary, with airplane tickets to the Yucatan, she felt a moment of pleasure, but then became angry that he did not consult her about her schedule and where she wanted to go. In fact, the time he had chosen was very inconvenient for her work, and she did not like hot places. She felt his behavior was controlling and that he was insensitive to her needs, though she refrained from expressing these feelings.

Likewise, in the beginning, Zack really appreciated Rina's taking charge of their social life. She was helping him to open up and be more at ease with people. He liked her friends and their acceptance of him. He found it exciting and stimulating to go out with interesting people. Later on, however, he resented her pushing him into social evenings when he really wanted to stay at home and read, listen to music, or work on a composition. Socializing began to feel like it always had—a tedious waste of time and energy. He began to balk at her plans. Though he did not openly refuse to participate, he would forget arrangements, forget to provide expected help, and sometimes become withdrawn at a dinner party.

How and why does this kind of major shift in attitude occur? Rather than feeling loved and more connected by the partner's taking charge, each feels controlled, discounted, and resentful. It is as though the loving, caring partner has turned into a controlling parent.

Paralleling child development, the early "in love" phase of a relationship activates the link between control, care, and connection. The subsequent phase of disappointment in the partner and need to become more separate activates the childhood link between parental control and loss of autonomy. With resurrection of this conflict, feelings of being controlled stimulate anger and resistance. In this sense, the second year (or month!) of a love relationship bears some resemblance to the second year of life, when the two-year-old wants to be more separate from mother, and assert autonomy and dominance.

In the development of the mother–child relationship and the adult love relationship, the wish to be more separate and autonomous goes hand in hand with disillusionment in the previously idealized mother and mate. In each situation, the discovery is made that neither mother or mate can fulfill all one's needs, nor can fantasies of oneness be very easily sustained, as differences become increasingly apparent. In this circumstance, doing what the partner wants no longer primarily feels like being loved and cared for, because the partner, who is now perceived as a controlling parent (or child), appears to be operating in his or her own interests instead of in behalf of the merged "We" of romantic love.

In the early phase of romantic love, partners often try to view their wants and needs as the same or similar. In this later phase, their differences become highlighted, even exaggerated. The adult partner, like the feisty two-year-old, wants his or her power and individuality not only recognized and applauded but also to be the dominating force in the relationship. As these feelings intensify, relationships may enter a phase characterized by self-assertion, opposition, and battles for control.

However, development can become stalled or stopped at this point, before full-blown expression occurs. A couple can become frightened and guilty about the negative, angry, self-assertive feelings generated in this phase and make great efforts to squelch their expression. In this event, the relationship becomes more distant in order to keep anger in check, and struggles for control go underground, becoming cloaked and indirect. Extreme forms of this reaction result in a collusive idealizing relationship, as occurred with Lola and Max.

Often a selfless kind of facade can develop, wherein each partner refrains from expressing his or her own needs and goes overboard to do what the other wants. When couples take this tedious and unrewarding route, they often find themselves going places, eating food, and seeing movies in which neither one ever had the slightest interest. Both partners of a couple I know humorously described finding the other one dropping off and snoring at a Wagner opera that neither wanted to see but both were sure the other would like. When a problem of this kind reflects a temporary developmental stall or regression, therapy can effectively be addressed toward exposing and understanding each partner's underlying fears of becoming more assertive and separate.

CONTROLLING TO FOSTER AUTONOMY: BATTLES FOR CONTROL

When therapy succeeds in promoting both partners' greater self-assertion, the partners are strong enough to fight for recognition of their thoughts, feelings, and wishes for their own way. For some couples, there are lots of fireworks, but for others, just a few intense disagreements occur before mutual understanding and working out a satisfactory power balance is achieved. For Rina and Zack (as for Eva and Sid, and Lola and Max), this phase was intense and prolonged because of the reenactment of the partners' control conflicts stemming from their childhood experiences.

When needs for self-assertion and autonomy predominate, each partner strives to be validated by the other for his or her unique individuality, desires for control, and power. In therapy, intensification of these wishes is easily recognized in the couple's characteristic form of interaction—parallel talking and courtroom-style argument. In parallel talking, both partners talk at the same time, usually rather loudly, without the least attempt to listen to the other. Each partner vies to be selected by the therapist as the right or smartest one, though this wish seems secondary to the sheer compulsion to blow one's horn so loudly and effectively that the other is drowned out.

In courtroom-style arguing, the aim of both partners is to prove him- or herself right and the other wrong, whatever the subject matter. Each one says in a multitude of ways: "We should do it my way, because my way is the right way, and yours is wrong, irrational, or stupid for a host of obvious reasons." The courtroom battling style appears more civilized in that the partners appear to listen to each other. However, this listening is primarily geared toward finding the weakness in the other's position, as a prosecutor or defense attorney would do. Distinctively lacking is the desire to understand the other's position, needs, or feelings.

When difficulties in listening and the need to interrupt are pointed out and examined, the partners' fears of losing autonomy and self-definition can be exposed. When Rina was confronted with her refusal to listen to Zack, she said: "I guess I don't want to listen to what he has to say, because if I start to listen, I can feel myself losing track of the point I'm trying to make. He's much more articulate and persuasive than I am." At another point, she revealed her fear of listening to Zack, especially when he detailed how and why she was wrong. Being wrong, we came to understand, made her feel inadequate and worthless. These reactions revealed Rina's insecure sense of self that underlay her self-confident, know-it-all exterior.

The Controlling Parent and the Oppositional Child

Underlying these self-proclaiming communicational styles of interaction is the resurrection of past struggles with parents and siblings. A certain kind of marital transference is often activated. One or both partners may act like a controlling parent. Each also perceives the other as the controlling parent and feels like a child struggling for autonomy and validation. To fend off the partner's control and avoid submission, the child/partner may become oppositional and uncooperative. The kinds of accusations delivered reveal the fears of losing autonomy through submission to a controlling parent: "You're trying to control me!", "You want me to act like a puppet on your string", "You make me feel trapped", "You want everything your own way", "You won't accept me for who I am", "You always have to be right!"

Often these roles flip-flop, sometimes even in the same argument. When one partner is in the position of the controlling parent, accusations toward the partner–child sound like the following: "You disagree with everything I say just to be contrary"; "You don't know how to cooperate"; "You just do what you want, like an irresponsible child"; "You're like a stubborn two-year-old."

When control battles reflect mild levels of disturbance, therapy can usually be brief. Such couples will often be highly responsive to the following kinds of therapeutic interventions: (1) exposing each partner's wishes and fears regarding control, dependence, and independence; (2) underscoring the normality and universality of control wishes and fears; (3) the therapist's neutrality and recognition of each partner as a separate, unique individual through validating each one's thoughts and feelings; (4) briefly exploring family-of-origin experience pertaining to control and autonomy, dependence and independence; (5) communication training geared toward helping the partners respectfully listen to, understand, and validate each other's perceptions, individuality, and autonomy, followed by training in negotiation and compromise.

However, with couples like Rina and Zack, who are stuck in pervasive control conflicts, more in-depth therapy is usually required. Although the interventions suggested here should initially be tried and will likely reduce the intensity of conflict and increase positive feelings, the couple's attempts to move forward developmentally will continually result in backslides to the apparently safer groove of control battling. Repetitive backsliding often indicates that a couple's power struggles have become primarily defensive. Along with the need to reenact continually painful control struggles from childhood for purposes of mastery and revenge, significant fears of change and intimacy are also usually involved.

The Therapist in the Role of Controlling Parent

Often, the partners' deeper fears and motivations are not clarified until the therapist becomes involved in the couple's control drama. Sooner or later, the therapist becomes cast in the role of controlling parent, whose authority must be opposed and thwarted. The goals of therapy often need to be defied as well.

In many ways, the process of therapy parallels the couple's development in the control domain. In the opening phase, many couples relate to the therapist as an ideal parent. Sometimes, if the opening transference is negative, the therapist will be seen by one or both partners as a critical, controlling parent. If the therapist has a rigid, authoritarian style, this negative transference is more likely to be stimulated. However, if the therapist is respectful, evenhanded, and quietly in charge, he or she will most likely be initially idealized for a short period of time. When the therapist is idealized in this manner, the early childhood association between parental authority and parental caring is activated in the couple. With the partners looking to the therapist to show them the "right" way, give the "right" answer, or assign homework, it is easy to fall into responding like a benevolent authority dispensing wisdom, advice, and helpful suggestions from on high.

This honeymoon comes to an end when the partners discover that the therapist's advice or interpretive wisdom does not solve their problems, does not make one partner less controlling or the other more compliant. The therapist begins to feel increasingly deflated when it becomes clear that one or both partners are not really cooperating with the program. This resistance will occur no matter what therapeutic approach is undertaken. However, a therapist with a strictly behavioral or a very directive approach will activate resistance much sooner than will therapists with less directive styles and approaches. A struggle for control between therapist and couple, or one partner, is then likely to occur, although this struggle may remain covert and unacknowledged for a time before it blossoms into an overt struggle. As frequently happens between partners in marriage, a covert power struggle between therapist and couple (or the "resistant" partner of a couple) can go on indefinitely if the therapist colludes to avoid open expression.

There are certain clear clues to this transference–countertransference enactment. When I find myself becoming overly talkative, giving advice, lecturing, or arguing to make a point, I know I have been drawn inside the couple's control collusion (marital transference or mutual projective identification system). Sometimes couples begin to seem like defiant toddlers or adolescents, or one partner in particular seems to be thumbing his or her nose at me behind a smiling, agreeable facade. I can sometimes sense the secret satisfaction derived by both partners when one of them really gets my goat. And then there is my telltale flash of intense anger that only a child's defiance can evoke in a parent or teacher (or a therapist who is feeling like a parent).

Therapy with Rina and Zack followed this general progression. They entered treatment very distressed but committed to each other and highly motivated to improve their relationship. They were insightful and very likeable. For a while, we all seemed to work quite well together. My elevated status as the wise one gave me the clout to effect certain progress with the kind of approach and interventions described earlier. They seemed particularly responsive to my validation and support of each one's thoughts and feelings, present and past. Working on their conflicts about giving and receiving nurture also contributed to their progress in the control domain, since patterns of nurturing and control are highly interrelated. Their control struggles subsided in the areas of parenting, social life, and their sexual relationship.

However, their cooperation was not stable and with any external stress, backslides continued to occur. Backslides also followed any period of greater intimacy. Although they graciously accepted my interpretation that they used their battles to keep a safe distance from each other, fearing greater closeness, this intervention and others I attempted resulted in token exploration but no lasting change. My former influence and power seemed to be slipping away. Treatment progress had slowed to a crawl, and they politely resisted any further help, which was now perceived as controlling intrusion. I felt irritated and stymied.

A periodic source of conflict was Rina's intense disapproval of Zack's smoking. While Zack had complied with Rina's demands that he improve his health care with a better diet, regular exercise, and less alcohol consumption, he would not give up smoking, though he agreed that smoking was a danger to his health. This battle followed a certain pattern. The smoking issue would receive intense focus in one session, exploration of feelings would occur, and, finally, some agreement would be made that usually involved Zack's promise to cut down or quit and Rina's agreement to back off from carping and monitoring. This issue would then recede for quite a while, apparently resolved or forgotten, but then suddenly resurface with great intensity. It was during a session focused on Zack's smoking (during this stall in treatment) that I found myself reacting angrily, like a thwarted parent. My underground power struggle with both, but particularly Zack, was finally flushed into the open.

RINA: I know I'm going to sound like the teacher reporting on a bad student, but I don't know how else to say it. Zack has not quit smoking as he promised he would. I caught him smoking on the patio last night. I just feel . . . I don't know . . . so furious and helpless.

ZACK: So I haven't totally quit. What's the big deal. I'm keeping it out of the house and away from you and Eliza [their little girl].

RINA: That was only one of my complaints. The big issue for me, as you well know, is your health. How can you even sit there and say, "What's the big deal?" You're in total denial.

ZACK: (*mocking*) I'm not an alcoholic. I can't be *"in denial."*

RINA: No, you're a drug addict *in denial.*

ZACK: Smoking a few cigarettes is not drug addiction.

RINA: Yes it is, when you can't stop, and you know the amount you smoke always increases. I've watched you go from a half a pack a day to two and half packs in three weeks. (*She turns to me for support.*) Nicotine addiction is considered to be worse than heroin addiction, isn't that right?

I felt pressured to take her side, but I thought it was essential that I stay neutral. I sympathized with Rina's position, but if I supported her, Zack would feel ganged-up on. His resistance would then stiffen, making exploration a meaningless exercise. However, if I did not support Rina, she would feel I was failing her, just like her mother always had. Although Rina was also enacting her general need to control Zack's behavior as the major way of taking care of herself, this motive did not seem accessible to exploration at this point. Her needs to assert herself, to be understood and validated, were too overwhelming. It also seemed untimely to address the partners' use of this repetitive conflict to create anger and distance in order to manage their fears of intimacy. When couples are in the heat of a deadlocked control battle, I have found that each partner's position and experience in his or her role must be addressed and understood before other motives are accessible.

In addition, I had my own feelings about smoking clouding their issues. I had been a smoker who had great difficulty quitting, so I felt quite sympathetic with Zack on that score. Yet I also had a mother who died from lung cancer because of smoking, making me very sympathetic to Rina's fears. Rina's favorite brother had been a heavy smoker who also died from lung cancer. I thought briefly about sharing my personal understanding of each one's position. But I was unsure of my motivation and whether such an exposure would really help them. Once that card was played, it was played for good. There was too much risk that they would feel burdened or exploited by my self-disclosure. I tried to keep my response as neutral as possible and throw the problem-solving ball back to them.

SHARPE: That's been said. But do you think it would help you to get into another debate about the hazards of smoking?

ZACK: Absolutely not. We'll just have the same old argument about it that goes nowhere.

RINA: (*sounding frantic*) What do I do? I don't know what to do. Why won't you just stop?

ZACK: (*sighing in exasperation, rolling his eyes*) Do we really need to go over all that again? We've already discussed the reasons so many times.

RINA: Well, where else can we go with this? Why don't you contribute something positive for a change, instead of controlling everything with your resistance and negativity.

ZACK: Like what? I already agree with you that I *should* quit.

I decided to try focusing on why their agreement had come apart, since broken agreements were a major problem for this couple and continually generated great anger.

SHARPE: What about your original agreement? What happened to that?

RINA: Didn't you hear Zack agree to quit smoking right here in this room?

SHARPE: Yes, that's my recollection. Is that your memory, Zack?

ZACK: I don't remember actually agreeing to quit. I agreed that I *should* quit.

RINA: No. You said you would quit. Remember? You said you knew how to do it, and it wouldn't be that hard.

ZACK: I honestly don't remember that I committed to that. (*He looks at me innocently.*) Do you remember what I said?

RINA: (*howling with throttled anger and anguish*) Ooh! This is so frustrating. We make these agreements, and then you don't do your part, and then you say we really didn't make such an agreement. It was all my imagination.

I had to work to contain my mounting anger toward Zack. I felt identified with Rina in her role as the defied mother, trying to hold onto some authority with a rebellious kid. She was absolutely right about his behavior. I felt like scolding him for his passive defiance, cavalier denial of the risk to his own health and to Rina's particular sensitivity on this subject. I tried to get past my parental reaction and inside Zack's skin. I knew I had once been where he was now.

SHARPE: Zack, I have an idea what happened. You did agree to stop smoking, but I think your heart wasn't fully in it. It may have seemed the best thing to do at the time to get Rina off your back. There's also a part of you that really thinks you should quit smoking, but another part that doesn't want to, and then a third very insistent voice that says, "No one's going to tell me what to do."

ZACK: (*too agreeably*) It's a plausible theory. I can't argue with it, since I don't remember what happened.

SHARPE: Not remembering is a part of this kind of defense. [I could hear the sharp edge in my tone.]

ZACK: (*sounding offended*) You're saying I deliberately forgot.

SHARPE: Not deliberately. I'm talking about an unconscious forgetting as a way to protect yourself. If you remembered making the agreement, then I think you'd feel more obligated to honor it, or clearly say to Rina that you were not going to honor it.

RINA: I'd rather he'd said straight out he wasn't going to do it than let me think he's sincere about quitting and then let me down again and again.

ZACK: Well, I do agree that I should quit. It shouldn't be that difficult. I should just do it. Screwing around with cutting down is just a waste of time.

SHARPE: All of those *shoulds* sound very burdensome, Zack. Your intentions are laudable, but what's to keep the same thing from happening again? What's to keep us from playing this same scene again in three months?

ZACK: Play it again, Zack, we could call it. (*No one smiles. He shifts back to ingratiating.*) No, I won't let that happen. I'll really do it this time.

RINA: Your word has no credibility.

ZACK: (*shrugging*) What else can I do?

SHARPE: We could try understanding this interaction better . . . why you each get stuck in the same role over and over.

Rina, in response, said that she saw herself acting as a mother trying to take care of Zack, who refused to take care of himself. She was familiar with this role, since she had taken considerable care of her two younger brothers in childhood. They had driven her crazy by mocking and defying her control. However, she felt, she had more power with them than with Zack, because she was backed by her parents' authority. She also felt more desperate with Zack, since she was dependent on him for her well-being.

I suggested Rina try stepping out of the thankless role of nagging mother and just talk about her fears without anger and accusation. She then spoke of her fears of Zack dying from smoking as her brother had. She worried much of the time about losing Zack and being left alone. Zack looked increasingly guilty and deflated by this straightforward description of Rina's feelings. When she was finished, he responded with more sincerity.

ZACK: I don't want to be doing this to you. I don't want to be making you feel so unhappy and scared. I feel awful.

RINA: I wish that feeling would make you quit.

SHARPE: (*Before another argument can get underway, I intervene.*) Zack, I'm wondering about the role you get into with Rina?

ZACK: I guess if she's the mother, I must be the child.

SHARPE: (*Squelching my irritation at his dopey smile, I press on with my interpretation.*) I think the role you get into with Rina puts you in a difficult bind. If you go along with what she wants, you'd feel like you were submitting, and possibly lose your self-respect. But if you don't submit, you risk losing her love. So to solve that dilemma, you try to play it both ways.

ZACK: (*smirking*) You mean to say I become a sneak. Actually, I have a much simpler view. I know I should quit smoking, but I procrastinate on doing it, because it will be very unpleasant. That's it.

SHARPE: (*I feel like arguing with him but realize how important it is for me to support his open disagreement.*) That's a good point. Quitting smoking is very difficult. Anyone would want to avoid that pain. (*I continue to encourage his expression of disagreement and underlying anger.*) I was wondering if you've picked up a bias on my part about your smoking.

ZACK: Sure. You think I should quit. I really don't hold that against you. (*He smiles unconvincingly.*) Anyone would feel that way. Smoking is a self-destructive activity.

SHARPE: Yeah, but I'd think you might feel pretty alone and ganged-up on if I've been so transparent in my bias.

ZACK: You've been better at staying neutral on other subjects.

SHARPE: It's true, I've had a hard time being neutral on the smoking issue. I, too, feel concerned about your welfare. However, I do believe it's your body and you have a right to be in control of your own body. I think it's impossible to make a decision about smoking just for someone else's peace of mind, even for someone you love. It has to be for your own welfare.

ZACK: I wish I was selfless enough to do it for her.

SHARPE: You have accepted Rina's influence in a number of important ways—on getting regular exercise, reducing your drinking, on working less. You may feel you've done enough compromising . . . compromising that could feel more like submitting. Maybe smoking has become a symbolic issue at this point, like Zack's last stand against being completely taken over by Big Brother.

ZACK: Big Mama, you mean.

SHARPE: (*chuckling*) Right. (*then theatrically*) Big Mama is watching you.

ZACK: (*paling*) Actually, that's a scary thought.

SHARPE: Oh?

ZACK: I'm reminded of my mother coming into my bedroom when I was a kid to watch me fall asleep. I would pretend to go to sleep fast, so she'd go away. She wasn't there to comfort me like some parents. She was there to keep me from masturbating.

This session succeeded in opening up the door to more meaningful exploration of both partners' struggles for autonomy and control in their original families and the reenactment of those conflicts in their marriage.

Reworking Control Conflicts from Families of Origin

Whatever the intensity of power struggles, past experience plays a role in each partner's particular needs, fears, and expectations. Couples can and do work out of negative family influences on their own. When the grip of the past is not too strong, the process of separating past from present can occur spontaneously through partners' discussing their reactions to each other and clearing up distortions. When some perspective is achieved, couples can more easily grasp the importance of each partner's need for control and to be respectfully heard and validated, even though they may disagree.

Like many couples, Rina and Zack needed help to understand the impact of their relationships with parents and siblings. Exploration revealed significant conflict for both in the areas of control and nurturing. Zack, an only child, described his mother as critical, domineering, and intrusive. His father kept his distance from an unsatisfying marriage by spending most of his time working and passively complying with what his wife wanted. With Zack, he was alternately critical and gruffly affectionate.

In relation to his mother, Zack had to struggle to maintain his masculinity as well as his autonomy. He learned to keep her at bay and preserve his sense of self by appearing to submit to her authority, then doing what he wanted behind her back. This may be the most common pattern that develops in children who are overcontrolled by a parent and are too fearful to do open battle. Parental love and care are ensured by surface compliance. Reinforcing this passive–aggressive response was Zack's identification with his father's similar role in relation to his wife. Zack responded to Rina's control in much the same way he had with his mother, by appearing to accommodate while conducting a quiet but persistent rebellion.

In contrast, Rina experienced minimal control and insufficient nurturing. Her mother was anxious, needy, overburdened, and frequently ailing. Her father was also rarely present, preoccupied with running a demanding business. When he was present, he was critical, irritable, and depressed. Rina, the oldest of three children, was needed to help her mother with the care of her younger brothers. From the age of three, she became mother's good little helper. Consequently, she did not feel safe unless she was in control of everything, having never been able to rely on anyone else. She was left with a legacy of needing to be omnipotently in control, conflicting with deep longings for someone else to take care of her and take charge. In her relationship with Zack, she acted out her familial role of responsible, in-charge caretaker while suppressing her needs to yield control and be passively nurtured. Resentment always accrues with this solution to such an internal conflict.

When these aspects of Rina's and Zack's family experiences were explored in depth, both were enabled to refrain from automatic, past-driven responses to each other and could begin trying out more constructive positions. Rina was able to recognize her excessive need to control Zack's behavior, especially his self-care, as a means of fulfilling her own needs for a caretaking parent and alleviating her own anxieties about feeling out of control. Understanding the influence of gender stereotypes on their fantasies, behavior, and role conceptions also contributed to reworking the control aspect of their relationship.

Overcoming Gender Stereotypes

In heterosexual relationships, gender differences are relevant in how men and women characteristically go about getting control and power. Historically, men assume and seek power more blatantly and women more subtly and indirectly (Person (1988). However, in recent years, this conception more aptly describes the older generation, or those men and women who have traditional relationships modeled on the patriarchal ideal. Increasingly, over the last two decades, women have become much more direct in expressing their power in relationships, and men more comfortable ceding some of their power.

However, the dominant man–submissive woman stereotype still appears in cultural expressions and in the fantasies of both men and women—patients and nonpatients alike. The persistence and pervasiveness of this fantasy is documented in Nancy Friday's books on women's sexual fantasies (1973, 1991) and in Ethel Person's book *By Force of Fantasy* (1995). The 1975 movie *Swept Away* (directed by Lina Wertmüller) begins with scenes on a yacht of a rich woman whose main pleasure in life is dominating, humiliating, and symbolically castrating both her husband and a male servant. The exercise of such power makes her increasingly strident and dissatisfied. But when she and this servant are swept away on a small boat to a deserted island, she finds true love, erotic ecstasy, and happiness in submitting to his total domination (though she resumes her former role upon returning to civilization).

The notion that a woman is more fulfilled and made sweeter when dominated by a man is the theme of many stories, such as Shakespeare's comedy *The Taming of the Shrew*. However, I have found it difficult to find recent examples of this theme in popular culture. Not surprisingly, stories of this kind do not seem to be as acceptable as they used to be.

The fantasy of women dominated by a strong man dovetails with men's favorite fantasy of having a wife or a mistress (or both), who is willingly and happily under the man's total control. This fantasy is chillingly portrayed in Ira Levin's best-selling novel *The Stepford Wives* (1972) and movie (1975). In this story, the men of a small town, Stepford, conspire to create android wives who are programmed to comply with their every wish. Their real wives (who are much too independent) are then killed and replaced with these look-alike wives. Everyone in this town then appears blissfully happy and content. Becoming a "Stepford wife" is the nightmare of many modern-day women.

This relationship of a submissive woman and a dominant man totally fulfilling each other seems to wield as much power as does family-of-origin experience. Many couples, like Rina and Zack, have parental models that are quite contradictory to this stereotype. One might speculate that these stereotypes and persistent fantasies originally come from biological necessity for survival of the species. In prehistoric times, men needed to be physically strong and dominant and women needed their men's strength and protection in order to survive and bear children. Thus, both men and women may have been quite fulfilled with this dominant–submissive division of power and responsibility.

While, in reality, a woman no longer needs a strong man to survive, nor does a man need submissiveness in a woman to ensure sexual relations and caretaking, the model of a dominant man and a submissive woman persists as an ideal in our culture. Although the way boys and girls are socialized to fulfill gender stereotypes is changing, boys are still influenced by culture and their parents to be dominant, aggressive, and self-assertive and girls to be passive, submissive, and nurturing. While many claim that this kind of relationship is only a male fantasy forced on women by men throughout history, this explanation is simplistic and does not account for why so many women have similar fantasies in spite of their wishes for equal power with men, as well as their achievement of actual power in the workplace and on the home front.

In addition to understanding influences from original families, it is very helpful for partners to recognize the influence of culture in shaping their control conflicts. Whatever the family experience, many modern heterosexual women experience conflict between wishes for a strong, powerful man who will take charge, take care of them, and to whom they will submit in erotic ecstasy, and the desire for a sensitive man who will recognize their needs, their individuality, and respond to their wishes and demands.

Because there is a conflict, fulfillment of either wish does not necessarily produce the expected satisfaction. If a man comes close to fulfilling the fantasized dominant role, women are often angry about not having equal power, being treated as an inferior, and discounted as a unique individual. On the other hand, if a man tends toward sensitivity, passivity, and will cater to their needs, women often berate this man for his weakness, lack of power, and masculinity. Therapists are familiar with the woman who insists that her emotionally reticent man open up and share his feelings so they can have a more intimate, meaningful relationship. But when the man is finally helped by the therapist to let down his hair and express his needs and fears, the woman becomes alarmed and repulsed by his "neediness" and "weakness" and will overtly or covertly discourage this expression.

Rina was aware that she had fantasies of having a strong, powerful man to lean on. However, as soon as Zack would show signs of taking charge, she would fight against his control and set about stripping him of his power, shaming him into submission with critical attacks. On the other hand, when he would appear to submit passively to her demands, she often accused him of being weak and irresponsible, always leaving her with the hard work and tough decisions.

ACCEPTANCE AND MODULATION OF WISHES
TO DOMINATE AND SUBMIT

Bringing these conflicting wishes and behaviors into awareness led Rina to examine her conflicted feminine identity. In order to feel like an attractive woman, she wanted Zack to take charge of their sex life, to actively demonstrate wanting her, and to initiate sex. However, when Zack took charge in any area, she felt anxious, demeaned, and fearful of being exploited and abandoned. These reactions derived from both the model of her mother, whom she perceived as a downtrodden, masochistic, and self-effacing, and cultural ideals of masculinity and femininity.

Since she felt unable to express her needs directly, she could only ensure her autonomy, importance, and power by seizing control and criticizing. Suppressing direct expression of her needs for nurture was also tied up with her concept of femininity—a good woman should meet the needs of others and not her own. When these conflicting feelings and their sources were clarified, she was gradually able to construct a more integrated feminine identity and masculine ideal that allowed both herself and Zack to be not only powerful and active but also passive and submissive.

Zack revealed his fantasy of a submissive woman who was constantly available and on call to meet all of his needs. She would look up to him as exceptionally competent, especially as intellectually superior. He had more difficulty admitting to his wish for a woman to take care of him in a motherly way. This wife–mother would take care of all the daily chores and petty responsibilities, leaving him free to pursue the important things in life—his music and other interests. Although in this fantasy, his mother–wife would take charge of everything mundane, he would be the final authority, the delegating general.

Since Rina was rarely submissive, he never got the opportunity to test out his dominance fantasy in reality. He imagined if he could dominate in this way, he would feel like an insensitive brute and very guilty. In acting out his passive, submissive fantasy that frequently occurred with Rina, he had mixed reactions. When Rina took charge of daily life and told him what to do, he would feel cared for but also invariably threatened—like a little boy with an emasculating mother. To counteract this threatening image, he would become resistant, passive–aggressive, or try to seize control from Rina.

Both partners' understanding of their conflicting wishes to dominate and submit as derived from family experience and cultural influence gradually freed them to resume development in this area. They became able to construct consciously their own versions of being a competent, effective man and woman. Their aims evolved similarly. Each wanted to be comfortable at all points on the power–control scale, from taking charge when needed to being able to "submit" by choice and allow the other to take charge.

Modulation of dominant–submissive wishes and perceptions are an important part of this process. This modulation comes in perceiving one partner's "dominance" as a taking charge or taking responsibility that could be agreed upon by both partners as desirable for the relationship, rather than the exercise of selfish, unilateral power. If both partners truly agree that one should be the leader, the initiator, the one in charge of something (planning a trip, planning the evening), then this leadership is no longer perceived as an act of domination—an exercise of power that coerces the other to submit. Similarly, taking a submissive position is also transformed into an active choice to give the other the leadership or his or her way about something. Optimally, what used to feel like submission to a higher authority becomes cooperation between equals to temporarily, and in context, play "unequal" roles.

Feeling that either position could be chosen enabled Rina and Zack to modulate and integrate dominant, passive, and submissive wishes and behaviors into their masculine and feminine self-images. By actively taking charge of reworking their own identities, they could develop greater personal security. This ongoing process fundamentally involves more consciously selecting and eliminating from the myriad of influences (past and present, familial and cultural) those aspects that will contribute to forming the kind of person (man or woman) one wants to be.

Understanding family and cultural influences helped Rina and Zack to gradually relinquish their dysfunctional role relationship and defensive control battling. Greater understanding of their control conflicts enabled them to become more direct about feelings they could not previously express for fear of being rejected. Zack's decisive response to Rina's attempts to take over his driving (reported in the opening exchange) was an early step in this direction. Rina's recognition of her bossiness, fears of being out of control, and wishes to rely on Zack allowed her to modulate and restrain urges to take over. Her shutting up in the car when Zack decisively confronted her inappropriate bossiness was a dramatically different response for her.

Later on in that session, she reported feeling anxious but also relieved just to let Zack take charge of the driving. Gradually, she became able to ask directly for his help and feel appreciative. In response, Zack became more reliable and emotionally supportive. With the reworking, modulation, and integration of their feminine and masculine identities, Rina and Zack became increasingly able to share power and cooperate more consistently.

CONTROLLING IN THE SERVICE OF COOPERATION

As implied in the previous discussion, in order for a couple to develop a workable balance of power, partners need to be relatively secure in their identities and gender roles. This security then enables each to feel connected with the other, without losing a sense of being a separate, autonomous individual.

It would seem that the exercise of control has come full circle from fostering a strong relational bond at the beginning of a relationship to becoming a means for partners to define themselves as effective individuals, to then being used again as a means of connection. However, the meaning and experience of control evolve in this process. Initially, the partners share the aim of seeing the other as like the self, of forging a merged identity, a sense of "We" that overpowers their differences and separateness as individuals. Each partner's attempts to influence or control the other contains the assumption that the other is an extension of the self who wants what the self wants. If Zack wanted to go to the Yucatan, he assumed that Rina wanted that too. Hence, no discussion was necessary to make a decision.

In this last step, the partners understand clearly that they are separate, distinct individuals who have many differing needs. Discussion, even arguing, is desirable for the expression of each other's needs and wants. Decisions are a result of both partners' input. Negotiation and compromise are possible, though the couple may need training in these skills. Each partner aims to effect a desired outcome, but with the shared assumption that the overall good of the relationship is the highest priority. Thus, control becomes a function of both separateness and connection—representing the "I" and the "We." Controlling is no longer primarily an expression of merger, domination, or submission, but has evolved into the desire and ability to cooperate.

Competing

"Anything You Can Do I Can Do Better"
—IRVING BERLIN (1950)

CHAPTER 15

Who's Better and Vying for Love

Tyler and Julia, a classy-looking couple in their mid-forties, married for twelve years, sought help because Julia had discovered Tyler's affair with another woman. Although Tyler ended the affair, Julia insisted on couple therapy to understand what had gone wrong between them. She was unusually sensible and psychologically sophisticated. From the first sessions, it was apparent that competition played an important role in their relationship. The following exchange occurred during the second joint evaluation session:

JULIA: The only good thing about Tyler's affair is that it's forced us to talk more openly about our feelings.

TYLER: We're closer now than we've been in a long time.

JULIA: I feel in such a strange, split state. I go back and forth—I feel so hurt and angry that I want to throw him out and never see him again. And then, all of a sudden, I feel such intense love that I want to hold him close and melt right into him.

TYLER: Julia's very articulate. She can describe how she feels much better than I can.

SHARPE: Sounds like you feel at a disadvantage in here.

TYLER: Well, this isn't my territory. I'm at home in a laboratory, with an electron microscope and a computer.

JULIA: You're just as verbal as I am.

TYLER: Not really. I can learn this insight work, but it doesn't come naturally. Taking action, getting the job done right are what counted with my father.

279

SHARPE: (*too enthusiastically*) That's insight you just demonstrated!

TYLER: (*jokingly*) I'm a fast learner, I've had to be. . . . Julia requires a worthy competitor.

JULIA: Me? You're the one who's competitive.

TYLER: Not me. I'm the one who's right.

JULIA: (*smiling*) Oh, yeah? About what?

TYLER: (*teasing*) So, you want to play who's smarter than who in here?

JULIA: You mean . . . who's smarter than *whom*.

TYLER: No, I don't think so. The correct statement is, *who* is smarter than *who*.

JULIA: You sound so sure of that, and pompous.

TYLER: I am sure. My father was a stickler for correct grammar. You use *who*, not *whom*, when both of the *who*'s are the subjects and have equal value.

JULIA: (*sighing*) Tyler beats me at Scrabble too, even though I'm the literary one. Tyler always wins.

TYLER: (*suddenly turning serious*) Not always. Not when it really counts.

SHARPE: What really counts?

TYLER: Julia, the girls . . . uh . . . my work . . . (*His voice trails off, the sparkle fading from his bright, blue eyes.*)

COMPETING FOR SUPERIORITY
AND COMPETING IN LOVE TRIANGLES

This exchange illustrates the two major patterns of competition that occur in love relationships—*competing for superiority* (dyadic competition) and *competing in love triangles* (triangular competition). Usually, competition is discussed as a single kind of behavior with varying motives. However, the two forms should be distinguished from each other because they are not only different in form but also have different underlying motivations. *Competing for superiority* (dyadic competition) is a two-way interaction that occurs when one partner tries to prove him- or herself superior to the other partner in some way. Increasing a sense of personal power, particularly in terms of competence, is the primary aim.

Competing in love triangles (triangular competition) involves a three-way interaction in which two people compete for the love of a third. At the same time that Tyler and Julia were dyadically competing about who was smarter, they were also in a triangular competition for my favor. The two forms are often interrelated. In competing for superiority, the major prize may be the love of a third party. In reverse, winning a triangular competition for the love of a third person may also involve winning a dyadic competition to prove superiority.

An example of both would be medieval knights engaged in a jousting match in which the competitors are motivated to win the contest to demonstrate superior skill as well as the love of their lady who is watching. A modern-day equivalent of this behavior would be two men at a party, one-upping each other in conversation. Both wish to prove their greater wit and higher status in relation to the other, but each also wants to win the admiration of the desirable woman standing nearby.

Triangular and dyadic forms of competition are distinct but frequently intertwine during the life of a relationship. Like other relationship patterns, both forms ideally evolve in constructive ways but also frequently become defensive and harmful.

CHAPTER 16

Winning, Losing, and Gender

Irving Berlin's duet "Anything You Can Do I Can Do Better" (from the musical *Annie Get Your Gun*) expresses the central aim of dyadic competition. The couple singing this duet is Annie Oakley and Frank Butler, two competitive, on-again-off-again-lovers just about to engage in a momentous shooting competition. Both are expert sharpshooters. The subject matter of their duet ranges from who can sing better, softer, sweeter, or higher, to who can shoot more accurately.

CONSTRUCTIVE COMPETITION

In the interaction just presented, Tyler and Julia competed about their intellectual abilities. On the surface, their verbal jousting seemed primarily playful, like the bantering duet between Annie and Frank. They appeared to enjoy the one-upmanship game, getting pleasure out of exhibiting competence, sharpening their wits, winning a point, feeling admired, but also admiring the other's scoring a point. In these senses, their competition is constructive. Personal power is gained from exhibiting their strengths, winning a round, and being admired. Additionally, affection and humor are shared. Hostility and envy are modulated and sublimated.

The positive, developmental aims of dyadic competition are to feel empowered as a unique person with special skills, attributes, or achievements, and to gain the partner's admiration. Tyler and Julia's relationship was enriched by this playful competition. These interactions fostered their connection, while, at the same time, their individuality was supported. Ideally, constructive competition advances both connection and separateness.

282

However, competition can easily become harmful in relationships, and it often does. Destructive competition, in overt and covert forms, frequently appears in couples who come for therapy. Tyler and Julia were selected as a case example, in part, because they demonstrated both positive and negative forms of dyadic competition. The damaging aspects of their competitiveness do not directly appear in the kind of dialogue presented except in the sense that this overt competitive bantering masks (and partially expresses) an unacknowledged covert competition. Tyler alluded to this undercurrent when he indicated feeling unlike a winner in the work arena.

Like the developmental aspects of devaluing and controlling, competing is another means of becoming a more defined, powerful individual in the relationship. In the normal evolution of any close relationship, competitive behavior occurs in many forms with varying motives (as detailed in Chapter 16, 17, and 18). However, serving as a means to greater self-definition and power is possibly competition's most well known positive role in child and adult development. Like the other relationship patterns, competing has its own developmental course that intertwines with all of the other patterns in the life cycle of a relationship.

DESTRUCTIVE COMPETITION

Partners can become frightened by the emergence of open competition and sometimes come to therapy for this reason. More often, couples come for therapy when they are stuck in repetitive, hurtful, competitive interactions that diminish each partner. Like Tyler and Julia, couples are often unaware of the harmful effects of their competitive expressions. They are more easily aware of being put down and devalued, without identifying the competitive component. If competition is seen as a problem, it is usually viewed as the partner's problem.

In destructive competition, the primary aim shifts from an exhibitionistic display of competence and superiority to a predominance of hostility and envy, acted out through devaluing and defeating one's partner. In the positive form, the aim of competitive behavior is to prove oneself competent and superior. In the negative, defensive form, the aim is to prove the partner inferior. If this motive predominates, a couple's connection weakens and individuality is discouraged.

In literature and the movies, the champions of degrading, competitive interaction are Martha and George from Edward Albee's play *Who's Afraid of Virginia Woolf?* (1983). Most couples only attain their degree of pain infliction for shorter intervals and are less creative in finding ever more hurtful routes to their partner's jugular. Possibly, the sadistic (and masochistic) pleasure experienced by partners interferes with desires for positive change, making them unlikely candidates for couple therapy.

Warming up early in the first act for an all-nighter of game playing, Martha attacks George after he has sexually rejected her (pp. 16–17).

MARTHA: You pig!

GEORGE: (*Haughtily*) Oink! Oink!

MARTHA: Ha, ha, ha, HA! Make me another drink . . . lover.

GEORGE: My God, you can swill it down, can't you?

MARTHA: (*Imitating a tiny child*) I'm firsty.

GEORGE: Jesus!

MARTHA: (*Swinging around*) Look, sweetheart, I can drink you under any goddamn table you want . . . so don't worry about me!

GEORGE: Martha, I gave you the prize years ago. . . . There isn't an abomination award going that you . . .

MARTHA: I swear . . . if you existed I'd divorce you. . . .

GEORGE: Well, just stay on your feet, that's all. . . . These people are your guests, you know, and. . . .

MARTHA: I can't even see you. . . . I haven't been able to see you for years. . . .

GEORGE: . . . if you pass out, or throw up, or something . . .

MARTHA: . . . I mean, you're a blank, a cipher . . .

GEORGE: . . . and try to keep your clothes on, too, There aren't many more sickening sights than you with a couple of drinks in you and your skirt up over your head, you know . . .

MARTHA: . . . a zero . . .

GEORGE: . . . your heads, I should say . . . (*The front door bell chimes.*)

In this interchange, Martha and George devalue and compete to retaliate and protect themselves from experiencing certain painful feelings. At the most obvious level is the eye-for-an-eye, immediate retaliatory response to one another's insults. Less obvious here, yet clear in the full play, is their use of competition as a projective means of coping with personal feelings of inadequacy and envy. Fear of rejection is also managed by this kind of pathological distancing interaction. Normal wishes to exhibit competence and be admired have become warped into one kind of destructive contest, expressed in their theme song: "I can humiliate you better than you can humiliate me."

While all of these defensive responses can occur normally in the course of a love relationship, they usually do not become pervasive, entrenched, and increasingly bitter. Martha and George overtly compete at a destructive extreme, while Julia and Tyler exemplify couples with a competitive problem in the moderate range of severity and treatment difficulty.

Overt and Covert Competition

Competitive themes and interaction can be expressed overtly or covertly. In general, hidden competition is more damaging than overt competition because the hurtful elements of the interaction remain unrecognized. Each partner is only subliminally aware of vicious circles of stabbing and being stabbed. The wounds cannot be stanched, because the source of the wound is unseen. In open competition that is hurtful, the wounds are visible to both parties. George and Martha were well aware of the injuries they inflicted on each other (and this is the only remotely positive aspect of their interaction). Because of their obvious warfare, there is at least the possibility that their wounds can be tended, treated, and potentially healed. Covert competition, on the other hand, saps a relationship like an ulcer bleeding internally.

There can be multiple layers of hidden competitive themes, each one concealing another, even more anxiety-provoking theme. For example, Julia and Tyler openly competed about intellectual competence, and this interaction was relatively harmless, especially earlier in their relationship. However, this competition concealed another, more painful covert competition. The playful sparring about smartness that Tyler always won defensively expressed, in reverse, the underground serious competition about who was more successful professionally. Woven within this career competition was another competition about gender—envy of the other's gender and a wish to defeat the other as a representative of men or women. Interwoven with professional and gender rivalry was yet another contest—to win parental admiration for being an especially competent little girl or boy.

The therapist's task is to work gradually through the layers of meaning expressed in a couple's competition, exposing and understanding each theme as it emerges more clearly. Once a competitive theme is openly acknowledged and understood, it can gradually be eliminated or modulated. Ideally, covert competition never takes root, because competitive feelings are openly expressed and utilized in positive ways by the partners.

General causes for a couple's development of multiple layers of covert competition stem from a combination of cultural and developmental influences. Everyone is affected by certain attitudes about competition, indicative of our culture and child-rearing practices, combined with a child's normal developmental processes. In addition, one or both partners may have suffered more pathogenic experiences in childhood. Partners who have experienced their parents as competitive and as favoring themselves or a sibling often contend with particularly intense competitive problems in their adult love relationships.

CULTURE, CHILDHOOD, AND COMPETITION

In the process of growing up, most of us are bombarded by a conflicting array of attitudes about exhibiting our competence, competing, winning, and losing. On the side of exhibitionism and competition is the following set of attitudes conveyed to us from mainstream culture and our families:

We should show off our abilities and feel proud of ourselves for our accomplishments. We should strive to be the best and win competitions in games, in school, and in the world. We should feel proud of winning. If we lose, we should lose gracefully and work harder to win the next time around.

Competition as portrayed in the Olympic games is the ideal model for these attitudes about exhibiting competence, competing, winning, and losing.

There is tremendous support from our culture to compete openly and win. Winning almost any kind of competition is rewarded—games, contests, grades, scholarships, jobs, business contracts, elections, wars. Winning a prized love object is also cause for celebration, admiration, and envy—a man winning the love of a beautiful woman, a woman winning love and marriage with a powerful, handsome man. Winners get gold stars, awards, trophies, money, praise, admiration. If we win really big, we get thunderous applause, fame, fortune, and power.

Many of us remember hearing our parents quote a version of Grantland Rice's famous line (to paraphrase): *It doesn't matter if you win or lose but only how you play the game.* If we look at the times when this sentiment was expressed by an elder, it was usually when we needed to be comforted for losing at something. Compelling as this piece of wisdom may sound (coming from the Great Scorekeeper in the sky), it made little impact compared to the glowing pride we saw on our parents faces when we won. What may take priority in our minds is coach Henry (Red) Sander's motto: "Winning isn't everything—it's the only thing!"[1]

While exhibiting, competing, and winning are applauded, they are also strongly discouraged in various ways and forms. This conflicting set of messages, also passed on to us by our culture and filtered through our parents, can be summarized as follows:

We should not show off our abilities; we should downplay, even conceal our accomplishments; we should avoid competition; wishes to show off, compete, and win are base, vain, and selfish, and should be suppressed. Furthermore, if we find ourselves engaged in a competition, we should demonstrate our goodness by letting the other person win.

The self-effacing person will eventually be rewarded in heaven, if not on earth. These attitudes, imbued in us especially from the Christian aspects of our culture, are more strongly instilled in girls but are also conveyed to boys, especially through their mothers.

In normal development, exhibitionism and competition are interrelated behaviors children use to build a sense of pride in themselves, their gender, and their abilities. Admiration from parents for all sorts of displays of prowess—from turning a cartwheel to winning a game—is internalized by the child and transformed into a growing sense of personal power and competence. However, young children's normal exhibitionism and pride in their competence and gender may be quickly deflated by unadmiring, critical, or competitive parents.

Deflation of self-esteem also normally occurs when a child discovers gender differences—the discovery that the other gender has certain attributes that oneself lacks. At the time of this discovery, children also become aware of the differences between their own attributes and those of their parents and older siblings. Envy develops of what the other gender and grown-ups have. Girls envy the boy's penis. Boys envy mother's breasts and ability to have babies. Boys envy their dad's bigger penis. Conflicting wishes emerge—to be one's own sex but to also be the other sex, to have it all and be bisexual (see Tyson & Tyson, 1990, for a more detailed discussion of these aspects of child development).

Children compete in constructive and destructive ways with those who are admired and envied—brother, sister, mother, father. Displays of power and superiority are used not only to advance development of com-

---

[1]This statement is usually attributed to the famous Green Bay Packers coach Vince Lombardi. However, the Library of Congress credits Sanders, who coached at Vanderbilt and UCLA. Lombardi said his statement was "Winning is not everything—but making the effort to win is."

petence, but also to allay anxiety, insecurity, and envy, warding off feelings of smallness, powerlessness, and inferiority. Admiring and confirming responses from parents not only fulfill developmental needs but also help a child cope with feelings of envy and inadequacy. Admiration from our spouses in marriage fulfills the same kind of functions.

Parents' responses to their child's early exhibitionism and bids for admiration are crucial to general self-esteem and particularly important for the child's developing pride in his or her accomplishments and gender. Feelings of pride, competence, and gender adequacy are necessary for developing the strength to compete openly and effectively. Feelings of shame and inadequacy lead to an avoidance of open competition, a suppression of competitive impulses, and tendencies to compete covertly.

Many parents interfere with their children's optimal development of exhibitionism and competition because of attitudes, beliefs, and their own internal conflicts in these areas. I have the impression, from observing many families, that parents are more comfortable admiring their very young children's exhibitionistic displays, but this support is often withdrawn as the child grows older. One reason for this withdrawal of enthusiastic admiration may be that a child's exhibitionistic expressions begin to include competitive, aggressive behaviors. Additionally, as children approach school age, parents become more invested in teaching, correcting, and criticizing to encourage certain kinds of performance and achievement.

Exhibitionistic displays can be difficult for parents to receive positively, particularly if they were not admired in this way as young children or, worse, were actively shamed for showing off. A child's competitive behavior, especially when expressed in relation to a parent, may be even more difficult to manage appropriately with good-humored acceptance. Many parents feel threatened by their child's competitiveness and development of competence. Such anxiety may lead a parent to squash competitive expressions through disapproval—"Nice girls/boys don't show off, brag, or compete." More potentially damaging are parents who react competitively to their children's showing off and competing. A child's normal expressions may incite their own narcissistic needs to show off, win, and be admired. Feelings of envy and inadequacy may be stimulated, leading some parents to react competitively.

Tyler described his father as needing to show off, instruct, and take over almost every activity he engaged in as a child. Playing sports was a particular ordeal for Tyler, because his father constantly had to teach and instruct him on how to throw or kick the ball the right way. One of the reasons he gravitated toward science was because his father left him alone with his chemistry experiments, having no interest or knowledge in the area. Science was a wonderful haven for Tyler to develop his abilities, because he did not have to contend directly with his father's needs to be competitively superior and admired.

Julia's description of playing chess with her father is another example of a competitive parental reaction. Her father, she said, always took delight in beating her. He never made any allowances for her being a child, never modified the rules or gave her any help. One day, when she finally beat him for the first time, he accused her of cheating. He became sulky, withdrawn, and less interested in playing chess with her after that.

When a child's optimal development of competence and competitiveness is discouraged by parents, a strong prohibition is internalized: *Don't compete with Mom and Dad, because we are bigger, better, and smarter than you are. We will be hurt and won't love you anymore if you compete and surpass us.* These same parents may also vigorously support their children, especially their boys, to compete aggressively with others *outside* of the family—in school, sports, and the work world.

Competition and the Marriage Relationship

This prohibition from our parents, conveyed in greater or lesser degrees, is carried with us into marriage and can have deleterious effects. First, eliminating all competition between married partners is impossible, since competitive feelings are most intensely experienced with those we love the most. Second, these impulses become more intense—more hostile and aggressive—when their open expression is prohibited. Third, because competition was likely discouraged in relation to our parents, many adults are looking for a corrective experience in marriage. We secretly hope for a mate who will admire, love, and support us in victory and defeat. With our partner, we hope to feel free to show off, compete, win, or lose and still be loved, accepted, and admired. Damaging covert competition tends to develop as a result of conflicting wishes to conceal and reveal these feelings, spoiling a couple's relationship like an unrecognized debilitating illness. The idea that open competition is harmful or even dangerous to a marriage relationship is also strongly reinforced by our cultural attitudes and expressions.

Open competition between men and women in the workplace is now becoming increasingly acceptable. However, open competition between men and women in love relationships continues to be discouraged, unless such expression is circumscribed and tamed into playing games with rules—such as tennis, cards, or golf.

Looking to the movies as reflective of mainstream cultural attitudes, there are very few American movies that centrally focus on the theme of competition in heterosexual marriage. When this subject has been undertaken, competition is almost always portrayed as destructive. The marriage is portrayed as seriously troubled, or worse, as in *Who's Afraid of Virginia Woolf?* (1966) and *Cat on a Hot Tin Roof* (1958); the relationship ends in alienation and/or divorce (as in *Gone With the Wind* [1939], *The Way We*

Were [1973], *Kramer vs. Kramer* [1979]); or the relationship ends with the alcoholism and suicide of the loser partner, as we torturously witness in the three versions of *A Star Is Born* (1937, 1954, 1976). In the marital horror movie *War of the Roses* (1989), the brutal competition between the divorcing partners results in their death. It is the unacknowledged covert gender competition between the partners that progressively erodes and eventually destroys this couple's relationship.

There is one old Spencer Tracy–Katherine Hepburn romantic comedy, *Adam's Rib* (1947), that portrays competition between the lawyer/married partners in a more appealing, less destructive light. However, even in this comedic, liberal-minded rendition of married partners openly competing in the courtroom, the marriage becomes insupportably strained, and the husband leaves his wife (albeit briefly) after she defeats him and wins the case.

When the partners are unmarried lovers or about to become lovers, there are many more movies that present hero and heroine competing in various ways as a preamble to their falling in love. Some of these better known movies include the musical *Annie Get Your Gun* (1950), *House Calls* (1978), *The Competition* (1980), *Romancing the Stone* (1984), *The Big Easy* (1987), and *I Love Trouble* (1994). The outcomes of these competitive romantic preambles to commitment or marriage are fairly predictable. Once the couple admits to being in love or marries, the competition appears to end. Often, the woman yields, or pretends to yield, to the man's superiority or need to feel superior. One message conveyed by most of these movies is that it may be acceptable to compete with your prospective mate before marriage, but such behavior should be given up at the time of marriage, especially by the woman.

Another, perhaps equally disconcerting theme that emerges from a study of these movies is that if the woman wins a competition with a man (especially in terms of career success), she seriously risks losing the man, as occurred in *Adams Rib, Annie Get Your Gun,* and *The Competition.* Alternatively, the man will totally fall apart and abandon the woman through alcoholism and suicide, as he did in *A Star Is Born.*

In order to get the man back, it is necessary for the woman to let the man feel he has really won or is superior. By giving this message, the movies simply echo what many mothers may still be advising their daughters—"Let the man win!" For example, in *Adam's Rib*, a humiliated and enraged Spencer Tracy only returns to the victorious Katherine Hepburn when he finds a way to prove her wrong and thus reestablish his superiority (which she then wisely appears to accept). In *Annie Get Your Gun,* Frank falls in love with Annie but leaves her because she is the better sharpshooter and more successful in their show. In order to win Frank's love back, Annie pretends she is not as good a shot as he and lets him win the shooting contest.

This brief foray into marital competition in the movies is very pertinent to the problems of Julia and Tyler, and those of many other real-life couples, for in this marriage, the partners were covertly competitive about their careers. The serious threat to the marriage came from the unacknowledged competition and the conflictual feelings in both partners, evoked by Julia surpassing Tyler professionally.

Exposing Covert Competition

The professional aspects of their covert competition are gradually exposed in the following excerpt from an early therapy session. The subject under discussion is the couple's decision to settle in California for the benefit of Julia's career.

SHARPE: How did you make this decision—to stay here for Julia's career?

TYLER: Julia had worked hard for the position she was offered, and it meant a substantial increase in our income, which we needed at the time. We have the girls in an excellent but expensive private school.

JULIA: (*defensively*) It wasn't just that. This is also a great place to raise children, and they're both very happy in their school and with their friends. To uproot everything didn't seem a good idea for them. (*looking anxiously at Tyler*) At the time, you said you were happy in the company.

TYLER: Yes, in the sense that I like the work and the environment. The problem was, and still is, that there is no place for me to advance. Also, we don't know from year to year whether we're going to get the funds even to survive.

SHARPE: This sounds upsetting.

TYLER: (*shrugging*) Two years ago, I had a good job offer, but neither of us could face moving to Dallas, Texas. The job wasn't particularly appealing, though it paid a lot more and there might have been better opportunities for the future.

SHARPE: How does your future look now?

TYLER: My future . . . well . . . if our company folds, I would likely have to teach entry level math or physics in a junior college or a community college, in order for us to stay here.

JULIA: We won't let that happen. We'll move somewhere else.

TYLER: I don't mind teaching. I used to be good at it. I foresaw that possibility when we made the decision to stay.

JULIA: We can always change that decision.

TYLER: You love your job.

JULIA: I can find another job I love.

TYLER: (*bitterly with a tight smile*) A lot more easily than I can.

His resentment had suddenly popped into the open. A tense silence followed. Julia looked stricken, and Tyler's face went blank.

SHARPE: This is a difficult subject, isn't it? I can see you both trying very hard to be fair.

JULIA: We've never talked enough about this. It seems too loaded.

SHARPE: It is loaded. You have to contend with the issue of who's career comes first and then deal with the emotional fallout from whatever decisions you make.

JULIA: I don't think we're dealing with the emotional fallout very well.

TYLER: I object to that metaphor. Fallout sounds like an atom bomb has exploded, and we're suffering from radiation poisoning.

SHARPE: Sorry to be so dramatic. But, you know, when certain feelings don't get expressed—like anger, hurt, disappointment—the atmosphere in a marriage can become poisoned.

TYLER: (*sounding irritated*) Frankly, I've lost the thread here. What are we talking about?

JULIA: About our careers. How we've coped with that issue.

TYLER: (*defensively*) I think we've coped well with that issue. We've discussed it and made the best decision we could, given all the factors. We're not tied to out-of-date values.

SHARPE: What values do you mean?

TYLER: The values from our families, like the man's job comes first.

JULIA: In my family, the man came first in general. Men were more important than women. My father was more important than my mother, and my brother was more important than me. We moved around the world because of my father's career. He led my mother around by the nose, and she didn't even know she minded.

Her description led me to think of my own behavior as a young, married woman. I, too, followed my husband and his career across the country, without giving a thought to doing anything else. It was what we women did, or most of us, three decades ago.

SHARPE: In your situation, you've done the opposite, gone against how you were raised. That takes considerable courage. But I think you'd be left with difficult feelings to work through, like resentment (*looking at Tyler*) and guilt (*looking at Julia*).

JULIA: (*nodding*) I feel guilty about being so ambitious and selfish. I feel guilty a lot of the time, especially when Tyler looks unhappy.

TYLER: But I'm not unhappy. Maybe something doesn't work out at the lab, and I have a bad day like everyone else, so I'm a little down.

JULIA: If you were happy with me, you wouldn't have had an affair.

TYLER: (*groaning*) Haven't we talked enough about that? I felt I was losing you. You were so busy, I hardly ever saw you. You were too tired at night to make love. And, I suppose I came to resent being left with so much care of the girls.

SHARPE: How about resenting your career being put second?

TYLER: I agreed to that.

SHARPE: That doesn't mean you don't also feel resentful and disappointed that your own career is not taking off in the same way Julia's has. (*He doesn't deny this.*) I think you try hard not to have these feelings.

TYLER: You're right about that. I don't like your implication that I envy or begrudge Julia's success. I'm proud of her. I really am. She's gifted in her field. She's worked extremely hard, and she should be rewarded.

SHARPE: Yes, that's true, but what about you? Haven't you worked hard too? Shouldn't you also be rewarded?

TYLER: Yes, yes . . . if life was fair. But life is not fair. And I chose a very narrow, out-of-vogue branch of physics to specialize in.

JULIA: (*proudly*) Tyler is also gifted in his field, more gifted than I am. He won a National Science Foundation postdoctoral fellowship. They're only awarded to the best graduate students in physics.

TYLER: (*looking acutely embarrassed*) That was a very, *very* long time ago. I know you mean well, but please don't do that sort of thing. It makes me feel like a small boy whose lost a game and needs bucking up.

SHARPE: Yes I see that, and now the winner is trying to comfort you. (*Tyler flinches in pain*)

JULIA: I'm sorry. I'm really sorry. I didn't mean to come across like that.

SHARPE: I think you feel very guilty about your success and are trying to make it up to Tyler. [I didn't add, at this point, that the condescending flavor of her praise also suggested some pleasure in his "losing the game."]

TYLER: It's called shoring up the frail masculine ego.

JULIA: I don't see you that way. You're not frail. I've always seen you as strong.

TYLER: That's a myth you know, that men are strong. Women are much stronger than men. They live longer for one thing. I don't like spoiling your illusion, but I'm afraid I haven't lived up to it.

JULIA: Yes you have. It's me that's failed you.

TYLER: That's nonsense. You're the best thing that's ever happened to me.

With this mutual beating of the breast and reassurance, it was clear that they had become frightened by the surfacing of less than honorable feelings toward one another. I had not gotten as far as I hoped, but it was a good beginning, especially with partners who hid their anger, disappointment, and envy behind well-honed idealizing, intellectualizing, and civilized competing. The door to their covert competition had at least been cracked open.

One of the results of women's liberation is the increase in the number of women who are surging ahead of their men in the workplace. Most couples are not yet prepared to handle the arousal of competitive feelings in an arena where the man has always ruled supreme. As was the case with Tyler and Julia, the negative effects of a wife's success on a man's self-esteem and masculine identity are so often managed by a couple's joint denial—a pretense that no competition or problem really exists. Tyler only proclaimed his pride in Julia and support of her achievements. The injury to his masculine self-image, envy, and anger were concealed even from himself.

If a couple does not openly acknowledge and process these feelings, the man is likely to compete covertly with his wife. In seeking to restore his lost power and masculine pride, he may unconsciously even the score by having an affair, sometimes soon followed by leaving the marriage. This attack on his wife's feminine desirability seems equal to the blow she has delivered to his masculinity and gender-role adequacy. Hell hath no fury like a man unmanned!

This is a reversal of competitive patterns appearing in the more traditional gender-role relationship, wherein the wife is selflessly devoted to care of husband, children, and home. Even though she may work part-time or even full-time, her jobs are understood to be less important than the husbands. Therapists are very familiar with women patients who feel depressed and suppressed as individuals in this role. Competition with a more important, powerful husband is often expressed covertly through undermining his masculinity in the bedroom (through disinterest or dissatisfaction) and his authority on the homefront by forming alliances with the children.

In traditional marriage, competitive feelings of the partners may not be as easily incited as in equal-partnership marriages, because each partner has a clearly demarked and separate area of work and achievement. Additionally, in the traditional or patriarchal ideal, both partners supposedly agree that the husband is more important and powerful, especially in terms of major decisions. In equal-partnership marriages, it is more difficult to avoid awareness of competitive feelings because the partners share every important domain of functioning and achievement.

While women who work and achieve success in their careers have been increasingly supported in the last two decades, most women are still conflicted about openly competing and winning. Although Julia vigorously competed to advance in her career in linguistics, she seemed subliminally aware of the negative impact of her great success on Tyler. Her insistence that he was always the winner of their word games seemed exaggerated, reminding me of deeply imbedded instructions to let the man win, or let the man *think* he's winning.

Julia, like other middle-aged women, grew up during the time when our culture strongly discouraged openly competitive behavior in girls. She learned the social lesson that men will reject and leave a woman who wins too much. Annie Oakley recognized this reality when she sang "You Can't Get a Man with a Gun." The old and the new cultural ideals of femininity created intense internal conflict for Julia, as they do for most women who are desirous of having a career. The feminine role passed down from mother to keep the man as a strong, powerful protector of a weak, "feminine" self conflicts with pressure from the women's movement to be independent and realize one's potential no matter what the cost.

The ideal of femininity now confronting women from outside and inside says that a real woman should be able to do it all—be the family's nurturer, a winner in the world, and as good as or better than a man. Expectations of men are equally conflictual and grandiose. Men feel great pressure to do and be everything. The ideal of masculinity is to still be a competitive, successful breadwinner and the family's strong, tough protector, but now it is also necessary to be emotionally expressive, a sensitive nurturer—an ever available Mr. Mom.

As life progresses, it seems to become more complex and daunting for both sexes to fulfill ideals of what it takes to be adequately masculine or feminine and to meet various internal and external expectations of gender roles—man, woman; husband, wife; mother, father; daughter, son.

Some say the job is more difficult for men, yet women tend to feel that they are the more burdened with impossible role expectations and standards of "feminine" attractiveness.

The therapist's first aim in working with these problems is to help the partners become aware of their underlying conflictual feelings relating to competition and gender-role expectations in connection with their current life and relationship history. Articulating the normality of competitive feelings between spouses and encouraging their open expression is important and necessary in order to counteract strong prohibitions from childhood and society. The therapist's grasp of our current cultural climate of confusing and grandiose gender-role expectations for men and women, husbands and wives, needs to be a consistent and explicit aspect of the therapeutic work.

It is essential to understand a couple's gender-role relationship—each partner's expectation of what a man and woman should be/do in the relationship—and how this relationship may have changed. So often, couples founder when one partner has deviated from a previous role. One of the common shifts in gender role occurs when a wife who functioned as a homemaker goes back to school, begins working, or becomes invested in building a career. Exploration of each partner's feelings about such a change is a necessary first step.

The shift in the gender-role relationship can be more subtle, as it was with Julia and Tyler. Both partners had always been career-oriented, and theirs was an equal-partnership marriage from the outset. However, their decision to stay in California for Julia's career reflected a fundamental shift in this relationship—from the couple's former conception of Tyler's career as the number-one priority to Julia's career as the priority. Tyler had become the follower instead of the leader—less important and less powerful in both partners' eyes. Their relationship suffered greatly in the aftermath of this change.

If Julia and Tyler had possessed the capacities to process competitive feelings at the outset, such action may have prevented these feelings from going underground to fester and corrode the relationship. Possibly, their relationship would have become closer and stronger instead of more distant, hurtful, and plagued by infidelity. *The Competition* (1980) is the one movie I have seen that portrays open expression and processing of competitive feelings, resulting in a heartening outcome to a similar story.

In this movie, the young lovers (played by Amy Irving and Richard Dreyfuss) are pianists who are fiercely competing for first place in a piano competition. The young woman almost withdraws from the competition, because her lover needs to win more than she does, for financial and self-esteem reasons. However, with his encouragement, she does compete; she performs spectacularly and wins. He comes in second. There is a wrenching scene in which it becomes clear that he cannot handle her winning and must withdraw from the relationship. It had never occurred to him that she could possibly be better than he.

He leaves her but in the final moment shows up at the celebration party. We are left with the implication that he loves her enough and has become man enough to stay in the relationship in spite of her winning and superiority as a pianist. There is the unusual portrayal in this story of lovers who openly compete, develop, and become strengthened by their competition. Their relationship, though stormy, becomes much closer.

Unfortunately, the movie does not show us the aftermath of these events. We are left to wonder how long Richard Dreyfuss could really take following Amy Irving around on her first prize concert tour to twenty cities—not very long without major difficulties, most would predict. Certainly, multiple problems beset Julia and Tyler, whose story with competition did not have such an easily won, positive outcome.

CHAPTER 17

Competing for Superiority
Development and Common
Treatment Problems

Competition may enrich a love relationship or effectively destroy intimacy. By contributing to the partners' sense of competence, it may strengthen their collaborative efforts. However, when one or both partners' needs for power stem from pervasive feelings of envy and insecurity, competitive interaction usually becomes destructive, derailing forward development.

Ideally, a couple needs to allow competition into the relationship but also be able to recognize and curtail destructive expressions. Some of the highlights of an optimal developmental process are outlined as follows:

- Competing as courtship play
- Competing for admiration and superiority
- Competing to cope with envy and inadequacy
- Acceptance of needs to compete (in self and partner)
- Modulation of competitiveness
- Competing to enhance collaboration

As with the other relationship patterns, this evolutionary process proceeds in a recapitulatory rather than a linear fashion. Partners revisit and rework the steps and their associated tasks many times during their relationship. Additionally, there is much overlapping and simultaneous occurrence of the psychological events and processes. Regressions and stalls in development normally occur at various points of difficulty, which will differ in kind and quality for each couple.

298

Competition may first emerge as an aspect of a couple's courtship, although many lovers repress these feelings toward each other. When partners work toward becoming more separate and self-defined following the romantic phase, exhibitionistic and competitive impulses may surface for the first time or become more strongly expressed. If one or both partners are conflicted about their competitive feelings or do not admire one another's displays of competence and superiority, competition may become overtly or covertly hurtful. Wounding competitive interaction also often appears as an expression of partners' initial and subsequent disappointments in each other. Additionally, in losing the partner as an ideal extension of oneself, one or both partners may become more aware of feeling inadequate and envious. Competing with the partner may be used to cope with these feelings. Pervasive destructive competition often reflects the partners' reenactment of injurious childhood relationships with parents or siblings. Partners' parents may have been experienced as unadmiring and competitive, resulting in lifelong feelings of inferiority. Parental favoritism of a sibling may have also contributed to low self-esteem and competitive envy.

Ideally, a couple works through all of these aspects of competition, including desires to feel powerful, superior, and competent, as well as those aspects that are motivated by disappointment, injury, inadequacy, hostility, and envy. When a couple can accept the need to compete and modulate competitive expressions, this mode can vitalize the relationship and enhance collaboration. Figure 8 outlines the main steps and associated tasks in the development of competing, along with the common problems encountered by many couples.

COMPETING AS COURTSHIP PLAY

As described in the previous chapter, competitive interaction between a man and a woman is often portrayed as a central aspect of their courtship dance. In their duet ("Anything You Can Do"), Annie and Frank are clearly competing, but they are also obviously falling in love. Their competitive interaction can be understood as not only showing off their individual prowess in the sense of a courtship display but also expressing their fears of falling in love. As previously discussed, the merging aspects of falling in love are threatening to many people for many reasons. Competitive behavior (like controlling behavior) effectively protects many lovers from fearful loss of their autonomy. Keeping competition alive, but playful, is a way to preserve individuality while gradually allowing a deeper connection.

The exchange between Tyler and Julia at the beginning of Chapter

Steps in Development of Dyadic Competing	Tasks for Couple/Guide for Therapy	Common Problems (Points of Regression and Derailment)
Competing as Courtship Play	Engaging in mutual exhibitionism and admiration Competing playfully to connect, while preserving separateness	Competitive feelings toward partner massively repressed
Competing for Admiration and Superiority	Defining and empowering oneself through exhibitionistic competing Responding to partner's competition as need for admiration of unique attributes Recognizing hurtful competition as a reaction to disappointment and injury Understanding the role of the past in perception of partner as an unadmiring, competitive parent	Competitiveness repressed and expressed covertly Withholding admiration and criticizing partner Continual denial of overtly destructive competition Reenactment of competitive parent–inferior child role relationship
Competing to Cope with Envy and Inadequacy	Understanding destructive competitiveness caused by inadequacy and/or envy Recognizing and working through gender envy and inferiority	Devaluing forms of competing used to manage feelings of envy and inadequacy Stalled in gender envy and inferiority
Acceptance of Needs to Compete	Recognizing competition exists in relationship	Existence of competition denied
Modulation of Dyadic Competing	Accepting superiority, competencies, and inadequacies of partner and oneself Channeling aggressive competition to playful expressions and games	Unable to construct realistic images of partner and oneself Competing used to prove oneself superior and the partner inferior
Competing to Enhance Collaboration	Recognizing and using each partner's strengths to solve problems effectively	Collaboration does not use each partner's strengths Need to prove partner inferior takes precedence over collaborative relationship

FIGURE 8. The development of dyadic competing (for superiority).

15 is an example of a similar kind of mutually entertaining competition. Although this interchange occurred twelve years into their marriage, the lighthearted atmosphere was stimulated by a brief honeymoon period following the trauma caused by Julia's discovery of Tyler's affair. In this interaction, the quality of competing is similar to that engaged in by many couples during their original courtship phase. This exhibitionistic, mutually admiring form of competition often does not last in a purely playful way as the full range of each partner's strivings and conflicts become expressed in the relationship.

Since competitive behavior is often threatening to a romantic attachment, many couples in the courtship and early phase engage only in mutual exhibitionism and admiration. In this common event, competitive impulses are repressed by the couple. The partners may displace these impulses by competing with others instead of each other. This management of threatening feelings has the potential to cause problems if repression is massive and competition emerges in covert forms.

COMPETING FOR ADMIRATION AND SUPERIORITY

As partners move out of romantic merging toward reestablishing themselves as separate individuals, an upsurge of exhibitionism and competitive expressions may appear more strongly as a normal aspect of individualizing themselves. By exhibiting competence and competing, the partners hope to prove themselves to be competent, but each also needs the other's admiring support. In the ideal relationship, partners recognize and admire one another's particular competence or superior skill. The hostile, aggressive aspects of competition are ideally channeled into competitive sports or games played either together or separately. However, as discussed in the previous chapter, there may be many obstacles in the way of one or both partners' being able to openly exhibit abilities, compete, win, lose, and accept the other or oneself as superior in certain areas but not so competent in other areas. Admiration of the partner or oneself as superior or a winner may also be impeded by feelings of inadequacy, envy, shame, or guilt.

Competing as a Reaction to Disappointment and Injury

Competition often makes its first appearance in a relationship in a harmful rather than a constructive way. With the fading of romantic love and becoming more separate, partners usually experience some degree of disappointment in each other. Since the partner is seen as less ideal and often devalued to some extent, withdrawal of admiration and an increase of criticism frequently occur, causing injury to each partner. When partners are unable to discuss their disappointments, they may express themselves in denigrating competitive interaction. Vicious circles can develop in which each partner copes with feeling hurt, angry, and rejected with the kind of competitiveness that is increasingly tainted by devaluing. Competition used to express injury can occur at any point in the life of a relationship. Certain events will cause a disappointed reaction and trigger another round of deidealizing, which in turn may be expressed in hurtful forms of competing.

Julia and Tyler were mutually disappointed about their career successes and failures, followed two years later by the traumatic rupture of Tyler's affair. Competitive interaction used to cope with such injuries is illustrated in the following excerpt from an early-phase therapy session. This exchange also indicates that the brief honeymoon period the couple experienced at the beginning of therapy is now over.

TYLER: I didn't feel that good about our interaction last night. I thought you put me down rather sharply in front of the girls. [The couple had two daughters, ages nine and eleven.]

JULIA: Oh, did I? I'm sorry. I was just so tired and feeling impatient with everything.

TYLER: This happens a lot. We get into these set-tos about words and minor points of trivia. It's like we put on a little competition for the girls, each of us trying to look smarter. It used to be fun. But now, I think it's gotten out of hand. I feel you actually get mad at me if I correct you, and you make nasty remarks.

JULIA: I don't know why I'm so irritable lately. But I think you're more critical of me, too. I remember now. It seemed like you were mocking me last night. Your tone and expression were saying, "how could you make such a stupid remark?"

TYLER: I wasn't aware of that. If I did that, I'm sorry. But I think we should avoid these word games for awhile. The girls are getting upset by us.

SHARPE: Maybe this competition is the way you're trying to cope with feeling hurt—you know getting the other back by one-upmanship?

TYLER: (*nodding*) I can see Julia being hurt when I score a point, and then she puts me down.

JULIA: (*sarcastically*) Oh, so it's all me? You're just an innocent bystander?

TYLER: (*attempting to joke*) That's right.

JULIA: I know you think I start these things by my responses. But a lot of times, I feel you're sort of out to get me as soon as I walk in the door.

TYLER: Oh, really? (*sounding surprised, he's thoughtful for a moment, then speaks hesitantly*) Well, I guess I could sometimes be annoyed about how late you are getting home. I'm there a couple of hours before you are. I've had to deal with the girls and their homework and get dinner going.

JULIA: Yes, I know, and I've had the sense that I'm not very welcome. You don't smile, and you aren't very affectionate when I arrive.

TYLER: (*sharply*) Well, neither are you. You're scowling when you come in the door. And you immediately notice what's not been done, rather than all we have done.

Julia looked wounded and did not respond. Tyler turned inward, his eyes glazing over. I presumed he was feeling quite anxious about his unusual directness and criticism of Julia. I broke the tense silence.

SHARPE: These kinds of receptions must feel pretty bad.

JULIA: (*softly*) I know I feel hurt. But I can't blame Tyler. I'm so guilty about being late. I know when I'm late he's had to do more work. I'm on edge and snappy because I'm guilty. (*She grimaces in self-disgust.*)

TYLER: We're both reacting to each other in negative ways, and it just gets worse when we get into these word games. Let's quit it. Surely we can. It's not an addiction, after all.

Although, in these instances, the couple's competing was prompted by mutual feelings of rejection, a deeper cause of injury stemmed from their disappointment in each other over career and role changes (which came to light later in this session).

Denigrating competitive behavior as a reaction to disappointment and rejection is also well illustrated in the dialogue between Martha and George, reported in Chapter 16. Martha's immediate response to George's rejection of her sexual overtures is to call him a pig. She then quickly adopts a superior, challenging attitude: "Look sweetheart, I can drink you under any goddamn table you want. . . . " George copes with being wounded by Martha in the same way. His retaliatory put-downs seem more devastating because they are more complex, devious, and delivered with greater detachment.

Unlike Julia and Tyler, Martha and George never moved beyond their initial experience of disappointment in each other (and in themselves). In

Albee's play, Martha's disappointment in George is particularly empha-sized. She repetitively harps on his failure to achieve distinction in acade-mia, become as powerful as her father, or act in any way like an adequate male. From a developmental view, this couple never moved beyond their initial disillusionment in each other, which they expressed by punitively competing. Their hopes and ideals were maintained through the creation of an imaginary child.

Competing in Response to Loss of Admiration

A common reaction to partners' mutual withdrawal of admiring attention is the development of a competitive struggle to win back the partner's lost admiration. Each one demands of the other in effect, "Look at me! Ad-mire me!" The other responds, "No! You look at *me*! You admire *me*!" It seems as though the well of admiration has dried up, and there is not enough to go around. Each partner views the other like an unadmiring, critical parent from childhood, while feeling like a child who cannot get the parent's approval. Each longs to recapture the admiring parent–spe-cial child role relationship that was a fulfilling aspect of their romantic love and mutual idealization.

In addition, as partners develop their individual capacities, each wants acknowledgment and admiration for special abilities and achieve-ments. Global kinds of admiration, indicative of romantic love—"You're the most wonderful woman (or man) in the world"—are no longer suffi-cient. More differentiated kinds of admiration are sought, and it is with the emergence of these specific needs that partners often disappoint each other. Couples in this state of need will often look to the therapist for re-storative acknowledgment and admiration.

In a continuation of the same session with Tyler and Julia, they reveal feelings of disappointment and loss of each other's admiration. Tyler has just suggested that they simply stop their competitive behavior as a solu-tion to their wounded feelings.

SHARPE: It might also help to look at why this as happening.

TYLER: Aren't we doing well enough to say how we feel? (*He says this lightly, but I sense he feels criticized and wants acknowledgment.*)

SHARPE: Yes, very well. I think it's great that you're saying how you feel, when you don't like something.

TYLER: Julia should also be praised.

SHARPE: Yes, indeed. You've both made a lot of progress in communicat-ing more directly. I know it's not easy for you to complain about each other. (*They both beam like children, soaking up my praise like needed nutrients.*)

JULIA: Neither of us does very well with criticism. Tyler's right. We're too critical of each other. It comes out most obviously in this game playing we do.

SHARPE: Do you have any idea when these interactions became more hurtful?

JULIA: I don't know. It was better for a little while lately, but then it got worse again. It's been gradual over the past couple of years.

TYLER: I'd say it tracks back to our decision to stay here and your promotion to associate. (*turning to me*) That's when I began to feel I was losing Julia . . . her presence, as well as her respect.

JULIA: You haven't lost my respect. I admire you more than any man I know.

TYLER: I just don't feel it's there like it used to be.

JULIA: Well, I feel the same way (*her eyes tearing up*). There's no glow in your eyes when you look at me. I used to feel beautiful and sexy and smart when you'd look at me. Your whole face would light up. Now, you look at me like I'm a worn out piece of furniture cluttering up the room.

TYLER: Oh, Julia, for God's sake. That's so ridiculous . . . and it's just not true.

JULIA: Don't get mad. I'm just trying to describe how I feel.

TYLER: I'm not mad . . . just . . . frustrated. I see you as more beautiful, sexy, and intelligent than when we first fell in love. I just don't convey these feelings as well as I did earlier on . . . I felt more positive and hopeful about myself when I was younger. You've changed, too. I don't exactly walk on water for you anymore. I feel you look at me, more often than not, as an annoying little boy.

Behind their feelings of hurt and anger about the accrual of day-to-day injuries and resentments lay deeper feelings of rejection, most acutely felt in the loss of one another's admiration. Their supportive admiration of each other, often expressed in the context of competition, had been a major component of their well-being as a couple and as individuals. Withdrawal of admiration and devaluing forms of competitiveness sometimes follow episodes of disappointment. These occurrences are normal, provided that they are temporary. Optimally, a working through of disappointments occurs, resulting in greater acceptance of the partner (and self), accompanied by the return of mutual support and admiration. However, in the case of Tyler and Julia, feeling deflated, unadmired, and increasingly competitive in hurtful ways were not temporary events. Accumulated injuries had resulted in a gradual distancing in the relationship, culminating in Tyler's affair.[1]

The Competitive Parent and the Inferior Child

This kind of derailment is often linked with the exacerbation of the partners' childhood wounds, which are often caused by competitive parents who provided inadequate mirroring and admiration. Admiration from the partner is particularly important when there was an inadequate or indiscriminant supply in childhood. The partner's withdrawal of this nutrient is then experienced as intolerably hurtful and rejecting. In exploring Tyler's and Julia's childhood experiences, we found that they hardly remembered admiring praise from their parents. As so often appears in the family histories of couples who are markedly competitive, both partners experienced one or both parents as critical, competitive, and unable to provide supportive admiration of their accomplishments and gender.

Tyler and Julia had parents who looked to their children for mirroring and admiration instead of being able to provide these functions. Tyler had a highly competitive father who favored his sister, and Julia's mother competed with her, while favoring her brother. The competitiveness of their parents squashed both partners' normal childhood exhibitionism and open expressions of competition. Additionally, these parents' preference of a sibling resulted in lasting hostility and envy, adding fuel to each partner's shame and need to bury rivalrous feelings.

This couple attempted to make up for these deficits by allowing competition into their relationship and displaying strong admiration for each other. During the early years, they could circumscribe and sublimate their more hostile feelings in verbal games. However, when Julia attained greater success, their competition became more hurtful than supportive.

From Tyler's viewpoint, in the early years of their marriage, Julia represented his childhood self that desperately needed support and admiration. He acted as an admiring parent, encouraging and nourishing her career development. When she began to surpass him, this comforting role relationship gave way to the one he had been attempting to repress and repair—that of Julia in the role of his critical, competitive father and him-

---

[1]Hurtful competition is only one kind of motive for infidelity. The reader is referred to Brown (1991), Pittman (1988), and Pittman and Wagers (1995) for the assessment and treatment of other motivations for affairs.

self cast back in his childhood role of the inadequate son, a secretly competitive son who wanted to surpass his father but feared losing his love.

In the early years of their marriage, Julia viewed Tyler as the admiring, supportive parent she longed for but never had, and herself as the adoring student. As she gained greater self-esteem, confidence, and success, her envy of Tyler came closer to consciousness. She began viewing him (transferentially) as her self-centered father and brother. She wanted to defeat both of them, thus proving herself more competent, powerful (and therefore more lovable) than any man. Like Tyler, her wish to triumph over men was laden with envy, guilt, and fears of losing love.

Intellectual competence was Tyler and Julia's main arena of competing. Since intelligence is highly valued in our culture, "who is smarter than who" is a central theme for many couples. Intelligence is particularly likely to be a focus of competition with those partners whose parents valued intelligence and academic achievement more highly than other attributes. For these partners, intellectual performance can become their lifelong way of gaining self-esteem and love.

COMPETING TO COPE WITH ENVY AND INADEQUACY

With the couple's recognition of being more separate and ordinary, feelings of inadequacy are resurrected, along with feelings of envy—envy of the partner's desirable attributes that can no longer be psychically annexed as parts of oneself. In the romantic phase, when merging is at its peak, a partner is viewed as an extension of oneself; thus, ownership of the partner's desirable traits is experienced. With a greater sense of being separate, ownership of those aspects of the partner that have been particularly admired is lost (along with his or her less desirable traits). This loss leaves us vulnerable to envying our partner. Envy is more likely to be destructively acted out if feelings of inadequacy are pervasive and lifelong.

In addition to feelings of inadequacy that may accompany the initial phase of becoming more separate, other life experiences will evoke feelings of failure and low self-esteem that may, in turn, arouse acute feelings of envy. Our own deficits may come into sharper focus with a perceived rejection or failure, or we may feel generally deficient in comparison with our mate, who appears to be more successful. He or she may have a more important job at a higher income, may be more self-confident, better looking, more intelligent, well-liked, or self-satisfied.

Competitive behavior is a common way of coping with these feelings and is an attempt to restore a sense of competence by besting one's partner (especially in the areas of felt inadequacy). If one feels particularly stupid because of making a mistake, one may try to restore self-esteem by scoring a point of superior knowledge with the partner. Julia and Tyler's intellectual debates were in part motivated by feelings of inadequacy and envy. As long as each allowed the other to feel some success, this interaction had a reparative effect.

Tyler came to view himself as a failure in his career. This recognition occurred slowly, over time, as the doors to his imagined career success shut one by one. Tyler's professional feelings of failure were managed by the couple's collusion to make him the winner of other competitions, such as their word games. However, these positive efforts became increasingly infected by Tyler's unrecognized envy of Julia, and Julia's envy of him. Tyler's envy of Julia's professional success was more apparent than the reasons for Julia's envy of Tyler. Her envy came to light later on in therapy.

Competitive reactions stemming from inferiority and envy always contain varying degrees of anger and hostility. At the center is the wish to punish the partner for having what we do not have, for being superior. These feelings will probably be acted out to a certain extent in most relationships. The greater our feelings of inadequacy and envy, the more likely competitive expressions will be hurtful and devaluing. If both partners suffer from vulnerable self-esteem, stemming from deeply wounding childhood experience, devaluing, competitive interaction may become the dominant mode of relating.

Gender Envy, Inferiority, and Competition

While Julia and Tyler's competitive problems were not nearly as destructive or pervasive as those of George and Martha, both couples shared feelings of gender inferiority, along with envy of the opposite gender. With Martha and George, gender inadequacy and envy can be inferred from their constant attacks on each other's masculinity, femininity, and gender-role adequacy. Throughout the play, Martha emasculates any man that comes within her range. This behavior suggests envy of men and feelings of inferiority as a woman.

Gender inadequacy, envy, and fear of the opposite sex are experienced by everyone to some extent. These feelings, like other feelings with a developmental history, can be viewed along a continuum from normal to pathological. Gender envy (and fear) is frequently managed by joking kinds of derision of the opposite sex. Women often bond by disparaging men, taking great pleasure in detailing male deficiencies, such as their self-centeredness, boyishness, insensitivity, addiction to watching football, and refusal to ask for directions. Men are famous for bonding though denigrating talk about women as sexual objects—"She has great tits" or "On a scale of one to ten, she's a zero." These behaviors are slightly more civilized versions of what occurred in the school yard, when girls would band together, ignoring or making fun of gross little boys, and boys would band together, teasing or hitting girls and running away. (These behaviors also reflect differentiation and solidification of gender identity.)

Couples also commonly deal with their envy and fear of the opposite sex by derisive joking and playful displays of male or female superiority. As in childhood, these methods are also used as means to preserve and confirm gender identity. Gender competition is expressed in a number of forms. Most common are variations on the theme: "Women are better than men" or "Men are better than women." Another form expresses superiority in gender role—"I'm a better woman than you are a man" or "I'm a better wife than you are a husband." A third version occurs in trying to prove oneself superior in the role of the partner's gender. For example, Martha conveys to George explicitly and implicitly throughout the play: "I'm a better man than you are. I wear the pants." Tyler and Julia also covertly expressed this competitive theme.

These expressions may be harmless or very harmful, depending on the delivery and the intensity of insecurity and hostile, envious feeling behind the delivery. Gender inadequacy and envy are destructive when one or both partners have a pervasive need to denigrate the other as an inferior male or female. Martha and George exemplify the pathological extreme. While Julia and Tyler's problems in these areas are much less severe and pervasive, they are more difficult to see and address. Both partners carefully hid these feelings because of the extent of their shame, guilt, and anger. Their feelings of gender inadequacy and envy were revealed to some extent in the following interaction taken from a midphase therapy session.

JULIA: We had a fight after we went to a play this weekend, and I know it was mostly my fault.

TYLER: You were so down on me for some reason. I couldn't do anything right.

JULIA: I did think about why, as we've been taught to do (*smiling at me graciously*). I noticed something about myself that surprised me. I realized I was anxious about going to the play, and that I'm often uncomfortable out in public, especially with you.

TYLER: Why? Am I not attentive enough?

JULIA: It's not that. It's that I feel small and insignificant. I wasn't wearing my heels that night, so I felt even smaller and more insignificant. You're very tall, and I'm very short, and the difference makes me uncomfortable. I really don't like my body.

TYLER: But you're very attractive. I don't understand this. So what if I'm tall and you're short? I thought you liked that I was tall.

JULIA: I do. It's me being short I don't like.

SHARPE: You envy Tyler his size?

JULIA: Yes, his size and his presence.

TYLER: I don't understand this. You're a perfect size and shape.

JULIA: You command attention, and I don't. People ignore me. Maitre d's, waitresses, and clerks. Even ticket takers and ushers. They seat you, not me. I feel invisible.

TYLER: I never would have guessed this was the problem.

SHARPE: These are difficult feelings to talk about. I'm impressed, Julia. Say more, if you can.

JULIA: I wish I didn't feel inferior and envious. It just adds to my feeling of smallness.

We spent time on the origin of Julia's body inferiority. Envy of men in general and her own internalized disparaging attitudes toward women came up. These traced back to feelings that her mother undervalued her and preferred her brother.

JULIA: I remember wishing I was a boy. I was lucky, I guess, that my father liked me better than my brother, because I was smart in school. My mother has just never appreciated me for who I am. She doesn't value intellectual achievement or women having careers.

SHARPE: Maybe you feel, if you'd been a boy, your mother would love and value you more?

JULIA: I think that's definitely so.

TYLER: I don't think that's true at all. I think she can't support you because of her own envy. I think she envies you . . . your intelligence and accomplishments. After all, what has she accomplished?

JULIA: She knows how to be feminine and genteel.

TYLER: (*sarcastically*) Some accomplishment! I don't know why you won't see it, but she's in awe of you and intimidated. Her carping about manners is the way she's trying to be important, to count for something in your eyes.

SHARPE: You see her as competing with Julia because she feels inferior and wants to impress her.

TYLER: Right.

JULIA: (*shaking her head vigorously*) Oh, I don't think so. She thinks I'm deviant. She thinks a woman should be at home catering to her man.

TYLER: (*grinning*) Well she has a point there.

Tyler was doing an excellent cotherapy job, but I also was aware that he tended to focus on Julia to avoid dealing directly with his own feelings. It was tempting to pursue Julia's resistance to the idea of her mother's envy, but it seemed more important to get Tyler focused on himself. I knew inadequacy and envy were problems for him as well, and saw a chance to try and involve him.

SHARPE: I think that's an important point you're making about Julia's mother feeling competitive with her. I was wondering if you had any of those feelings too . . . about Julia. [He looked ready to leap to a denial. I realized he wouldn't want to be like Julia's mother. My approach was too direct and threatening. I quickly tried to find a more palatable entry.] Julia's been talking about how she envies certain attributes of yours, so I was wondering if there are things you may envy about her.

TYLER: I can easily talk about feeling proud of Julia. Envy doesn't seem right.

JULIA: Envy is too base a feeling for Tyler to have.

TYLER: That's right, I have a better class of feelings than Julia does.

SHARPE: Start with being proud. Maybe we can work up, or is it down, to envy.

TYLER: I'm proud of her about so many things.

JULIA: You know, when you talk only about being proud of me, it makes me feel like a child, like you really don't consider me as an equal.

TYLER: Well, I don't think of you as a child. I consider you better than my equal. You've accomplished more than I have. You've managed your career much better than I've managed mine. I actually think you're smarter than me in a lot of ways.

SHARPE: You admire Julia, but without *any* envy or resentment. [I hoped he'd see this unlikelihood for himself.]

TYLER: Well, I can't absolutely rule out the possibility. But I'm more aware of being bothered about not measuring up to my own standards.

SHARPE: Go on.

TYLER: If my father were alive, he'd say, I told you so. That I never should have gone into physics, never should have gotten the PhD. He said I'd end up in some small midwestern college teaching introductory physics and earning a pittance.

JULIA: I'm the one who's ended up in a college watching freshman yawn at my lectures, not you.

TYLER: Yes, but you're a renowned linguist. I'm not a renowned physicist.

JULIA: But you've always avoided doing the kind of research and politicking necessary for that.

TYLER: True. I've always had to do my own thing in my own way, and now I'm not happy with the outcome.

SHARPE: You're a little young to be talking about outcomes. It's not to late to change direction if you want to, is it?

TYLER: Actually, it is in my field. It would take too long to tell you why, but it's too late. I think I just have to come to better terms with what I've done.

SHARPE: I'm wondering about your father's voice in this. It sounds so condemning and as though it's his expectations, his hopes that you feel you've failed.

TYLER: I could never please my father. Even if I succeeded at something, he found fault or had to take it over, so it was really his success. I can see the competitiveness in Julia's mother because my father was so competitive with me, with everyone . . . except my sister. My sister was spared . . . maybe because she had no special gifts—intellectual or otherwise. And she always did what my father wanted.

SHARPE: And . . . she was a girl.

TYLER: Meaning what?

SHARPE: I'm not sure. Maybe a girl was less of a threat to him.

TYLER: It's possible.

SHARPE: Sounds like your dad was very conflicted—like he wanted you to succeed but only under his tutelage. And he was also threatened by your surpassing him.

TYLER: Well, he wouldn't have to worry about that now. I haven't surpassed him.

SHARPE: Maybe that's been a factor in how things have gone.

Julia's feelings of smallness in body and as a woman were paralleled by Tyler's feelings of smallness professionally, leading him to feel unsuccessful as a man. Each felt inadequate and unsupported in their genders by the same-sex parent. Identifying and working through their shared feelings of inadequacy and envy as these feelings related to their family experience substantially helped them to refashion more realistic and acceptable self-images. As themes of triangular competition were also identified and understood (reported in Chapters 18 and 19), the couple had less need to compete in hurtful and covert ways.

ACCEPTANCE AND MODULATION OF NEEDS TO COMPETE

From a therapeutic viewpoint, the desired outcome to competitive problems is not elimination of competing, but rather a transformation of the couple's need to compete destructively. A first step is to identify a couple's competitive patterns and bring covert forms of competing into the open. Enabling the couple's acceptance of competitive feelings is necessary for therapeutic work in this area. The heart of therapy is the therapist's understanding with the couple of the many forms and meanings of their competitive patterns, from cultural, relational, and developmental viewpoints.

In working with destructive competitive expressions, couples are encouraged to delete from their communicational repertoire any disrespectful devaluation of the partner, along with grandiose assertions of superiority. Instead, respectful, modulated expression of one's abilities, ideas, and thoughts are strongly encouraged. Tyler and Julia tended to be the kind of partners that automatically modulated themselves once they were made aware of hurtful aspects of their communications. With more reactive couples, therapeutic focus in this area may need to be extensive (described in the treatment of serious devaluing and blaming behavior, Chapter 12).

When sufficient understanding of competitive patterns and modulation of expression are achieved, couples who pervasively compete can be encouraged to channel competitive needs into more appropriate arenas (i.e., from the bedroom to the tennis court). A therapist aims to promote the developmental process of sublimation, gradually transforming a dog-eat-dog approach to life and love into playing civilized games with rules. With couples like Martha and George, who are addicted to competitive, destructive games, therapy can be a long and difficult. For couples like Tyler and Julia, the therapy journey is more circuitous in that civilized forms of competitive expression already exist, but these games with rules mask other competitive processes that are more quietly eroding the relationship.

In normal development, many rounds of competing unsuccessfully and successfully are necessary for competition between partners to evolve in ways that strengthen the individuals and the relationship. Periods of disrespectful and grandiose competitive interaction will likely be a part of this process. Learning how to win and lose gracefully with each other and in life is not a quick or easy achievement. When partners are able to compete constructively, the relationship can provide a safer testing ground in which both can learn to manage competition more effectively in the outside world. (A safe haven and training ground for competitive expressions likely did not exist in either partner's original family). In the crucible of their competitive interaction, partners gain intimate knowledge of their own and the other's competencies and weaknesses. Integration of this knowledge is crucial to their modulation of grandiosity and its opposite, self-devaluation, thus aiding in the development of realistic perceptions of oneself and partner.

COMPETING TO ENHANCE COLLABORATION

I am reminded of the long struggle I had with my husband about landscaping our yard. In the first round, early in our marriage, we each thought our positions were superior in every way. I saw my husband as narrowly obsessed with trivial practicalities such as drainage, quality of the soil, position of the sun, and prevailing winds, while I embraced the larger, aesthetic vision of attaining a sense of beauty, serenity, and charm. He thought my ideas were absurdly impractical. We had many intense fights. Because we really did not know our strengths, our attempts at compromise resulted in a remarkable dovetailing of our weaknesses. I chose many of the plants, and he determined the overall design. Somehow, we ended up following gender-role stereotypes in which the man makes the big decisions and the woman decorates. The yard emerged as ugly and impractical.

For ten years, I watched my plant selections grow out of control or die one by one, because the practicalities of soil, sun, drainage, and growth pattern of the plant were not sufficiently taken into account. He came to realize that the yard lacked any distinction or charm. In fact, he found it unpleasant. I lamented that I should have listened to him—his practical judgment was of immeasurable value; he acknowledged that he should have listened to me—I knew how to make things look good and feel right. Fifteen years later, we tried again. We still struggled, but this time we were able to dovetail my superior aesthetics with his superior practical judgment. We made a beautiful, efficient yard.

When partners understand and accept each other's areas of superiority and inadequacy, their capacities to maximize their strengths and minimize weaknesses are greatly enhanced. In this sense, competition leads to more effective collaboration. This point is also nicely illustrated in the story of the real Annie Oakley.

In my research of movies depicting competition, I came across the true story of sharpshooters Annie Oakley and Frank Butler. In reality, Annie Oakley did not give up or conceal her superiority as a sharpshooter in order to win Frank. In fact, they were married (in 1876) shortly after she won the big shooting competition. Subsequently, she became the star of their Wild West show and Frank, proud of her unsurpassed skill, became her manager. Their professional collaboration was extremely successful, reportedly, as was their marriage of fifty years. So it seems that Annie did get her man with a gun.

CHAPTER 18

Competing in Love Triangles
Development and Common Treatment Problems

Of all the relational patterns that couples experience, triangular competition may arouse the most intense passions. Many relationships are forged in the excitement of a competitive love triangle, and many others are destroyed by one partner's attachment to someone or something outside the relationship. Like Tyler and Julia, couples often come for therapy in crisis over the discovery of one partner's infidelity, a betrayal that incites an array of difficult emotions—humiliation, rejection, rage, guilt, and acute fears of loss.

A partner's love affair with another person is considered by many to cause the most serious threat to the emotional integrity and actual survival of a love relationship. However, all couples in our society cope with love triangles of less dramatic kinds on a day-to-day basis. More subdued versions of the passions inflamed by adultery and its discovery are experienced by couples in their everyday interactions within and outside their families.

The safety and flexibility of a couple's boundary is persistently challenged by the ongoing task of including and excluding others in their relationship. In reverse, a couple's development of a strong, safe, but flexible boundary to protect their connection depends a great deal on how the partners learn to manage relating to third parties—especially those third parties that threaten their attachment, arousing insecurity and competitive feelings in one or both of them.

In contrast to dyadic competition, *triangular competition* involves a three-way interaction: the two partners and a third someone or something. Love triangles with couples take two forms. In the first, one partner competes with an outsider (a third party) as a rival for the other partner's affection. An obvious example is Julia's competition with Tyler's mistress as a rival for his love. Such obvious love triangles usually also represent hidden triangles from each partner's past love relationships. The current cast of characters is often found to represent previous lovers, partners, and original family members.

In the second form of love triangle, one partner competes with the other as a rival for the love of an outsider. The partners act like siblings, competing for the love of a third person, who is cast in an idealized, parent-like role. Julia and Tyler's competition for my preference is an example of this adult edition of sibling rivalry that I term *partner rivalry*. Partner rivalry frequently occurs in relation to parents, children, friends—or with any valued outsider, such as a couple therapist.

THE DEVELOPMENT OF TRIANGULAR COMPETITION

The development of a couple's expression and management of triangular competition in both forms is the most complex of all the relationship patterns. Expressions of these patterns are so pervasive, multilevel, and multifaceted that it is difficult to tease out a developmental progression. My description of development in this domain reflects a cobbling together of observations, impressions, and suppositions, and reflects only a rough sketch of major events and processes.

In the course of managing triangular competitions, a couple optimally develops safety and intimacy as a twosome and the ability to comfortably regulate the inclusion and exclusion of outsiders. While these capacities may sound rather ordinary, they usually take considerable time, effort, and angst to develop.

When outsiders are permitted into a couple's relationship, the quality of partners' relating needs to change to accommodate the new person. Some couples do not accommodate to outsiders. In the presence of others, the partners continue focusing almost exclusively on each other. Such couples never evolve beyond the merged relating of the romantic phase, even though the reasons they remain riveted on each other no longer may have much to do with passion or sexual excitement.

Many people wish only to relate on a one-to-one basis and avoid the anxiety and complications of including others. Shutting out the world can seem to be the way to keep a relationship safe and secure. When a third party is significantly included, anxiety is usually triggered about an alliance forming between two persons that will exclude the third person.

When they have a baby, couples typically worry that the child and one partner will form a stronger, closer connection than the partners can sustain with each other. The fear of an alliance that leaves one partner out is also a universal anxiety of couples coming for therapy.

In these triangular constellations, some people fear their own wishes to compete and collude to leave someone out. Others fear being the favored one, whose allegiance is sought by the others. And still others experience all of these fears at one time or another. Being married is no safeguard against these fears.

While being alone with our partners may stimulate fears of merging or losing control of angry impulses, being in threesomes and groups is more likely to incite fears of being left out, rejected, competitive, and guilty. In threesomes, competitive triangles can easily arise, with one partner competing with the outsider to protect the couple connection, or the partners vying with each other for the third person's affection. In these events, partners may temporarily lose their primary connection to each other. Temporary experiences of these sorts are normal aspects of development. However, if a competitive triangle becomes entrenched, a couple's development in this area will be derailed.

Such entrenched competitive triangles are seen in those families wherein two members of the family compete for the love of a third. For example, a husband and a son compete for the wife/mother's love, or a wife and her mother-in-law compete for the husband/son, or a wife and daughter compete for the love of their husband/father. When such a dynamic comes to dominate a family, almost every interaction expresses some nuance of the triangle. In the movie *Cat on a Hot Tin Roof* (1958), based on the Tennessee Williams play, one brother's competition with the other for Big Daddy's love dominates three generations of a Southern family, including the brothers' wives and their children. The fact that Big Daddy is dying seems only to intensify this rivalry.

If partners can weather and sustain themselves as a couple within the competitive triangles that typically arise in their lives, they will gradually develop a strong, but also flexible, couple boundary and a secure feeling of connection with each other. The *couple boundary*, as previously described,[1] is a psychological boundary constructed by the two partners that keeps them an intact unit in relation to the outside world. Like any other psychic structure, the couple boundary needs to develop, becoming more effective and appropriately flexible at varying times. Over time and experience, partners learn to maintain themselves as a unit, while also being able to relate comfortably and closely with others—parents, children, and friends.

---

[1]See Chapter 3, p. 44 for definition and further discussion.

In order for this boundary and level of safety to be achieved, most partners will need to experience and successfully manage a number of competitive triangles—universally occurring with parents, in-laws, children, friends, and careers. Sometimes these triangles will involve competing *for* the partner and *with* the partner for the love of another. Most couples will also need to contend with the hidden love triangles, carried over from childhood relationships with parents and siblings, that may be reenacted in their current life situation.

In normal development, partners go through many phases of being too closed and potentially isolated as a couple and then swinging to the opposite extreme of overincluding outsiders. They eventually work out an agreement (their couple boundary) about when, how much, and for whom to open and shut their doors to the outside world. Outsiders may provoke temporary feelings of threat and rivalry, but the partners will have developed ways to reassure one another of being the most important and best loved person. Ideally, they become able to discuss their insecure, jealous, and competitive feelings with each other as they arise. Distorted perceptions can then be corrected and reassurance gained.

One of the important aims of couple therapy is encouraging partners to verbalize feeling left out, insecure, or jealous in their interactions with others. Mutually sharing and understanding such feelings are the most effective ways to prevent partners from acting out destructive urges to retaliate because of feeling rejected. The cruel provocation of jealousy in one's partner or having an affair can cause great and sometimes irreparable damage. An effective way to facilitate this verbalization is to focus on the partners' reactions in the love triangle of couple therapy. In the ideal relationship, the need to compete for love becomes unnecessary, because the feeling of being reliably first with the partner has been securely won.

The developmental steps, associated tasks, and common problems many couples experience as they engage in the love triangles of their lives are outlined in Figure 9.

COMPETING *FOR* THE PARTNER

Threatening third parties in competitive triangles come in all shapes and sizes. This rival can be an actual or imagined lover, an in-law, a child, a friend, a boss, or a pet. A partner's attachment to certain activities or objects—such as work, a hobby, sports, drugs, alcohol, the telephone, the television, the computer—can also take on the status of a rival. "He's really married to his work," has been commonly said by many wives. Now, many husbands are likely to say the same thing about their wives.

The pager and the cell phone appear to be the latest technical rivals

Steps in Development of Triangular Competition	Tasks for Couple/Guide for Therapy	Common Problems (Points of Regression and Derailment)
Competing *for* the Partner	Competing with rivals to win partner Excluding outsiders in initial and later romantic phases Forming a secure couple boundary	Avoidance of competing for partner Overinclusion of outsiders Early entrenchment of a love triangle Failure to form a secure couple boundary
Competing *with* the Partner	Deidealizing the couple relationship Idealizing and including outsiders Vying with partner for preference by others Creating flexibility in the couple boundary	Couple remains overly idealized and exclusive Too fearful to include outsiders; competition avoided Partner rivalry destructive to intimacy Couple boundary too rigidly closed or open
Reworking Past Competitive Triangles	Recognizing transference of love triangles with parents and siblings onto couple Distinguishing past victory or defeats from present	Reenactment of an oedipal triangle or oedipal sibling triangle: Destructive provocation of jealousy in partner Competing to avoid intimacy
Regulation and Modulation of Competitive Triangles	Discussing insecure or jealous feelings with partner to gain reassurance Appropriately competing for partner when the relationship is threatened	Acting out rather than verbalizing jealousy and rivalrous feelings Too insecure and angry to modulate jealousy and competitiveness Too fearful to compete appropriately
Winning First Place with the Partner	Valuing partner and relationship before others Achieving security with partner in all constellations (twosome, threesome, etc.) Feeling reliably first with the partner Supporting partner's activities and relationships with others	Other people or activities valued more than partner Insecure in triangular constellations Not feeling first with the partner Too insecure to support partner's outside activities or relationships

FIGURE 9. The development of triangular competition.

for a partner's focused attention. I used to hear more about the television and computers, but now the cell phone is a more omnipresent intruder. Partners regularly irritate each other by responding to their pagers or answering their cell phones in the midst of a conversation, taking a walk together, having a romantic dinner, and at the beginning or end (or sometimes even in the middle) of making love. There seems to be no getting away from the pager or cell phone. Being small and portable, they can go anywhere, interrupting a couple's intimacy anytime, anyplace. As I watch people holding, fondling, examining, or securing these objects to their midsections, the attachment seems umbilical.

At the same time the cell phone acts as a rival, it also may act as a means for more frequent connections with one's partner. Like an umbilical cord, it keeps partners constantly in touch—on the freeway, in the supermarket, in the shopping mall, on the airplane. It also acts as a comforting transitional object when not in actual use, representing instant connection with a loved one.

This use of pagers and cell phones points up how rivals, in general, can be used by a couple to create distance in the relationship, when intimacy may seem too threatening, and for creating greater closeness.

Competing in the Service of Connection

Love relationships often come into being because one partner has competed with a rival third party for the love of the other partner. Tyler fiercely competed to win Julia away from a man with whom she lived at the time they met. Julia also competed to win Tyler away from his first wife and family. After marriage, competing with outside rivals is also often necessary to protect the integrity and intimacy of the couple relationship. Children challenge this bond, as well as parents, friends, or anyone who too strongly intrudes or attracts one of the partners. At times, it is necessary for us to intervene with partners to pull them away from attachments with others that may seriously jeopardize the relationship. Competing can be an effective method of bringing the partner back into closer connection.

When Julia discovered Tyler's affair, she competed like a tigress to win him back. This reserved, gracious woman went on the warpath, threatening to "gouge the bimbo's eyes out." She quickly put her demanding job on the back burner and focused her attention and reawakened passion onto Tyler. Long after the affair had ended, she continued to feel wary and watchful. For months, she closely monitored Tyler's behavior and activities. If Julia had not competed in this situation, she would have risked losing Tyler, who briefly imagined he was in love with this woman. By vigorously competing, Julia reassured him of her love, her need for him, and his desirability. Her impassioned, decisive action rather quickly eliminated this external threat to their relationship. Their boundary restored, the couple was then able to work toward strengthening the damaged connection.

Many people flirt or act conspicuously interested in a third party in order to incite a neglectful partner to take notice and pay more attention. A jealous, competitive reaction may also be wanted and inspired. The conscious or unconscious wish is to provoke our partner to compete openly and display his or her love for us in the hope that we then feel reassured and more secure.

Tyler had turned to another woman because he felt Julia had emotionally left him for her career, his biggest rival for attention. Feeling like a loser in this "love" triangle, he sought to restore his damaged self-esteem and assuage feelings of rejection by an affair with an adoring younger woman, with whom he was the first priority. While Tyler did not openly compete to win Julia away from her other preoccupations, his infidelity provoked her to compete for him.

Couples often appear to regulate their closeness and distance to each other by creating these kinds of triangles, with and without infidelity. One partner provokes jealousy (by flirting, paying a lot of attention to another) and the other partner reacts with an open display of jealousy and rivalry. This "game" is also used by couples to rekindle passion. If used with much frequency, this game can be destructive, becoming more of a vehicle to express anger. Injury and distance, rather than greater closeness, are continually created.

Competitive triangles of this kind, repetitively enacted, are used by partners collusively to protect themselves from being intimate. George and Martha (from *Who's Afraid of Virginia Woolf?*) demonstrated this pattern, wherein Martha would provoke George's jealousy and retaliation by outrageously flirting with and seducing younger faculty members. George retaliated by rejecting her sexually, along with other forms of punishing devaluation. In this way, the couple made sure they kept a constant and great distance in their relationship.

Most of us are aware of the quality of our partner's attachment to other people and alert to signs that may pose a threat. An alarm goes off when we perceive our partner to be more attached in some significant way to a third person than to us. When he or she seems unusually enthusiastic about meeting an attractive person of the opposite (or same) sex, we may feel suddenly possessive and competitive. Feelings of anxiety and rivalry may increase if an old girlfriend, boyfriend, or ex-spouse of our partner reenters our social sphere.

There are other kinds of threats to the couple bond. We can feel strongly threatened and competitive about our mate seeming to prefer the companionship of someone else, even when there is no question of erotic or romantic feelings being involved. Many husbands have been incited to jealous rage by their wives talking with women friends on the telephone. Our partner's nurturing care of someone else may be experienced as a threat, including care of our own children or an ailing parent. Our spouse's perceived attachments to parents often provoke rivalrous feelings and behavior that may develop into painful, ongoing love triangles.

The common thread linking all of these third-party threats is the perception that someone or something else is (or might be) preferred to oneself in one or more roles—as a lover, a companion, a partner in parenting, a parent, a child. It would seem that most of us want to feel first in most, possibly all, areas of affectionate attachment. This may be a defining factor of a couple's unique bond— feeling first with each other in most domains, most of the time. Ideally, once the feeling of being first is *reliably* attained, we are secure enough to encourage our partner's outside activities and attachments.

In the opening, romantic phase of a relationship, a couple ideally shuts out the rest of the world to a great extent, in order to focus on each other and become intimate. The needs and demands of outsiders and potential enmeshments in love triangles are not as likely intrude on a couple's intimacy. Our society also sanctions this exclusive, mutual focus of lovers. We therefore have permission to keep out the world and put our lover first. In this way, society provides an external shoring up of the nascent couple boundary.

With commitment, marriage, and day to day living, this focused concentration on each other gives way to the inclusion of others and the demands of the outside world. As outsiders come knocking on the door, a couple is called upon to figure out how to regulate the frequency and intensity of others' presence in the relationship. At this point, a couple may first experience triangular competition. If a partner is not really separated from his or her family of origin, this developmental lag will appear and intrude on the couple's relationship. This partner's overattachment to parents will become apparent as he or she allows parental needs and demands to come before the spouse and the couple relationship. Allowing parents limitless access to the couple's time and domicile is a common symptom of this problem.

In this frequent event, the other partner may begin to feel threatened, left out, rejected, and competitive. A love triangle may form, in which the excluded partner competes with the in-laws for the love of his or her mate. Often, such a triangle instigates the first disappointment and deidealizing of the spouse and relationship. The presenting problem of Alex and Marla involved Alex's continued childhood attachment to his parents, causing Marla to feel threatened and competitive. Treatment focused on exposure of the painful triangle and its harmful effect on their relationship (see pp. 205–207).

This same underlying dynamic can occur with other people acting as parent surrogates or symbols—overattachment to a friend(s) to a boss, or overinvestment in school or work.

When this kind of problem reflects a normal phase or mild lag in relationship and individual development, treatment is often straightforward and short term. The partners will likely need to confront and understand the influence of their familial attachments at some point in the early years of marriage. When such a problem reflects embedded conflictual attachments to parents, a deeper understanding and working though of childhood conflicts may be necessary.

Oedipal Triangles and Competition: The Legacy from Childhood

Our first romantic quest for the love of our parents involves the famous Oedipus complex and love triangle (named by Freud after King Oedipus, who murdered his father and married his mother, albeit unknowingly, in Sophocles' great play, *Oedipus Rex*). This quest also involves an important phase in child development, the oedipal phase. Our particular experience of this drama and phase is thought to impact profoundly how we love and experience being loved in adult life. Although in psychoanalytic developmental theory, the oedipal quest is restricted to a specific phase of development, I use this term more broadly to refer to a person's general felt experience about competing for the love of each parent and associated conflicts.

When a three- or four-year-old child experiences and enacts wishes to win one parent's love away from the other, he or she has entered the oedipal phase of relationship development. A child in the oedipal phase views one parent as the desired love object and the other as a rival, and competes for the desired parent's love. Each parent is viewed as the desired parent and the rival parent at different times (or possibly simultaneously). In this phase, the child not only competes for a parent's exclusive love but has conflicting feelings of love and guilt toward the rival (for a more detailed description, see Chapter 3, this volume; Tyson & Tyson, 1990).

In theory, we are supposed to resolve these competitive feelings substantially and give up these wishes by the age of five or so for the following reasons:

1. We give up this quest because neither Mom or Dad will be seduced away from remaining first with each other—"first" in the sense of their romantic/erotic bond.
2. We give up because we love the rival parent and our hostile wishes toward that parent cause us too much anxiety and guilt—anxiety about this parent's retaliation (anger, withdrawal of love, castra-

tion) and guilt about wanting to triumph over, displace, and even destroy this parent.
3. We love both our parents and want them to stay united, so we can continue to feel secure in their ability to take care of us as little children.
4. We learn from our parents in their transmission of the incest taboo that it is wrong, even sinful, to have erotic desires for parents or other family members.

These factors supposedly enable us to accept our defeat, give up competitive wishes and behavior, and accept our realistic position as a loved little child (thereby relinquishing grandiose notions of our power). We can accept feeling left out of our parents' love relationship because we still have their special love for us as children, and we are presumably given the hope of marrying someone like Mom or Dad when we grow up. Oedipal wishes and impulses go underground until they are resurrected in adolescence to be reworked and resolved by the end of adolescence if all goes well.

In any close observation of human emotions and relationships, especially couple relationships, a final resolution does not really occur in late adolescence. Every new love relationship appears to involve the reworking of past love relationships—the same themes, deficits, and conflicts. In adulthood, oedipal-like conflicts continue to be stirred up in any love relationship or triangular situation of emotional intensity. While winning the love of our chosen mate is supposed to represent the longed-for oedipal victory (we have won a mate presumably as desirable as Mom or Dad), oedipal feelings and competition are not so easily laid to rest.

Oedipal-like competition is reactivated when a third party threatens our position of being first. Feelings about our own past oedipal experience are also reactivated for another round of working through and partial mastery. In an optimal relationship, when competitive feelings arise, we gain the needed reassurance from our partners of our lovableness, desirability, and being first in their hearts. Repeated experiences of feeling threatened and then gaining the necessary reassurance make us increasingly secure in our relationship.

However, if we do not receive the necessary reassurance (perhaps because, in fact, our partner is overly attached to someone else), or the reassurance given does not allay feelings of jealousy and competitiveness (because we are too personally insecure), then competitive feelings and expressions can become destructive. Love triangles may form that tend to replicate childhood love triangles almost entirely, with all the raw intensity of childhood passions.

The partner who feels vulnerable to rejection and competitive feelings often appears to be the most insecure and troubled in the relationship. Yet the partner who apparently feels more loved and secure may carry hidden anxiety about losing this position and will often instigate competitive triangles in which he or she is the sought-after prize. In this way, this partner gains reassurance of being and staying in first place, while also inducing the spouse to act out his or her own feelings of insecurity (via projective identification).

It is hoped that such insecurity in love could be avoided if we were properly loved in childhood or had an optimal oedipal experience. An optimal oedipal experience would be having parents who receive our loving, wooing efforts positively but do not succumb to a romantic attachment, while continuing to love us as a very special child. The rival parent allows some expression of hostility and competition but insists on appropriate restraint, though not punishing or withdrawing love. The parents remain steady in their primary romantic connection to each other. They do not let their child win, but they also do not shut the child out with overly rejecting or punitive responses. They provide consistent love and understanding of their child's competitive wishes and conflicts. They encourage the child's anticipation: "When I grow up, I'll marry someone just like Mommy or Daddy."

This is an ideal most of us likely have not experienced. While every variant of how we experienced love in our original families affects our subsequent lives, those of us who become caught in painful love triangles usually have had a very distressing experience of winning or losing an *oedipal* competition for one or both parents' love. (Siblings may also play a part in a triangular competition for parents' love, as will be discussed subsequently.)

COMPETING *WITH* THE PARTNER: PARTNER RIVALRY

Triangular competition may take another form that most often promotes the partners' individuality and separateness. This pattern occurs when one or both partners views the other as a rival for the love of a third party. Partners often find themselves in this kind of triangle in which they are competing with each other for the preference of their children, a friend, a parent, or an authority figure of some kind—such as their couple therapist. This type of rivalry looks like sibling rivalry, wherein the third-party prize, even if he or she is a child, seems to be cast in the role of an idealized parent figure. This kind of competition can easily become destructive, eroding the couple's intimacy.

This aspect of triangular competition tends to emerge more strongly during the first and subsequent periods of disappointment and deidealization of our partners. During the first fall from grace, when our partner's idealized glow is waning and his or her faults seem to glare, relating as a tight twosome that keeps out the world becomes less desirable. In fact, outsiders begin to look more appealing, sometimes far more appealing, than the partner. Time spent with others starts to seem more exciting and rewarding than being alone together. To cushion the blow of disappointment and lonely feelings of being more separate, other people and other connections may take on the idealizing glow. Flirting with others may occur, along with feeling competitive with the partner for the preference of someone else—an interesting friend, a parent or other relative, another couple.

Couples will often manage this "letdown" period and feeling competitive with each other by falling in love with and "marrying" another couple with whom they do everything. In part, because this foursome is made up of two committed twosomes, triangular competition in either form does not seem to be a real threat. Nora Ephron gives a particularly good description of the cushioning role of the best-friend couple in her novel *Heartburn* (1983), also pointing out how such intense couple friendships help to make distant, unhappy marriages seem quite palatable. Of course, many of these intense couple friendships do evolve into love triangles, often double triangles, in which each couple swaps partners, as portrayed in the memorable sixties movie *Bob & Carol & Ted & Alice* (1969).

Another frequently attempted solution to this deidealizing of the twosome is to have a baby, in the hope of gaining a happier, idealized threesome. Unfortunately, babies are the most potent stimuli to incite triangular competition and reenactments of love triangles from our original families. The demand on the couple to move from dyadic relating to relating as a threesome requires a sizable developmental leap.[2] Babies incite both kinds of competition. At times, each partner feels threatened by the baby taking too much of the other's time and attention. At other times, each may experience wishes to be the baby's one and only love and to be rid of the partner. Competitive triangles forming with a new baby are a well-recognized cause of trouble for couples, though partners often do not address these problems until long after the baby's arrival.

Beyond babyhood, partners are at times rivalrous for their children's admiration and affection. Tyler and Julia competed to be most admired by their two daughters. Just as siblings try to outshine each other in the ways that are most likely to win the love and admiration of their parents, so do married partners have the same aim when they compete to win a

---

[2]The developmental shift from dyadic to triadic relating is extensively discussed in Chapter 13.

third person's preference or love. Tyler and Julia exemplified this joining of dyadic and triangular forms of competition in relating to me and to their daughters. As noted previously, their playful word games involved both the dyadic aim of proving superiority in relation to the other and the triangular aim of winning my admiration and preference. This combination of goals also occurred when they engaged in these interactions with their daughters, who were used as an admiring audience.

When we wish to win something for ourselves over our partner, whether it is a feeling of greater competence or the love of a highly regarded person, the developmental aim of this behavior is to build up and distinguish ourselves in some way as a separate person. Specifically, we aim to be considered more lovable than the spouse in the hope of gaining a greater sense of personal security. In constructive versions of this form, triangular competition promotes individual development rather than fostering the partners' connection.

Sibling Rivalry and Oedipal Sibling Triangles

The quality and intensity of partners rivalry with each other often stem from their experience competing with siblings in childhood. A spouse may be unconsciously viewed (transferentially) as a particular sibling, and thus has the power to stir up the same intense feelings of love, hate, and rivalry that occurred with that sibling in relation to his or her parents. In a therapy session to be reported, Julia's competitive reactions to Tyler were found to stem from her relationship with her brother.

When partners come to view each other as sibling rivals, great anger and distance can be created. With the occurrence of this kind of transference, each person needs emotionally to differentiate partner from sibling (as well as partner from parent) in order for the relationship to progress. Partners feel more secure and their relationship strengthens when sibling transferences are resolved. Therapists see this result frequently. Couples who do not come for therapy but also experience reliving sibling rivalry with a spouse (whether in mild or intense forms) may be able to find their own way out of these reenactments and ultimately attain greater mastery of rivalry issues in general.

Psychoanalytic theory, beginning with Freud, has ranked parent–child relationships as the most important in shaping our development and the quality of our intimate relating. The influence of siblings in our lives has only recently begun to receive some attention. In working with couples, competitive difficulties deriving from the transference of a rivalrous sibling relationship to the marriage appear as frequently and intensely (if not more so) as do the transferences of oedipal experience. In studying couples and individual patients who have been significantly affected by competition with their siblings, these love triangles have appeared to share most of the characteristics of oedipal triangles—ambivalent feelings of love and hate for the rival sibling, guilt about defeating a rival sibling, and a profound impact on adult love relationships (see Sharpe & Rosenblatt, 1994).

Destructive Partner Rivalry

Partners who constantly compete with each other for the love of someone outside their relationship can erode, even destroy, their identity as a couple, because the outsider becomes more important than the partner. In therapy, couples may exhibit these problems by flipping back and forth between competing *for* the therapist (in the oedipal sibling mode) and competing *with* the therapist for the partner (in the oedipal parental mode). A frequent factor in the backgrounds of couples with these issues is the existence of marked parental favoritism in the partners' original families.

Parental favoritism toward a sibling greatly intensifies envious and rivalrous feelings, particularly in the sibling who was not favored. For the sibling who was favored, guilt in its various guises is often more intensified. The literature is tiny in this vastly important but neglected area, consisting of three papers, authored by Bieber (1977), Bank (1987), Siegel and Robertiello (1987), and my own collaborative work (Rosenblatt & Sharpe, 1998). Partners who were unfavored or worse, actively disfavored, may need to compete with and defeat their spouses (who represent their sibling) vis-à-vis a third party to reverse painful childhood experience. Those partners who believed themselves to be the favored sibling may need to keep reasserting a favored position with important people in order to sustain the feeling of being loved and secure.

Tyler and Julia harbored both of these motivations. Each had one sibling of the opposite sex. Both felt favored over their siblings by the opposite-sex parent. Tyler's mother favored him over his sister, while Julia was favored by her father over her brother. However, each felt their siblings were favored over them by the same-sex parent. Tyler's father strongly favored his daughter, and Julia's mother strongly favored her son. The impact of the sibling triangle with her mother and brother on Julia and her relationship with Tyler is illustrated in the following excerpt from a midphase therapy session.

JULIA: We've had a disastrous week. My mother's been visiting, and things between us have not gone well.

TYLER: Julia's mother has been here for the last five days. It's caused . . . tension and a lot more work. She's not an easy person. She's very self-centered . . . narcissistic, I think you'd call it.

JULIA: She's very critical. She's always criticizing the girls' manners, and it makes me furious.

TYLER: She's even more critical of you, and then you take out your bad feelings on me when we're alone.

JULIA: That's not what our fight was about. Our fight was about you deserting me.

TYLER: Deserting you? You're the one that jumped on me for leaving my clothes on the floor, as soon as I walked in the bedroom.

JULIA: That wasn't the real problem. I told you I was bothered about being left to do the whole dinner myself, while you joked around and played cards with my mother.

TYLER: And I told you I was sorry for not helping. I thought I was doing the more important job of keeping her entertained and away from you. I'm not particularly enamored of her company, you know.

JULIA: Is that so? (*mocking*) You put on a great act. You play Mr. Charm and Wit so beautifully . . . and she just eats it all up. [Tyler and I were both taken aback. Julia had never before attacked so sarcastically.]

TYLER: What are you talking about? I don't get this.

JULIA: (*flushing with anger*) I was in the kitchen screwing with that damn goose, and I felt so angry I could hardly see.

TYLER: (*looking acutely uncomfortable*) Did feelings about . . . um . . . the affair get set off? [I could see the effort it took for him to address actively rather than avoid Julia's anger about his affair.]

JULIA: Well, I don't know. I hadn't thought of that, actually.

TYLER: (*quickly shifting subjects*) Maybe it was some kind of Cinderella feeling. You were left in the kitchen to do the scut work.

JULIA: (*considering this suggestion more seriously*) Maybe. At home, I always ended up in the kitchen or doing other housework because I was a girl. My brother had one job, taking out the trash.

SHARPE: I'm recalling that you felt your mother favored your brother. Maybe this scene was reminiscent of how it was with your brother, your mother . . .

JULIA: My mother more than favors my brother. I'm surprised she even came to visit us without his being here. (*She pauses.*) When I was in the kitchen, I had the thought that she wasn't here to see me or the girls, she was here to see Tyler.

TYLER: Oh, come on, Julia. That's utter nonsense.

JULIA: I don't think so. She thinks you're brilliant and charming. She thinks I'm an awful wife and mother, and she thinks the girls are like me, spoiled and mouthy.

SHARPE: You must feel terribly hurt and rejected by her.

JULIA: (*eyes tearing up*) I've never done anything right in her eyes. I'm not pretty enough or popular enough. I have no social graces. That's what matters to her. Carlton, my brother, has all the charm. It doesn't matter that he never amounted to anything.

SHARPE: You called Tyler "Mr. Charm."

TYLER: Surely you don't think of me as like your brother.

JULIA: Not in terms of character . . . not at all. Carlton is a con man. But you're charming and witty like he is. And you get along socially very well. You're very well liked.

TYLER: Well, so are you.

JULIA: No, I'm not. I've always been a wallflower. You and Carlton have always been popular, especially with women. How many girls were chasing you when we met?

TYLER: I really dislike this comparison. I don't think your brother is particularly charming or funny. He's a slick lounge lizard that tells off-color jokes.

JULIA: He can chat up an old woman and make her feel special. It's how he makes his living.

SHARPE: Maybe that's what made you so angry in the kitchen. Tyler seemed like your brother chatting up your mother, and you felt excluded from their little lovefest.

JULIA: (*groaning*) I always felt excluded by them. You're right. They're more like lovers than mother and son. I really envied my brother for what he had that made her light up like a Christmas tree whenever he walked in the room. She scowls when she sees me and finds something wrong with my appearance.

A therapist who understands that sibling rivalry is frequently reenacted in love relationships is in a better position to help couples become aware of this form of competition. Partners' feelings of having been favored or not by one or both parents are often important to bring into the open for therapeutic work. In this session, my interventions were primarily geared toward understanding Julia's anger with Tyler as, in part, fueled by her childhood rivalry with her brother. This rivalry had been markedly aggravated by her mother's favoritism of her brother.

Irving Bieber (1977), in his groundbreaking paper on the topic of favoritism, noted that adults who experienced cross-gender favoritism in their families (mother prefers son, father prefers daughter) are likely to feel insecure in their genders and have problems with intimacy. Tyler and Julia both experienced cross-gender favoritism. Their envy of, and competition with, each other, deriving from gender inadequacy, have been discussed. Their intimacy was further polluted by guilt feelings and desires for revenge, which are yet to be revealed here.

In order to help Tyler and Julia to access and understand all aspects of their past relationships played out in the present, it became important to acknowledge and work with the love triangle existing among the three of us. Moving into this emotionally fraught territory requires the therapist to engage more intensely with the couple and experience the passions of the oedipal triangle—at times feeling inflated in the role of desired love object or like a guilty rival for one partner's love.

CHAPTER 19

Love Triangles
in Couple Therapy

The couple therapy situation evokes the reenactment of all kinds of competitive triangles. Partner rivalry is usually the most apparent, because the therapist is in a parent-like role from the start. This kind of competition was evident from the first session with Julia and Tyler. I could feel each of them competing to win my favor. Each one vied with the other to appear more intelligent, insightful, witty, and charming. Their competition in this respect was well modulated and felt rather enjoyable, at least at the outset. Couples' displays of partner rivalry range from hardly evident to obvious but well-modulated, to extremely devaluing and omnipresent.

Competition of both types (competing *for* and *with* the partner) usually exists in all couples' repertoire, though these patterns may not be in the foreground or visible early in therapy. Usually, couples are more easily in touch with feeling and expressing competition toward a threatening third party, such as a partner's work, best friend, a lover or mistress, or intense involvement with a parent or child. Partners are less easily in touch with competitive impulses toward each other.

Likewise, therapists are more or less in touch with their own competitive feelings in their lives and with their patients. In general, therapists can more easily see overtly and covertly displayed dyadic competition between partners. They are less sensitive to the many forms of triangular competition provoked by the therapy triangle. Partners may conceal their competition with each other for the therapist's favor, but it is always there to a greater or lesser degree of intensity. Additionally, the therapy triangle may provoke one partner to become competitive with the therapist for the other partner's primary allegiance.

Therapists are also constantly reacting to the triangle and the conflicting feelings evoked by a particular couple. A universal conflict operating in all couple therapists (whether consciously or not) is the wish to help the partners stay together by improving their relationship, conflicting with the wish to ally with one partner and split the couple up. This conflict derives from childhood oedipal wishes to have parents who are a strong unit but also to win one parent away from the other, and so split them up. Since the triangle of couple therapy stimulates everyone's competitive wishes and fears, past and present, the therapist's awareness in this area is often crucial to successful treatment.

In the second session with Tyler and Julia (recounted at the beginning of Chapter 15), I found myself immediately reacting in powerful and conflicting ways to them. I was aware of liking them as a couple and as individuals, and wanting their admiration and affection. But a conflicting wish also intruded. I felt particularly drawn to Tyler. I found his candor, intelligence, and sense of humor very seductive. I was aware of feeling a little envious of Julia.

Later, I realized that my unconscious wish to win him away from Julia was revealed in my overly enthusiastic response to his display of insight in this session. I became uncomfortably aware that I did not respond to Julia with this degree of enthusiasm. This recognition made me feel a little anxious and guilty. Unprocessed at the time, these feelings were expressed in my becoming oversolicitous of Julia later in the session, in order to make up for my imagined crime. I liked and respected Julia very much, and I did not want to lose her affection or in any way interfere with their basically good relationship. On the other hand, I had the momentary competitive urge to do just that.

Staying alert to these kinds of reactions is very important to the success of treatment. The therapist's reactions to a couple usually give important information about the couple's dynamics, but they can also be potent and harmful to treatment if unrecognized and unprocessed by the therapist. In reviewing my own work and the supervised work of students and colleagues, I have noted that one of the biggest reasons couple treatment fails (assuming motivated partners) or stays on a superficial level, or ends prematurely, is because the therapist has not recognized his or her own involvement in the enactment of a competitive oedipal or sibling triangle.

The therapist's recognition of the reemergence of his or her own oedipal wishes in response to the couple should be sufficient to abort or at least, restrain acting out this countertransference. However, as noted earlier, it is important for the therapist to sort out which reactions are primarily set off by personal history and which are largely generated by the couple through projective identification. There may, of course, be considerable overlap. In my initial countertransference responses to Julia and

Tyler, and observation of their interactions, I was able to discern certain themes of their oedipal experience that had been activated and were currently undermining their relationship.

The seductive, competitive quality of Tyler's behavior and my attracted response suggested to me that he was, historically, an oedipal victor with his mother (or a partial one). He conveyed an aura of self-confidence, of knowing his way around women and liking them. This made me think that he was used to competing for women and winning, and, perhaps, *needed* to compete for women and win. In contrast, my countertransference to Julia suggested to me that historically, she was, an oedipal loser. Although Julia was a distinct personality and an engaging woman, I found myself noting a tendency to lose track of her reactions. In part, my response was evoked by her projected self-image of the left-out, rejected little girl. She conveyed this aura in subtle ways: her plain clothes; her quiet, controlled manner of speech; her tendency to hold herself tightly, making herself as small and unobtrusive as possible; her looking to Tyler to take the lead. The presenting problem of Tyler's affair also suggested the oedipal victor–oedipal loser dovetail (though this hypothesis is by no means always borne out).

As their story continued to unfold, these hypotheses, gleaned in part from my countertransference, were verified to a great extent. In the subsequent excerpts from mid- and end-phase therapy sessions, the hidden influence of both partners' parental and sibling triangles were exposed more vividly as we came to better understand how they impacted their marriage relationship in an ongoing way. Tyler began the discussion in the following important session:

TYLER: Things are going pretty well, but we had a curious interaction on the patio this weekend that's left us both feeling . . . tense. (*He looks to Julia for confirmation.*)

JULIA: (*snippy*) Well, you made that silly remark about my being all alone, and I was just reacting to that.

TYLER: You did look all alone and out in the cold.

JULIA: Well, I didn't feel that way. I was having a good time by myself.

TYLER: Maybe it was a wrong or silly remark, but why the hostility? Did you feel I should have been helping you clean the patio?

JULIA: No, I wanted to do it by myself. But I was irritated that you didn't appreciate what I'd done. (*pausing*) And then you just disappeared into the kitchen to gobble up a sandwich and run off to the game with Jason [Tyler's fourteen-year-old son from his first marriage].

TYLER: Why the scornful tone about my fixing and eating a lousy sandwich? I don't gobble food or make a mess. We cleaned up afterward. I don't get your anger.

JULIA: (*hesitating, looking inward*) Something about your manner bothered me, I guess. You seemed guilty and like you were trying to make up for being guilty.

TYLER: Guilty about what? That I was going off to the game and not helping you clean? Maybe I did feel a little guilty, but I don't see why that should be irritating.

SHARPE: (*to Julia*) Maybe your reactions had something to do with Jason's being there.

JULIA: Well, now that you mention it. I was thinking last night and this morning that Jason really isn't doing very well.

TYLER: What do you mean? He seems fine to me.

JULIA: Well, he doesn't seem fine to me. He seems so insecure. I don't think he has many friends. He seems very lonely.

TYLER: He does very well in school. I think he's doing better with friends than he was last year.

A discussion ensued about Jason's problems, which sounded like those of an exceptionally bright, nerdy, adolescent boy who is not good at sports. I intervened.

SHARPE: Maybe something in particular is getting to you about Jason's troubles.

JULIA: (*nodding*) The way he looks . . . it makes me feel so sympathetic. He reminds me a little of me at that age. And then I start to feel that awful gnawing guilt.

TYLER: Guilt? You haven't done anything wrong. You've been terrific about Jason, gone way beyond what's expected of a stepmother. And he's very attached to you.

JULIA: I think he misses you, and he's lonely for you. (*looking at me*) If Tyler had stayed with his original family, maybe Jason wouldn't be having these problems. (*She pauses, looking anguished.*) That's what I've been thinking about.

TYLER: So that's it. Now I get it. Why haven't you talked with me about this?

JULIA: It's hard to talk about . . . because I'm afraid I'll find out that you really feel the same way and wish you'd never left . . . that I'm not a big enough prize to make up for what you've lost.

TYLER: That's nonsense. I don't feel that way. I've never regretted marrying you.

Julia continued to look anguished. I sensed there were more layers to her guilt, and I searched for another way into her feelings.

SHARPE: I'm wondering about the scene of you alone on the patio, and Tyler hurrying to run off with Jason to the soccer game. Maybe you felt a little deserted and left out . . . that Tyler preferred to be with Jason, and all that means, than be with you.

JULIA: (*nodding slowly, taking this in*) It's funny how these things go. I was accusing Tyler of being guilty and indirect, and really it was me. (*She sits quietly for a moment.*) I've just never been able to get comfortable with our marriage being okay, that Tyler won't someday regret it, resent me, and want to leave.

TYLER: Oh, never. I'd never leave you. I love you.

Tyler, I noticed, always had the knack of saying the right thing at the right time, with the right amount of feeling. He was every woman's dream in this respect. But I was aware that his seemingly heartfelt declarations did not reassure Julia for very long.

JULIA: I know that, really. I just can't seem to feel secure, and I have these periods of feeling horribly guilty.

SHARPE: Say more about your guilt.

JULIA: I don't like myself for what I did. I went after Tyler, knowing he was married and had a child, and I still went after him.

TYLER: Well, so what. I went after you, too, and you were living with someone else. We weren't happy with our situations, and we fell in love. What's so wrong about that? I think it's a miracle that we found each other.

SHARPE: You competed for Tyler and won. Maybe that's what makes you feel guilty.

JULIA: Yes, I really went after him, and got him. It's always seemed . . . ruthless. I'd never behaved that way before.

TYLER: You're not ruthless. You're a kind and giving person. Besides, I prefer to think that I won you, not that you won me.

JULIA: Well, there you see. You really don't like the picture of me going after you, of trying to win you. It was ruthless, and I feel you don't approve of me for it.

TYLER: I just can't agree with your use of the term "ruthless." That you wanted something and went after it is a natural thing. For god's sake, I do that all the time. I did that with you. Do you think I'm ruthless?

JULIA: No, I don't think of you as ruthless. And it seems okay with me that you're competitive—up to a point. (*she smiles weakly.*)

SHARPE: But it's not okay with you that you're competitive, is it? It's especially not okay if you're the winner in this sort of competition.

JULIA: No, it's not. I feel like a bad person who should be punished.

SHARPE: Punished for winning, for putting your own needs first?

JULIA: Yes.

SHARPE: Since we're into words, "ruthless" is a word that makes me think of great anger. I wonder if you also feel guilty about the anger that may have fueled your competing to win Tyler—your anger about feeling so much rejection from your mother and father.

JULIA: Yes, I feel very angry about my mother and brother. We've talked about that. (*She pauses, deep in thought.*) But I was also angry at my father for leaving us, even though I knew their marriage was bad. I was asking Tyler to do the very thing I hated my father for doing. [Her father had left the family for a mistress when Julia was an adolescent.]

TYLER: So you're angry at me, too, for leaving them?

JULIA: No, not rationally. What I feel gets so confusing. I'm still mad at you about your recent affair, not the one you had with me twelve years ago.

SHARPE: It's not so easy to figure out what feelings belong to whom and when.

JULIA: Obviously, that's so. (*looking at Tyler*) So far, you've gotten it for my mother, brother, and father, and my own worst feelings about myself. I'm just wondering who I'm paying for, you know, from your side of things.

TYLER: I haven't got a clue about that. [He was safe in his proclaimed inability to remember his childhood.]

Therapy with Tyler and Julia was rewarding in many ways but also disturbing, in that Julia was the only one really to engage in most of the deeper work. Tyler slipped and slid around getting into the origins of his difficulties. I thought the marriage could probably chug along quite well, with Julia so much the wiser and the improvements Tyler had made in directly expressing his negative feelings to Julia. However, I thought that without greater understanding of Tyler's triangular conflicts, especially involving women, each would continue to be plagued with ongoing insecurity about the other's love.

I was aware that the only way to a deeper level with Tyler was to confront his competitive behavior as it occurred in therapy sessions. Then, he could not so easily avoid and intellectualize. For reasons that were unclear to me at the time, I had been unable to take this therapeutic action. I assume, now, that it had to do with my fear of losing Tyler's affection. I was also probably carrying Tyler's own fears of losing love, if one does not totally please the other person. As it happened, I had helped Julia enough to enable her to help me in confronting Tyler. This kind of collaboration is one of the great advantages of couple therapy over individual therapy.

Julia's perfectionistic overachievement came up for discussion early in a midphase therapy session, and she had demonstrated her ability to laugh about this trait in herself. In response to a joke she made about her perfectionism, I made a joke intended to expand her awareness. This was all right with her, and she laughed. Then Tyler made a joke, and he and I both laughed, but Julia did not. She suddenly looked injured and began to cry.

TYLER: What happened? I didn't mean to hurt you. I thought we were just kidding around.

JULIA: I know. I know. This is silly of me.

SHARPE: Obviously, you were hurt.

JULIA: (*regaining control*) Well, it was all right before Tyler made his remark and you both laughed. I'm not sure why. This is stupid.

SHARPE: Maybe our laughing made you feel ganged-up on and left out.

JULIA: Well . . . yes . . . I guess so. I hate to admit that. It's a childish reaction. Just for a moment, I felt that you and Tyler were laughing at me, you know, not with me, and that made me feel humiliated and left out.

SHARPE: I can see how that happened . . . how you were hurt. This is an old wound we've scraped open, isn't it?

JULIA: (*nodding*) And one I'm very ashamed of.

SHARPE: I'm glad you're speaking about it. Have you felt that way before in here?

JULIA: No, not really. Well, maybe a little bit. It's nothing you've done. But sometimes I have the feeling that a special connection exists between the two of you that I'm left out of. I think it's the old thing about my mother and brother . . . and me being the outsider. Usually, I can suppress that sort of feeling.

SHARPE: But our laughing made it difficult.

JULIA: That . . . and . . . the fact that Tyler is charming and funny, and I'm not. I can't make people laugh.

TYLER: That's not true. You're plenty charming and funny. You're also more insightful than I am and deeper. As for this special connection with Dr. Sharpe . . . well, that surprises me. Actually, I thought it was the other way around. It's the two of you that get into this groove about interpreting the past. I'm not so good at that. I can hardly remember my childhood.

SHARPE: So you've felt left out as well.

TYLER: (*looking taken aback*) Well . . . perhaps . . . at times, though I've never identified the feeling as such. It's not exactly a reaction I care to dwell on. I'm more aware of feeling competitive, being competitive . . . but I'd guess you'd say that's a way to avoid *being* left out.

JULIA: Oh, that's interesting.

SHARPE: Yes, do say more. [I felt a surge of excitement. This was as far into himself as Tyler had gone without a lot of leading and prodding.]

TYLER: Well, if you focus on competing to win and do win, you have to be noticed . . . reckoned with. You can't just be forgotten in a corner.

SHARPE: (*encouragingly*) That's very true. How might you do that in here, you know, make sure you're not forgotten in a corner? [I felt on edge, as if Tyler could slip away at any moment.]

TYLER: Well, it's probably obvious. I try to make sure I'm liked. I try to be pleasing.

JULIA: (*sharply*) To Dr. Sharpe?

TYLER: Well, sure . . . and to you. I try to please you both.

SHARPE: That sounds like a strain. (*Tyler neither responds nor denies it.*) Julia, did you have something in mind when you asked about his trying to please me?

JULIA: Well . . . I've felt Tyler competing with me in here . . . not in any blatant way. It's subtle . . . the way he curries favor.

TYLER: Curries favor? What a repellent description.

SHARPE: Are you aware how you might go about . . . let's call it . . . trying to please?

TYLER: By being responsive . . . and entertaining, I suppose . . . and a good student of this process about which I haven't the slightest knowledge or ability.

JULIA: (*pouncing*) There it is! It's a sort of winsome, self-deprecation that you do . . . and then, sprinkle in a few compliments, trump me with a great insight, and you get them eating out of your hand.

SHARPE: So you think he's got me eating out of his hand? [I could see Julia's anxiety about her implied criticism of my gullibility.] Do you see me then as being fooled by him?

JULIA: Not fooled really . . . I think it's more that you go easy on him, let him slide off the point . . . don't hold his feet to the fire.

SHARPE: You know, I think you may be right about that. Any ideas why that happens?

JULIA: It's not just you. All women are like that with Tyler, including me.

TYLER: I really object to this. You're both talking about me as though I'm not here . . . like I'm some sort of curious specimen. [He turned his anger on Julia instead of me.] Is your point to show me how it feels to be left out?

JULIA: Not intentionally. It just sort of happened. (*She hesitates.*) But it doesn't feel very good, does it?

TYLER: (*angrily*) I don't need a lesson. If you'd been listening, you might have heard me say I spend a lot of time and energy avoiding that position. I do so because I know very well it's a painful state. Believe me, I don't need any lesson from you.

SHARPE: From me either, I expect. [I offered to include myself in his anger.]

TYLER: (*giving me a quick glare*) From either of you.

SHARPE: You're right, Tyler, we were insensitive. But clearly, we struck a nerve, just like we struck a nerve with Julia earlier on.

TYLER: That you did. I felt very alone, small, and insignificant in those few moments.

SHARPE: Remind you of anything?

TYLER: Yes indeed . . . of being a very small child. (*He pauses, checking back and forth to ensure that he has our full attention.*) I think I felt very lonely growing up. I know I've said I was my mother's favorite, but it was hard work keeping her interest. She had a short attention span and was easily seduced.

SHARPE: Seduced by who?

TYLER: By whoever pleased her or needed her the most . . . my father, my grandmother, her friends.

SHARPE: So you had to compete.

TYLER: She was the only game in town—the only one around who thought I was anything special. Making sure I kept her approval was survival driven, I'd say.

SHARPE: If you lost her attention, you were alone.

TYLER: Early on, I think I felt alone a great deal.

JULIA: What about your sister? Where was she?

TYLER: She was there, but we were in different worlds. She idolized my father. They were very close, and I can't even describe what kind of close; I wasn't in on it.

SHARPE: That sounds painful.

TYLER: Well, I convinced myself that I didn't want to be in on it. I thought she was a silly nuisance, and my father was a bully and a bore. I suppose I consoled myself with the idea I had Mother.

SHARPE: Who you couldn't rely on.

TYLER: (*wryly*) You mean "*whom*" I couldn't rely on. [He found his way back to an old, familiar anesthetic.]

With Tyler's recognition of his childhood feelings, we could more meaningfully examine his relationship with Julia in light of his early triangular experience. His dependence and great anger at women both became apparent. The dimension of the affair not previously exposed was the central element of Tyler's huge, but largely repressed, anger toward his mother for her inconstancy and unreliability. Tyler's affair was meant to punish Julia, who had become the embodiment of his fickle, unreliable mother.

In another scenario, his need to upstage Julia, by making himself the more lovable one, involved his painful rivalry with his sister, a rivalry that he had also substantially denied. In yet another constellation, Julia took on the role of his father, whom he ambivalently loved and hated. In this role (the easiest to access), he also wished to defeat her but could not really permit that victory because of guilt and fear of losing love. Consequently, he slid into the backseat in the career arena much more quickly than was good for him.

When a couple's understanding of past and present love triangles diminishes their power to undermine the relationship, a stronger, safer bond of connection is created between the partners. This means that the gnawing or reactive kinds of insecurity about being truly loved and being first (or the defenses erected against experiencing such insecurity) no longer plague the couple in obvious or unseen ways. Outsiders are no longer a threat, nor are they viewed as tempting pawns to be manipulated by a couple compelled to reenact love triangles.

In therapy, this achievement most obviously shows in the diminution of competitiveness in the therapy threesome, in the partners' reduced need of the therapist, and in the therapist's loss of the halo of idealization. The idealizing glow shifts back to the couple relationship. Getting here is the point of therapy, but it usually leaves the therapist in a mixed state, with an uneasy blend of pleasure about succeeding and pain about the loss—loss of the couple and of being so important in their lives. The more intense the relationship with a couple has been, the more intense these feelings of satisfaction and loss. It had been emotionally intense with Tyler and Julia, and they had been an exceptional working couple. Being so strongly motivated and committed to each other, they were willing to be more open and go deeper than most couples.

I remember an affecting session close to the end of treatment, a session during which it dawned on me that we were very close to saying good-bye. Julia had greeted me with a radiant grin.

JULIA: Something really important happened this week, at least for me. [I noticed how stylish and attractive she looked. Every trace of dowdiness was gone. It was as though she'd left her role as the lead's best friend in a black-and-white movie to play the star in Technicolor.] My mother was visiting this weekend, and Tyler was fantastic. He stayed right next to me the whole time. Even when he wasn't there I felt him rooted there, beside me. And he did something else remarkable. He offered to cook the dinner, so that my mother and I could spend some time alone together. He told her that, and so we were sort of forced into it. We actually sat down alone together and had a decent conversation about something. She actually inquired about my work.

TYLER: (*beaming*) I'm glad you think I'm finally getting it.

JULIA: I think *we're* finally getting it. (*She reaches for his hand, and he pulls her into a hug.*)

As I watched the couple lovingly embrace, I now felt like the one who was being left out. Sadly, I also became aware that I'd better start getting used to it.

References

Ainsworth, M. D. S., Blehar, M. C., Waters, E., & Wall, S. (1978). *Patterns of attachment: A psychological study of the Strange Situation.* Hillsdale, NJ: Erlbaum.

Albee, E. (1983). *Who's afraid of Virginia Woolf?* New York: Signet.

Bader, E., & Pearson, P. T. (1988). *In quest of the mythical mate: A developmental approach to diagnosis and treatment in couples therapy.* New York: Brunner/Mazel.

Bank, S. (1987). Favoritism. In S. P. Bank (Ed.), *Practical concerns about siblings: Bridging the research–practice gap* (pp. 77–89). New York: Haworth Press.

Berman, E. M., & Lief, H. I. (1975). Marital therapy from a psychiatric perspective: An overview. *American Journal of Psychiatry, 132,* 583–592.

Berman, E. M., & Lief, H. I. (1981). A model of marital interaction. In G. P. Sholevar (Ed.), *The handbook of marriage and marital therapy* (pp. 3–34). New York: Spectrum Medical & Scientific Books.

Bieber, I. (1977). Pathogenicity of parental preference. *Journal of the American Academy of Psychoanalysis, 5,* 291–298.

Birk, L. (1984). Combined concurrent/conjoint psychotherapy for couples: Rationale and some efficient new strategies. In C. C. Nadelson & D. C. Polonsky (Eds.), *Marriage and divorce: A contemporary perspective* (pp. 157–167). New York: Guilford Press.

Blass, R. B., & Blatt, S. J. (1992). Attachment and separateness: A theoretical context for the integration of object relations theory with self psychology. *Psychoanalytic Study of the Child, 47,* 189–203.

Blass, R. B., & Blatt, S. J. (1996). Attachment and separateness in the experience of symbiotic relatedness. *Psychoanalytic Quarterly, 65,* 711–746.

Blatt, S. J., & Blass, R. B. (1990). Attachment and separateness: A dialectic model of the products and processes of development throughout the life cycle. *Psychoanalytic Study of the Child, 45,* 107–127.

Blos, P. (1979). *The adolescent passage: Developmental issues.* New York: International Universities Press.

Boszormenyi-Nagy, I., & Framo, J. (1962). Family concept of hospital treatment of schizophrenia. In J. Masserman (Ed.), *Current psychiatric therapies* (Vol. II, pp. 159–166). New York: Grune & Stratton.

Boszormenyi-Nagy, I., & Framo, J. (Eds.). (1965). *Intensive family therapy*. New York: Harper & Row Medical Department.

Bowen, M. (1961). Family psychotherapy. *American Journal of Orthopsychiatry, 31*, 42–60.

Bowen, M. (1966). The use of family theory in clinical practice. *Comprehensive Psychiatry, 7*, 345–347.

Bowen, M. (1978). *Family therapy in clinical practice*. New York: Aronson.

Bronte, E. (1981). *Wuthering Heights*. New York: Bantam. (Original work published 1847)

Brown, E. M. (1991). *Patterns of infidelity and their treatment*. New York: Brunner/Mazel.

Burch, B. (1985). Another perspective of merger in lesbian relationships. In L. B. Rosewater & L. Walker (Eds.), *Handbook on feminist therapy: Women's issues in psychotherapy* (pp. 100–109). New York: Springer.

Burch, B. (1987). Barriers to intimacy: Conflicts over power, dependency, and nurturing in lesbian relationships. In Boston Lesbian Psychologies Collective (Eds.), *Lesbian psychologies: Explorations and challenges* (pp. 126–141). Urbana and Chicago: University of Illinois Press.

Burch, B. (1993). *On intimate terms: The psychology of difference in lesbian relationships*. Urbana and Chicago: University of Illinois Press.

Cheever, J. (1991, January 21). Journals. *The New Yorker*, pp. 34–35.

Colarusso, C. A., & Nemiroff, R. A. (1981). *Adult development*. New York: Plenum Press.

Coyne, J. C., Kahn, J., & Gotlib, I. (1985). Depression. In T. Jacobs (Ed.), *Family interaction and psychopathology* (pp. 509–533). New York: Pergamon Press.

Dicks, H. (1967). *Marital tensions*. New York: Basic Books.

Duvall, E. M. (1971). *Family development* (4th ed.). Philadelphia: Lippincott.

Dym, B., & Glenn, M. L. (1993). *Couples: Exploring and understanding the cycles of intimate relationships*. New York: HarperCollins.

Ephron, N. (1983). *Heartburn*. New York: Vintage Books.

Erikson, E. H. (1959). *Identity and the life cycle*. New York: International Universities Press.

Erikson, E. H. (1963). *Childhood and society* (2nd ed.). New York: Norton.

Fitzgerald, F. S. (1934). *Tender is the night*. New York: Scribner.

Framo, J. L. (1973). Marriage therapy in a couples group. *Seminars in Psychiatry, 5*, 207–217.

Framo, J. L. (1976). Family of origin as a therapeutic resource for adults in marital and family therapy: You can and should go home again. *Family Process, 15*, 193–210.

Framo, J. L. (1982a). *Explorations in marital and family therapy: Selected papers of James L. Framo*. New York: Springer.

Framo, J. L. (1982b). Symptoms from a family transactional viewpoint. In *Explorations in marital and family therapy: Selected papers of James L. Framo* (pp. 11–57). New York: Springer. (Original work published 1970)

Framo, J. L. (1992). *Family-of-origin therapy*. New York: Brunner/Mazel.

Francis, C. A. (1997). Countertransference with abusive couples. In M. F. Solomon & J. P. Siegel (Eds.), *Countertransference in couples therapy* (pp. 218–237). New York: Norton.

Freud, A. (1963). The concept of developmental lines. *Psychoanalytic Study of the Child, 18*, 245–265.

Freud, S. (1961). Civilization and its discontents. *Standard Edition, 21*, 57–145. London: Hogarth Press. (Original work published 1930)

Freud, S. (1963). On narcissism: An introduction. *Standard Edition, 14*, 67–102. London: Hogarth Press. (Original work published 1914)

Friday, N. (1973). *My secret garden: Women's sexual fantasies*. New York: Pocket Books.

Friday, N. (1991). *Women on top*. New York: Pocket Star Books.

Gershenfeld, M. K. (1985). A group is a group is a group: Working with couples in groups. In D. C. Goldberg (Ed.), *Contemporary marriage* (pp. 374–419). Homewood, IL: Dorsey Press.

Goldbart, S., & Wallin, D. (1994). *Mapping the terrain of the heart: The six capacities that guide the journey of love*. Reading, MA: Addison-Wesley.

Gottman, J., & Silver, N. (1999). *The seven principles for making marriage work*. New York: Crown.

Gould, R. L. (1978). *Transformations: Growth and change in adult life*. New York: Simon & Schuster.

Haley, J., & Hoffman, L. (1967). *Techniques of family therapy*. New York: Basic Books.

Hoffman, L. (1980). The family life cycle and discontinuous change. In E. A. Carter & M. McGoldrick (Eds.), *The family life cycle: A framework for family therapy*. New York: Gardner Press.

Jacobs, T. J. (1986). On countertransference enactments. *Journal of the American Psychoanalytic Association, 34*, 289–307.

Jacobson, N. S., & Gurman, A. S. (Eds.). (1986). *Clinical handbook of marital therapy*. New York: Guilford Press.

Jacobson, N. S., & Gurman, A. S. (Eds.). (1995). *Clinical handbook of couple therapy*. New York: Guilford Press.

Kernberg, O. (1975). *Borderline conditions and pathological narcissism*. New York: Aronson.

Kernberg, O. (1976). *Object relations theory and clinical psychoanalysis*. New York: Aronson.

Kernberg, O. (1993). The couple's constructive and destructive superego functions. *Journal of the American Psychoanalytic Association, 41*, 653–677.

Kernberg, O. F. (1995). *Love relations: Normality and pathology*. New Haven, CT: Yale University Press.

Kirshner, L. A. (1998). Problems in falling in love. *Psychoanalytic Quarterly, 67*, 407–425.

Kohut, H. (1971). *The analysis of the self*. New York: International Universities Press.

Kohut, H. (1977). *The restoration of the self*. New York: International Universities Press.

Lansky, M. R. (1980). On blame. *International Journal of Psycho-Analytic Psychotherapy, 8*, 429–456.

Lansky, M. R. (1986). Marital therapy for narcissistic disorders. In N. S. Jacobson & A. S. Gurman (Eds.), *Clinical handbook of marital therapy* (pp. 557–575). New York: Guilford Press.

Levin, I. (1972). *The Stepford wives.* New York: Random House.

Levinson, D. J., Darrow, C. N., Klein, E. B., Levinson, M. H., & McKee, B. (1978). *The seasons of a man's life.* New York: Knopf.

Lindenbaum, J. (1985). The shattering of illusions: The problem of competition in lesbian relationships. *Feminist Studies,* 11(1).

Luepnitz, D. A. (1988). *The family interpreted: Psychoanalysis, feminism, and family therapy.* New York: Basic Books.

Mahler, M., Pine, F., & Bergman, A. (1975). *The psychological birth of the human infant.* New York: Basic Books.

Maltas, C. (1998). Concurrent therapies when therapists don't concur. *Journal of Clinical Psychoanalysis, 7,* 337–355.

McWhirter, D. P., & Mattison, A. (1984). *The male couple: How relationships develop.* Englewood Cliffs, NJ: Prentice-Hall.

Miller, M. V. (1995). *Intimate terrorism: The deterioration of erotic life.* New York: Norton.

Modell, A. (1976). The "holding environment" and the therapeutic action of psychoanalysis. *Journal of the American Psychoanalytic Association, 24,* 285–307.

Nadelson, C. C. (1978). Marital therapy from a psychoanalytic perspective. In T. J. Paolino & B. S. McCrady (Eds.), *Marriage and marital therapy: Psychoanalytic, behavioral, and systems theory perspectives* (pp. 89–164). New York: Brunner/Mazel.

Nadelson, C. C., Polonsky, D. C., & Mathews, M. A. (1984). Marriage as a developmental process. In C. C. Nadelson & D. C. Polonsky (Eds.), *Marriage and divorce: A contemporary perspective* (pp. 127–141). New York: Guilford Press.

Nelsen, J. (1995). Varieties of narcissistically vulnerable couples: Dynamics and practice implications. *Clinical Social Work Journal, 23,* 59–70.

Nemiroff, R. A., & Colarusso, C. A. (Eds.). (1985). *The race against time: Psychotherapy and psychoanalysis in the second half of life.* New York: Plenum Press.

Nemiroff, R. A., & Colarusso, C. A. (Eds.). (1990). *New dimensions in adult development.* New York: Basic Books.

Peglau, L. A., Cochran, S., Rosh, K., & Patesky, C. (1978). Loving women: Attachment and autonomy in lesbian relationships. *Journal of Social Issues, 34,* 7–27.

Person, E. S. (1988). *Dreams of love and fateful encounters: The power of romantic passion.* New York: Norton.

Person, E. S. (1995). *By force of fantasy.* New York: Penguin Books.

Piaget, J. (1950). *The psychology of intelligence.* New York: Harcourt Brace.

Pittman, F. S., & Wagers, T. P. (1995). Crises of infidelity. In N. S. Jacobson & A. S. Gurman (Eds.), *Clinical handbook of couple therapy* (pp. 295–316). New York: Guilford Press.

Renik, O. (1993). Countertransference enactment and the psychoanalytic process. In M. J. Horwitz, O. F. Kernberg, & E. M. Weinshel (Eds.), *Psychic structure and psychic change: Essays in honor of Robert S. Wallerstein, M.D.* (pp. 131–160). Madison, CT: International Universities Press.

Rosenblatt, A. D., & Sharpe, S. A. (1998, November 13–15). *Mother always loved me best–didn't she?: Favorites and their fates.* Paper presented at The Impact of Siblings Conference sponsored by New Directions in Psychoanalytic Thinking, a program of the Washington Psychoanalytic Foundation.

Ross, J. M. (1992). *The male paradox.* New York: Simon & Schuster.

Sander, F. M. (1979). *Individual and family therapy: Toward an integration.* New York: Aronson.

Sander, F. M., & Feldman, L. B. (1993). Integrating individual, marital, and family therapy. I. *Review of psychiatry* (Vol. 12, pp. 611–629). New York: American Psychiatric Press.

Sandler, J. (1976). Countertransference and role-responsiveness. *International Review of Psycho-Analysis, 43,* 43–47.

Sandler, J., & Rosenblatt, B. (1962). The concept of the representational world. *Psychoanalytic Study of the Child, 17,* 128–145.

Scharff, D. E., & Scharff, J. S. (1991). *Object relations couple therapy.* Northvale, NJ: Aronson.

Scharff, D. E., & Scharff, J. S. (1987). *Object relations family therapy.* Northvale, NJ: Aronson.

Sharpe, S. A. (1981). The symbiotic marriage: A diagnostic profile. *Bulletin of the Menninger Clinic, 45,* 89–114.

Sharpe, S. A. (1984). *Self and object representations: An integration of psychoanalytic and Piagetian developmental theories.* Unpublished manuscript, Fielding Institute, Santa Barbara, CA.

Sharpe, S. A. (1990). The oppositional couple: A developmental object relations approach to diagnosis and treatment. In R. A. Nemiroff & C. A. Colarusso (Eds.), *New dimensions in adult development* (pp. 386–415). New York: Basic Books.

Sharpe, S. A. (1997). Countertransference and diagnosis in couples therapy. In M. F. Solomon & J. P. Siegel (Eds.), *Countertransference in couples therapy* (pp. 38–71). New York: Norton.

Sharpe, S. A. (1998). "Defensive splitting in couples": Comment. *Journal of Clinical Psychoanalysis, 7,* 328–336.

Sharpe, S. A., & Rosenblatt, A. D. (1994). Oedipal sibling triangles. *Journal of the American Psychoanalytic Association, 42,* 491–523.

Siegel, E., & Robertiello, R. C. (1987). The favored child: A variation on the Cinderella theme in psychotherapy. *Journal of Contemporary Psychotherapy, 17,* 300–308.

Siegel, J. (1992). *Repairing intimacy: An object relations approach to couples therapy.* Northvale, NJ: Aronson.

Siegel, J. P. (1998). Defensive splitting in couples. *Journal of Clinical Psychoanalysis, 7,* 305–327.

Silverman, L. H., & Lachmann, F. M. (1985). The therapeutic properties of unconscious oneness fantasies: Evidence and treatment implications. *Contemporary Psychoanalysis, 21,* 91–115.

Silverman, L. H., Lachmann, F. M., & Milich, R. (1982). *The search for oneness.* New York: International Universities Press.

Silverman, L. H., Lachmann, F. M., & Milich, R. H. (1984). Unconscious oneness fantasies: Experimental findings and implications for treatment. *International Forum for Psychoanalysis, 1,* 107–152.

Slipp, S. (1988). *The technique and practice of object relations family therapy.* Northvale, NJ: Aronson.

Solomon, M. (1973). A developmental conceptual premise for family therapy. *Family Process, 12,* 179–188.

Solomon, M. (1989). *Narcissism and intimacy: Love and marriage in an age of confusion.* New York: Norton.

Stern, D. N. (1985). *The interpersonal world of the infant: A view from psychoanalysis and developmental psychology.* New York: Basic Books.

Terkelsen, K. (1980). Toward a theory of the family life cycle. In E. A. Carter & M. McGoldrick (Eds.), *The family life cycle: A framework for family therapy.* New York: Gardner Press.

Tyson, P., & Tyson, R. L. (1990). *Psychoanalytic theories of development.* New Haven, CT: Yale University Press.

Vogel, E. F., & Bell, N. W. (1981). The emotionally disturbed child as the family scapegoat. In R. G. Green & J. L. Framo (Eds.), *Family therapy: Major contributions* (pp. 207–234). New York: International Universities Press.

Waller, R. J. (1992). *The bridges of Madison County.* New York: Warner.

Wallerstein, J. S., & Blakeslee, S. (1995). *The good marriage.* Boston: Houghton Mifflin.

Wallerstein, J. S. (1997). Transference and countertransference in clinical interventions with divorcing families. In M. F. Solomon & J. P. Siegel (Eds.), *Countertransference in couples therapy* (pp. 113–124). New York: Norton.

Wile, D. B. (1985). Phases of relationship development. In D. C. Goldberg (Ed.), *Contemporary marriage: Special issues in couples therapy* (pp. 35–61). Homewood, IL: Dorsey Press.

Willi, J. (1982). *Couples in collusion.* New York: Aronson.

Winer, R. (1994). *Close encounters: A relational view of the therapeutic process.* Northvale, NJ: Aronson.

Winnicott, D. W. (1965). *The maturational processes and the facilitating environment.* New York: International Universities Press.

Wynne, L. C., Ryckoff, I. M., Day, J., & Hirsch, S. I. (1958). Pseudomutuality in the family relations of schizophrenics. *Psychiatry, 21,* 205–220.

Zilbach, J. J. (1968). Family development. In J. Marmor (Ed.), *Modern psychoanalysis: New directions and perspectives* (pp. 355–386). New York: Basic Books.

Zilbach, J. J. (1989). The family life cycle: A framework for understanding children in family therapy. In L. Combrinck-Graham (Ed.), *Children in family contexts: Perspectives on treatment* (pp. 46–66). New York: Guilford Press.

Zinner, J. (1976). The implications of projective identification for marital interaction. In H. Grunebaum & J. Christ (Eds.), *Contemporary marriage: Structure, dynamics and therapy* (pp. 293–308). Boston: Little, Brown.

Zinner, J., & Shapiro, E. (1975). Splitting in families of borderline adolescents. In J. Mack (Ed.), *Borderline states in psychiatry.* New York: Grune & Stratton.

Index